D1367134

VIBRANT HEALTH FROM YOUR KITCHEN

by
Bernard Jensen, Ph.D.

THE INFORMATION PRESENTED HERE WAS GATHERED DURING OVER 50 YEARS OF SANITARIUM EXPERIENCE, WORKING WITH DIET, EXERCISE AND THE NATURAL HEALING ART TO BRING PATIENTS TO A RIGHT WAY OF LIVING.

PUBLISHED BY: Bernard Jensen, Ph.D.
Route 1, Box 52
Escondido, CA 92025 USA

First Edition

Copyright 1986 Bernard Jensen
ALL RIGHTS RESERVED

BERNARD JENSEN, Publisher
Route 1, Box 52
Escondido, CA 92025 USA

AUSTRALIAN BRANCH ADDRESS:
LEON BROSNAN
143 NEWMARKET ROAD
WINDSOR, BRISBANE, QUEENSLAND
AUSTRALIA 4030

ISBN 0-932615-01-5

I Believe

I believe man wants to do what is right and will, if shown that doing the right thing will result in a better life.

I believe that we all have the right to pursuit of happiness, but the pursuit of happiness will never be fulfilled unless the pursuit of health goes with it. It is your privilege to seek them.

I believe that to attain health and happiness, a person's lifestyle must be approved by the universal God and must be in harmony with natural principles.

I believe in a universal consciousness of sharing, love, brotherhood and peace.

I believe we will have peace when people refuse to take a job that will harm another person.

I believe, given a choice of therapies, that the therapy closest to nature will produce the deepest and most lasting tissue correction.

I believe that the man who conquers his own hostilities does more than if he conquers a whole city.

I believe this book will be a "wayshower," an uplifting experience, bringing us another step toward our final destiny of health, happiness and the joy of living that all people desire.

—Dr. Bernard Jensen
April 1986

Preface

The Reason for This Book

In the past few years, so many of my patients and students have asked for a book that would summarize the food and nutrition classes I have that I finally put aside the time needed to do it. I feel there is an obligation on my part to share what I know about building good health through foods. So I come to you as an ambassador of goodwill, an ambassador with gifts to offer, gifts of health knowledge, of food knowledge—knowledge of the better things in life. In this book, I am giving you the very best I have.

Some of you may have ignored the path of health wisdom and have taken the easy way, the convenient way, the "fast track" in life. Maybe you just didn't want to make the effort. Sometimes it takes a serious health problem to bring us to the place where we are willing to pay attention; but I want to tell you, the wise person learns from the mistakes of others.

According to the National Research Council's Food and Nutrition Board, there is growing evidence of a link between diet and degenerative diseases such as cancer and heart disease. Yet, a survey by the National Research Council released in 1985 found that the average medical school teaches the future doctors of the United States too little about food and nutrition. Covering 45 of the country's 127 medical schools, the survey showed that the average medical school graduate has received only 21 hours of nutrition education in 4 years of study. Twenty percent of the schools surveyed provided less than 10 hours of nutritional studies and 60 percent provided less than 20 hours. The National Research Council recommends at least 25 to 30 classroom hours of nutrition education. Until doctors receive better and more thorough training in food and nutrition, it is up to the individual to find out how to eat right to stay healthy and to avoid the chronic diseases that are so prevalent in Western nations in our time. This is one of the main purposes of my book.

We don't always want to come into this health work, this nutrition work, but I want to say there is an extreme obligation on the students' part. Life is a school, and to do well in it, you need knowledge and wisdom. If you are in the 2nd grade, you have to learn; if you are in the 5th grade, you have to learn. There is always something *more* to learn, to get ready for the next higher grade. We are "in training" on this planet to do better things, not to make the same mistakes every day. We're here to follow the path of wisdom. This book is slanted toward the best health possible through nutrition.

Students have an extreme obligation to realize that there may be a better way than the one they are following now. We should have an inquiring mind. We should want to do the right thing. We should never slam the door on anything until we find out whether it could be a better way of life. They say "Opportunity is knocking at your door." Will it return if you slam the door in its face?

I think it is time we have a better communication with one another, person to person. We must learn from the mistakes of others because we just can't afford to make their mistakes all over again. I don't think we're going to live long enough to repeat all the mistakes that others have made. We might as well learn from one another. We might as well find out whether we have missed something we should know in order to have a more complete life.

My mother used to say, *"Health isn't everything, but without health, everything else is nothing."* She would also say, "You can lose your money and you've lost a lot; you can lose your health and you've lost still more; but if you lose your peace of mind, you've lost everything."

In the wholistic approach to health, nutrition is only part of a larger picture, only one aspect of the healthy life. I would like to teach about peace of mind, happiness, nature, relaxation, beauty and security—where our security really is. I would like to teach about wisdom and knowledge, and how to use them to serve others and live the good life. I would like to teach about true cure and how it takes place from the inside out, how we live on what we pour out.

If we don't have anything within—spiritually, mentally or physically, how can we express the worthwhile life?

We find that nutrition and foods are a good place to start for the average person. This will provide a foundation for getting into good health and not into treating disease. When we treat the patient on the other end of disease symptoms, building toward better health by taking care of the whole person, the symptoms are often left behind. Drugs may change the blood chemistry, but they cannot rebuild or replace tissue. *Only foods can do that.* This is why we need to know about nutrition and foods.

Many reasons can be brought out to explain why people eat the way they do, but lack of knowledge is the number one reason. We may have put our health in the hands of doctors who have never studied enough nutrition to offer advice to the family. We may have been following food traditions passed down through the family without considering a balanced food regimen. The family is considered the basic social unit of a healthy society, but we can't have a healthy society unless the family has the proper food knowledge to be healthy.

This book is a guided tour through the experiences I have had in taking care of thousands of patients through nutrition. It is meant to be practical, useful in food shopping, food preparation and in the kitchen. It represents a concerted effort to help every member of the family—no matter what age—come to a better level of health.

Teaching you these things fulfills my side of the obligation; learning them and enjoying better health will fulfill your side.

TAKING ON A NEW PATH

This book is an introduction to a new way of living. We cannot hold on to the old, otherwise the new cannot take its place. Coming into this health way is taking on a new path, a new direction, a new obligation and eliminating the old ways, the ways that cannot build good health. If we are going to build new tissue to replace the old, we have to clean out our pantry, we have to have new insight, new outsight and a new homesite. We have to move—we won't have the same address anymore. We are going to a new place, a new level in life.

We have to realize that until now, perhaps, doctors have made a living on your living. What kind of life is that? We find that *we have to live an entirely different kind of life.*

Taking on a new way of life isn't always going to be pleasant. When you leave sugared breakfast cereals behind and get into more natural whole grain cereals, you are not going to do it without some reluctance. And if I tell you to give up wheat, I can see your opposition coming up. *Many new things are automatically opposed.* You're not going to give up wheat until I show you a good substitute for it. When we talk about giving up regular cow's milk, I know you're going to say, "But I've had it all my life! I drink a gallon a day!"

We can make changes slowly. We don't have to do it all at once. If you will go along with me in this work, you will begin to understand that there are many facets of life we need to get into to complete our job of taking up a healthier way of living.

Consider it like getting into the ocean. We put our toes in first, and if the water isn't too cold, we get in up to our ankles. If that feels good, we may go in up to our knees. Maybe that's as far as we get the first day, but if we feel a little bit better for doing it, we will go in deeper the next day.

This path takes daring—it takes an adventurous mind to get into this health work. Getting well, working toward good health, is really a mental thing as well as a physical thing. I won't be with you physically to hold your hand while you are getting well, but I'll be with you mentally. I have given up a great part of my life to help others find a more healthy way of life, and I know what they go through because I've gone through it myself.

IT ISN'T EASY TO CHANGE

Taking certain well-loved foods away from the average person who is sick and ailing (or even those without symptoms) is like pouring ice water on a sunbather. There is some yelling, some opposition, some disagreement. I know. I've been there myself.

I was raised on Danish pastry and worked my way up to 20 cups of coffee a day. This started in my childhood and went on for many years. But I didn't know any better. These days many people have heard that pastry is hard on the bowel; that coffee is hard on the nerves, liver, gallbladder and breaks down the friendly bacteria in the bowel. But, you see, I have to find these things out, and I learned the hard way. I was what you might call a "chocoholic"— nothing tasted better than chocolate. I didn't realize what it was doing to my body—the chocolate, the Danish pastry, the coffee— until I got to the place where I didn't have the body to work with. I only realized that something was wrong when I reached the place where my health was almost gone.

I didn't want to give up the foods I loved, but when a person really gets desperate, he is ready to try anything. Then I was really ready to go into a health program.

We can get set in our ways. We don't want to move because we are comfortable. It's so easy to go to the "fast foods." It's so easy to snack on whatever we like whenever we like. It's so easy to shop for the commercialized foods, the "dollar foods" developed and sold to the consumer market by big business. Or didn't you realize that the business people in the food industry were interested in profits?

Now, here I am—77 years of age at this moment—trying to bring you through the pathway of change, and this is a most difficult thing. My business is to bring better health to you. I had to learn the hard way, and I am offering you a better way, an easier way to learn than through doctor bills and hospital bills. This is a very personal thing with me. I hope you can feel that.

FEELING GOOD IS NOT ALWAYS ENOUGH

Over the past 50 years, I have taken care of about 350,000 people in my classes and my sanitarium work, people who were able to use what I taught them, what I gave them, to regain or improve their health. Now I am trying to bring the same message to you, so you can have better health.

If you think you can be satisfied with sickness and disease, with doctor and hospital visits, with a body that has become bankrupt of energy and health, perhaps you aren't ready to learn. Sometimes it takes many years to build a disease before it comes fully into bloom with symptoms. A survey has shown that 9 out of 10 Americans say they "feel food,' even though 4 out of 20 have some chronic disease. Feeling good does not necessarily mean you are living or eating properly. Many diseases come gradually, insidiously, into full maturity without a sign of warning beforehand. They come in very slowly. If you want to learn how to prevent disease, how to reverse disease conditions and get rid of the old, you need to start learning now.

It isn't easy. I tell my patients it takes 6 months to a year to make a good body with proper nutrition and a healthy lifestyle. It takes time to break old habits and to get into a new way of doing things. We have to re-educate ourselves, change ourselves, turn our lives around. You may not have much company on the path to good health, and it can be a very lonely path, because we find that most of the people in this country are sick—one government study announced the figure to be 92%. That's a lot of people who are not well. Do you want to walk with them on the pathway to disease? No, it is better to walk the lonely path, knowing you are doing the right thing. My mother taught me, when I was a child, *that the more truth you have, the more alone you go.*

You know, if you don't realize the value of gold and diamonds, you will walk right past them if they're all around you. Yet, health is more valuable than gold and diamonds, because you can't buy it with money. You have to earn it. *You have to learn it.* You have to work for it, little by little, day by day. The value of health is in having the energy, strength and power to live right, to have a good marriage, to be a good parent, to do well at your job or in school. These are the things that bring joy and satisfaction into a person's life.

We hear about labor unions going on strike for better working conditions. Someone has to be willing to stand up and tell people there is a better way. Considering the air and water pollution, toxic waste dumps, refined, devitalized foods, and the effects of alcohol, cigarettes and drugs, someone has to stand up for living right.

I have tried to be fair and honest with you. If you want to prove whether I'm right or not, you're going to have to try my program. And, like my old teacher used to say when I first got started, *"The least you can do is try it; you can always go back to your old mess again."*

My obligation is to point toward the right path. It's up to you whether to walk it or not. We live by our beliefs; we live by our knowledge; we live by our wisdom. It is possible to change, no matter how old we are, no matter what our circumstances are. We find that the wise man does in the beginning what the fool does in the end. But, then, wise men are not born, they are made. In your development, I encourage you to seek the kind of knowledge, wisdom and beliefs that lead you to a better body, better health and a better life.

THE REASON FOR THE PICTURES IN THIS BOOK

For many years, people—ranging from housewives to health professionals—have asked about my sanitarium work and where I found the food ideas used so successfully in building health and preventing disease. The reason for most of the pictures in this book is to provide answers to these questions.

The pictures show what sanitarium life was like for the patients, the staff and for me. They show not only what our ranch looked like, but how we had our meals, exercised, worked and relaxed.

A large section of travel pictures show where I found many of my food ideas. I have traveled to over 55 countries, keeping an eye out for the best and healthiest foods and for health-building processes in each country and each culture.

Soil pictures are shown because the soil is the source of nutritional values in all our foods. How we use or abuse the soil of our planet has a vital effect on health and disease in man, because nutrient-rich soil and foods with proper balance and variety are the keys to healthy, disease-resistant bodies.

Every housewife should consider how to make her home into a "mini-sanitarium" for the good of her family, for better health and for the well-being of all family members.

CONFUSION IS NO SOLUTION

Many people are confused about health ideas, what to eat, how much to exercise, whether supplements are needed, what to give their children, menu planning and many, many other subjects. It is best to follow the ideas of someone who has a balanced health program, a balanced food program, proven over years of actual use by thousands of people. We should not follow confusion but wisdom in this matter. My patients have been my books, and I have developed most of my ideas by seeing what it takes, nutritionally, to bring a person out of a disease and into a balanced way of life. The same ideas that lead from disease to wellness will also prevent a future disease and keep your children from being raised to be doctor bills.

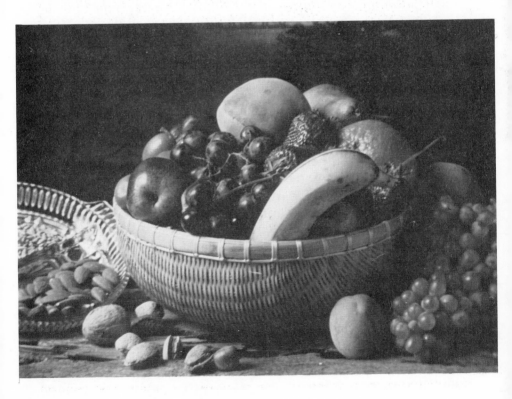

Nature, God, the Earth and the Sun have certainly been good to us.

Biography

Dr. Jensen has spent over 50 years in the field of natural health and nutrition, refining and organizing the best available information on foods and their relation to health. He has developed a program, as presented in this book, that most people can follow to feel better and reduce doctor bills. "If you want go get specific results," Dr. Jensen says, "you should follow a specific food program, and a specific direction, nutritionally. Taking a salad and a multivitamin tablet now and then won't do much for you."

During the early years of his training, Dr. Jensen studied with such great nutritional pioneers as Dr. John Harvey Kellogg, Dr. Bircher-Benner, Dr. V. G. Rocine and Dr. John Tilden, among others. He has traveled around the world, visiting more than 50 countries to study their oldest, healthiest citizens and discover their secrets to health and longevity.

"Each country offered me some highlight on nutrition, certain foods, certain insights, a certain philosophy of life," Dr. Jensen says. "I looked for ways to put these things together to help the average person learn to live right and avoid disease."

All over the world, the search is on for the best anti-cancer diet, the best diabetic diet, the best cardiovascular diet, the best catarrhal elimination diet, the best allergy diet and on and on. "Special diets may be useful for a short time but lead to imbalances and deficiencies in the body over the long term," says Dr. Jensen. "We need to get away from diets and into a right way of living. Too many people are jumping from one unbalanced diet to another." The greatest danger to health is when a person's food habits are dominated by only a few foods.

Poor food habits, assisted by fatigue, stress, environmental pollution and various lifestyle problems, lead to catarrh and catarrh is almost always found at the beginning of a disease. Many people n the United States live a disease way of life because no one ever told them how to eat properly, how to live right.

This book is invaluable for the person who wants to live the health way of life and prevent disease, for the person who is tired of doctor bills, *for the housewife who wants to take care of the nutritional needs of the whole family.*

Between the covers of this book, you will not find another diet, but a comprehensive program for living that includes balanced nutritional tips and guidelines. Dr. Jensen's thoughts on foods and food laws in this book are designed to provide the foundation you need for building a healthy way of life.

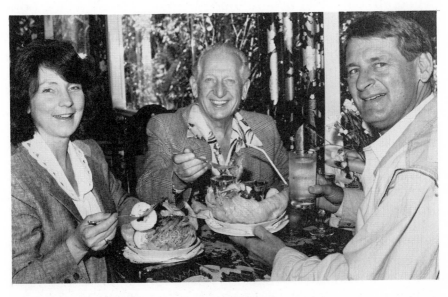

Good food for the body, mind and soul—nutritionist and author, Dr. Bernard Jensen, lunching with Anne Garms and Brisbane, Australia nutritionist, Leon Brosnan.

Introduction

In caring for ourselves and others in this day and age, it is necessary that we know enough about nutrition to keep ourselves and our families as well as possible. There's no reason we should be raising our children as doctor bills. We should know how to keep them healthy.

We have all heard, "You are what you eat," but I have discovered, *"You are also what you don't eat."* Neglecting to take foods needed by the body is just as bad as eating wrong foods, junk foods, "foodless foods." So it is necessary to make a new start by leaving behind foods that do not naturally nourish the body and by taking up foods that build the body. Before we can do the right thing, we need to learn the right thing.

We should know how to work toward a balance with natural foods, and to do this **we have to start at the kitchen table,** or even farther back, with the soil our foods grow from. We must realize, we are "the dust of the earth," and only if the soil is chemically balanced will our food be chemically balanced to build strong, healthy bodies.

Now we are going to analyze nutritional and diet ideas in this book and put them back together so that when you put them to work in your home you will know what you are doing and why. You should know how to tell what foods build health, what the proper proportions are, the acid-alkaline balance and the other basic food laws and ideas.

There is no reason why we should be producing disease from the kitchen table when, with the proper foods and preparation methods, we could be producing health for the future instead.

Everyone needs to understand that improper foods, wrongly prepared foods and unwise living habits contribute to catarrhal conditions, and we find that catarrh is in the beginning of every disease. Catarrhal conditions such as colds and flu are often suppressed with drugs and our lifestyle which drives the catarrh back into the tissues to develop into a chronic or degenerative condition later. This should not happen and does not have to happen when we make the right changes in our foods and manner of living. It is the purpose of this book to introduce you to ideas that will help you take a new and healthier direction in foods.

A 1984 survey by Louis Harris and Associates showed that 9 of 10 Americans say they are in excellent or good health, even though 1 out of every 4 of them has a serious chronic disease. Many times we go on with an unhealthy way of life because we "feel good," not realizing that many diseases can be at work in the body long before symptoms appear.

This book will benefit the whole family, not just by pointing the way to have healthier children, but by raising the health and vitality level of the mother and father as well. We find that we cannot have harmony in the home unless we have healthy bodies and minds, and we cannot have healthy bodies and minds unless we have harmony in the foods we take in. This is a book that teaches a harmonious way of eating and living so we can develop the best life possible.

MY GREATEST DISCOVERY

In this book, I tell about my work with wheat, milk and sugar, which I believe is one of the great factors for the declining health in America. The average American diet is 29% wheat, 25% milk and 8% sugar.

It is this "big 3" that cause so much trouble in America. The best of this is in the chapter, "Starting Out Right with Foods and Knowing Your Food Laws"; the next is, "Discovering the Good in Foods." This takes up the chemical intolerance of wheat, milk and sugar.

The "Wheat Story" and "Nutrition and Tissue Cleansing" have helped me to make the biggest changes with my patients.

I encourage you to read these chapters carefully and thoughtfully, and to follow the path of wisdom in how you respond to this food knowledge.

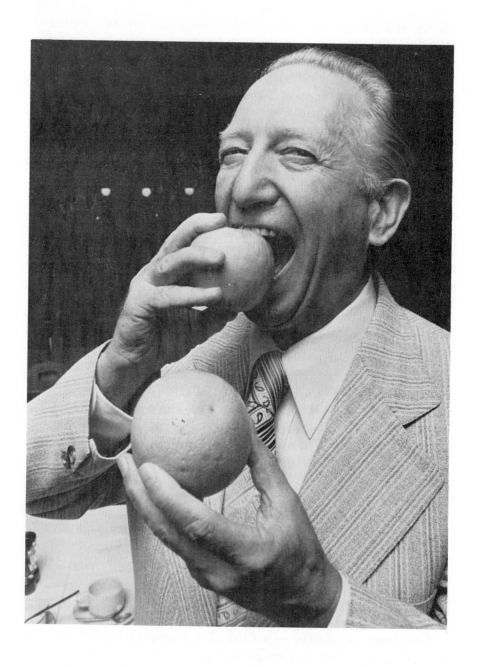

Replenishment time.

CONTENTS

1

Diets and a Healthy Way to Live

Now we would like to begin to take care of the body through nutrition. Many have said, **Whatever we eat today becomes our body tomorrow.** We find that practically every disease is a sign of a certain lack in our diet.

One of the things we have to be very careful with is that everyone seems to be **on a diet**—but we can't look to nutrition to cure everything. I think one of the first things we have to remember is to get our lifestyle straightened out. If you are tired and fatigued, you can't digest your food well. If you are working late hours or overtime and not getting enough rest, you could become disorderly from a mental standpoint, emotionally strained, and would not digest your foods well. We cannot digest our foods really well unless we are happy, refreshed and hungry.

You can't be well unless you're happy, and you cannot be happy unless you are well. **They go together.**

WHOSE DIET ARE YOU ON TODAY?

The first thing I would like to have you see in this work is that you must get off diets. A diet is, by its design, imbalanced. We must strive for a balanced nutritional program.

Now we have all kinds of diets. We have what is called the frankfurter diet, the grape diet, the carrot juice diet and more, and I've seen so many of these diets that it's unbelievable. Some of them are very good, as far as getting a balance is concerned. **Yes, I**

1

said balance. Where does balance come in? *Balance is probably the most important thing.*

There are many people whose body chemistry is imbalanced due to nutritional deficiencies caused by improper food habits or imbalanced diets. In my studies, I have looked into the person who is lacking calcium. The person lacking calcium doesn't have the power to repair and rebuild. Who is lacking magnesium? That's the person who can't relax. So we find now that these chemical elements all have a story to tell. Silicon is the magnetic element; whenever we have any skin trouble, nail trouble, hair trouble, nerve troubles and even gland troubles, we are lacking silicon. We know that we have to have iodine for the thyroid gland. When we have emotional problems, we can wear out the thyroid gland a lot faster than we can build it up with foods.

We should know that we have to get these chemicals from the **dust of the earth**, through the foods we eat.

Even a regular way of eating has to correspond to the kind of work we are doing, the kind of a marriage we have, even the kind of a person you are—the type of person. Those with a narrow chin are a mental type. And you find they would rather do mental work than physical work. They probably will need more protein in the diet. Those who work at physical jobs need more carbohydrates, more starchy foods, because carbohydrates give out the work energy they need. Under physical or emotional stress from the job or marriage, we need foods that bring in the B vitamins to protect the nerves, and iodine to support the thyroid, the **emotional gland**. Our eating has to correspond with what is going on in our lives.

We have to understand that many symptoms are signs of deficiency in certain chemical elements in the body. Phosphorus, for instance, comes from the Greek word meaning *the light bearer*. We find that we cannot carry the light of happiness and the light of upliftment in life unless we have enough phosphorus. The phosphorus-depleted person becomes depressed, morbid and develops mental symptoms. Likewise, we need sulphur for the life force in the body and manganese for our memory.

There hasn't been a single patient I have seen who didn't lack certain chemical elements. I have never seen a perfectly well person. But who wants to spend years studying deficiency symptoms and how to take care of them? Most people eat by taste.

2

Most people eat at pleasurable times. We find they eat what their mother and father had or what they've had in years past. But is it the right thing? Many people who think they are well have hidden problems that haven't manifested yet.

DO YOU KNOW WHAT A BALANCED WAY OF EATING IS?

What we all need is a program that provides a balanced way of eating, one to feed us all the chemical elements we need so we won't have to study deficiencies or worry about them.

It has taken many years with my sanitarium work to come up with ideas that will help you develop a healthy way of living. In using experience as a basis from which to work, I can tell you I have seen diets do wonderful things. Fasting has given wonderful results. Carrot juice has done wonderful things.

I have personally seen patients at my sanitariums get rid of life-threatening degenerative diseases through fasting, grape diets, carrot juice diets and other extreme programs. These are all good diets, but they should only be used under a doctor's supervision. What we need to do is to get off even *good diets* and get onto a healthy way of living. (The diet most in need of a doctor's supervision is the junk food diet so many are on.) **The** worst diet in the world is the junk food diet.

The elimination diets we have discussed, such as carrot juice, are good, but they are, again, diets. They are not going to balance the chemical composition of the body.

We need all the chemical elements. I wondered, *How can I develop a food program that has all these chemical elements, so we won't have to worry about chemical imbalance?* The key to the prevention of disease is a healthy way of living, and over a period of years, I developed my **Health and Harmony Food Regimen**, a program that is half eliminating and half building. The body is normally and constantly building and eliminating. That is the procedure we have to follow in a healthy living program. If you emphasize building and don't do enough eliminating, then you're going to have to go on an alkalinizing diet or elimination diet. My **Health and Harmony Food Regimen** will be presented in another chapter. *Remember, proper nutrition isn't everything, but without*

3

It, no other therapy will work to bring healing. Only foods repair and rebuild tissue.

You can't be like the young man who came to us at the Ranch one time. He said, "I've been three weeks on grapefruit, and, you know, my sinuses are a lot better. And," he added, "I hear you're using carrot juice here, so I'd like to go three weeks on carrot juice because I hear it's high in vitamin A, and it gets rid of catarrhal conditions." He went three weeks on carrot juice, but when he finished, he announced, "I believe I'll try three weeks on watermelon next. I hear it's very high in silicon." What's wrong with this **diet shopping** is that every time you focus on a single food or juice that is high in one element, you come up deficient in all the other chemical elements. Your body goes from imbalance to imbalance as you go from one diet to another.

For most people, it is hard to find a healthy way of life. They don't know what to do. However, I've formulated an approach to foods that has worked very well with my sanitarium patients and with those who have taken it home to live by. I think you will appreciate this because you are looking for a right way of living and if you can just get away from what you're doing now and follow this harmonious way, you will be all right. So after any extreme diet—even if it's a good one—you'd better get right onto my **Health and Harmony Food Regimen**. And, if you've been on pickles and chocolate or 36 flavors of ice cream, it's time you find out what a good healthy way of living is.

SNACK HABITS IN THE U.S.A.

Most snacks (76%) are eaten in the privacy of the home. Those most likely to snack are dieters. Those over 55 eat more brownies, pastries, cheesecake and ice cream than those under 55. Men prefer salty snacks. Women prefer healthy munchies. Women snack more than men from age 25-54. Four out of ten snacks are sweet; two out of ten are salty. Southerners snack less (by 10%) than other Americans, while those from the North Central states snack the most.

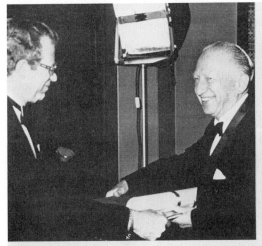
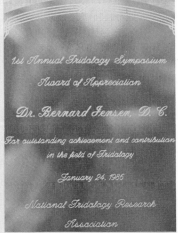
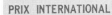

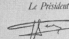
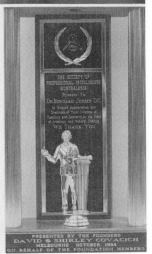

Upper left: Dr. Jensen receiving the Dag Hammarskjold Award (lower left) from a representative of the Pax Mundi Society, Brussels, Belgium. Upper right: Award from the National Iridology Research Association. Lower right: An award Dr. Jensen received from Iridologists in Australia.

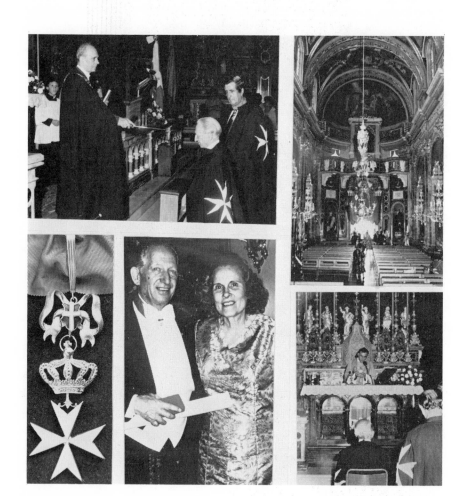

Top left: Dr. Jensen's knighthood into the Order of St. John of Jerusalem, Knights of Malta. Right (top & bottom): The church where Dr. Jensen was knighted on the Island of Malta. Lower left: The cross of St. John of Malta. Dr. Jensen is now a Knight Commander.

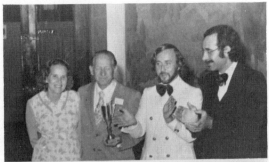

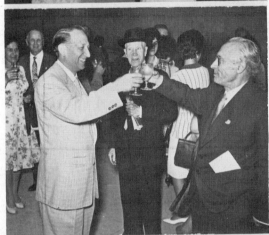

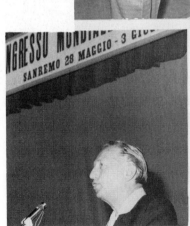

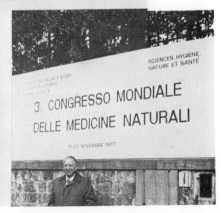

Top: An award for my film "World Search for Health and Long Life," narrated by Dennis Weaver. Middle: A toast with Dr. V. L. Ferrandiz in Barcelona, Spain. Bottom: Accepting the Iridology Gold Medal award at San Remo, Italy, during the World Congress of Natural Medicine.

7

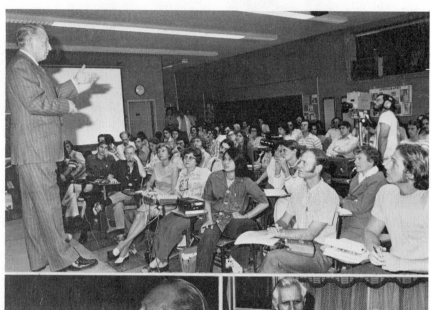

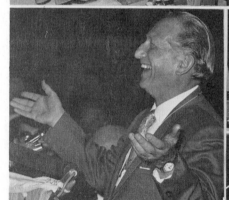

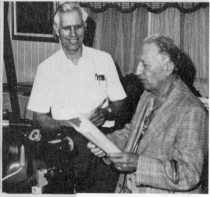

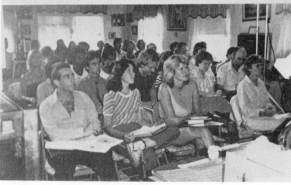

Why not choose to learn how to have vibrant health? Mid rt: Lynne Johnston, a long-time friend from Mesa, AZ, assisting Dr. Jensen in his many lectures.

8

THE WORLD IS HUNGRY FOR KNOWLEDGE OF RIGHT LIVING

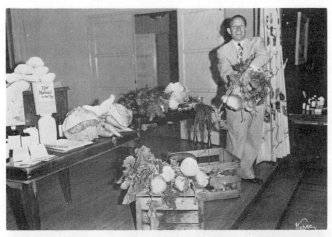

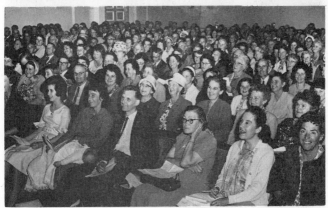

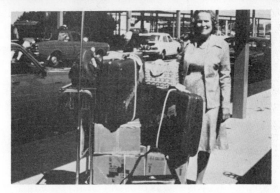

We have lectured all around the U.S. and around the world to wonderful people from many countries.

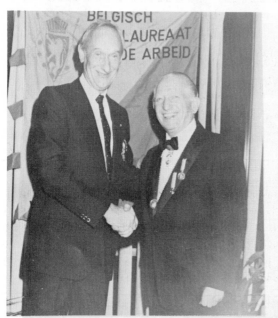
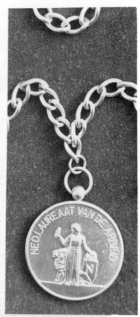
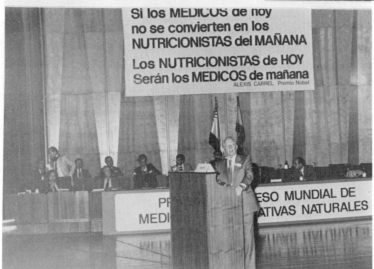

In Madrid, Spain, Dr. Jensen was presented with the Royal Netherland Labor Decoration created by King Albert of Belgium and now administered by Queen Juliana.

2

Starting Out Right With Foods And Knowing Your Food Laws

The word *health* comes from an old Teutonic word meaning *salvation. If good health is to be your salvation, you find that foods you eat have to be natural, pure* and *whole.* That is the first food law we should know. Let's take some time to find out what I mean by natural, pure and whole.

WE NEED NATURAL, PURE, WHOLE FOODS

What God makes for us—that's *natural.* You cannot pickle a cucumber and make it better than God made it for you. You can't bleach whole wheat flour and make it better than God made it for you. If God made it for human beings to eat, I don't think you can improve on it.

One example of an unnatural food is the cyclamate sweeteners used some years ago as a sugar substitute. They were found to be cancer-producing and were banned by the government. Saccharine, another sugar-substitute, was also found to be linked to cancer, but Congress overruled an FDA attempt to ban it because of objections by diabetics and others. Now we have *Nutra-Sweet,* another chemical sweetener, and time will tell what its side effects are. White sugar itself is not a natural food because it has been through a refining process that removes all vitamins and minerals. The only natural sweeteners are honey, bee pollen, carob, maple syrup and fruits.

What we have to consider about foods is that whenever man

11

handles the food, he nearly always does something that reduces the value in it. Through processing, salting, bleaching, heating and the additives he puts in, man creates foods so altered that we have every reason to be afraid of what many of them will do to the human body.

Most of our foods today are what we call "dollar foods." Most of those making foods for us know practically nothing about health. They are in business primarily for profit, and, yet, they are trying to feed you. One thing tells me we have to have a change. When I look at the average family, I see they are raising doctor bills. Their children are future doctor bills, and there's no reason for all this ill health among our kids. We need to learn the right foods to give them.

The average doctor is not going to teach you this. He has a treatment that he's trained to give. He's going to give you something to take care of your symptoms regardless of your bad habits, lifestyle and the things you don't know. Doctors make a living on your living. They make a living on your ignorance, and I think it's time for you to wake up a little bit to recognize that if you made the move to **whole, pure, natural foods**, you would make the first and best change that you could make in your health program.

Our nutritional program has to take in foods that are **pure**. Sprayed foods are not pure. We cannot call foods pure unless they are organically grown in a soil that is not chemicalized with artificial fertilizer. Pure foods cannot be called pure if they are pickled, salted or processed. They cannot be canned. You want to get away from those foods **as much as you possibly can.**

Fruits and vegetables are among the purest foods we can get, yet we have to be careful to wash them thoroughly. Not only do we find that pesticide spray residues may be on them, but also sulfite chemicals are often sprayed on them to make them stay fresher-looking and crisper, especially in salad bars. Many people are allergic to sulfite sprays, and a number of people have died after eating sulfite-sprayed foods. Many canned and packaged foods have labels that show chemicals have been added. None of these are pure foods.

Pure foods cannot be called pure if they are pickled, salted or processed. They cannot be canned. You want to get away from those foods as much as you possibly can.

Now we find that the third principle is **wholeness**. Some time ago, I discovered the value in this principle of whole foods. To begin with, I studied the work of McCollum and Simmons from Columbia University, in which they took away calcium from food given to animals and found they could not produce good bones. They found that if they took potassium away from the food, the animals' muscles weren't developed well. I know that many times the processed foods people use do not have certain chemical elements in them, and it is evident that they will develop deficiency problems.

In the Philippine Islands, they fed white rice to chickens, and after a couple of months, these chickens developed what we call "droop wing." They couldn't hold their wings in place. If they continued feeding them white rice, they would die. But they found that giving them brown rice, the whole grain instead of the polished rice, brought these chickens' wings right back into position in a few hours.

One of the big drug companies tried feeding pigeons exclusively on white rice, and in four days they lost the use of their legs and would flap backwards on the ground. But after receiving rice polishings, the pigeons were able to stand in three hours, and were completely recovered in twelve hours. Even at the point of death, the pigeons could be revived by feeding them rice polishings. The disease causing this and "droop wing" in chickens was beri-beri, the first deficiency disease discovered.

White sugar, white flour and white rice are all examples of "refined" foods, foods depleted of some or all vitamins, minerals and fiber. Such foods create deficiencies in the body, and deficiencies create conditions that lead to disease. I call these foods excoriated, foodless foods, because they no longer deserve to be called foods.

We can prevent deficiency problems by using **whole** foods, foods with nothing missing, altered or chemicalized.

When I discuss whole foods, I am including whole cereal grains, fruits, vegetables, whole milk, nuts and seeds. I include milk with some caution, because if you could see the way milk is often handled today, you'd thank God it was pasteurized. But we should be able to get raw milk that has been taken from cows milked under sanitary conditions, with the whole process subject to an

13

inspector. And we should be willing to pay an extra 10¢ a quart to get **raw whole milk**, because it is much better for us. We cannot live on depleted food. Dr. Pottenger gave cats pasteurized milk, and by the third generation, they could not reproduce. Pasteurized milk is not a whole food.

It is reported that some 27 elements have been reduced to a minimum after the refining of whole wheat flour. In other words, we are being cheated out of certain chemical elements our bodies need. The same principle can be applied to any food: *By having the whole food, we are going to build a whole body*. Can you understand now why some parts of your body may be underfed and some may be overfed? That's what happens in many different diseases in which certain organs break down from a lack of certain chemical elements. The thyroid breaks down from lack of iodine, the bones and teeth from lack of calcium, the muscle tissue from lack of potassium.

I received a letter a short time ago from a man who had Perthes' disease, where little holes develop in the bones. The man was 56 years of age, and the doctor told him it is very difficult to cure Perthes' disease at his age, almost an impossibility. But the man said that in a year and a half, by following my food regimen, those bones are much better. Is it possible? Yes, I see this often in taking care of the chemical needs of the body.

Remember, our first law is that foods should be natural, whole and pure.

THE LAW OF PROPORTIONS

The No. 2 Law is that we have to have the *proper proportions of foods*. The proper proportion law is lovely. After all, our body is proportionately put together with a certain amount of calcium, silicon, iodine—and we find that we should be able to feed this body proportionately.

Every day we should have 6 vegetables, 2 fruits, 1 good starch and 1 good protein. I don't want to be responsible for you if you don't eat any proteins. I don't want to be responsible if you don't have starches. I don't want to be responsible for you if you don't have fruit or vegetables. And, I don't want to be responsible for you if you don't have the right proportions.

In the proportions I've recommended, we find a good harmony that's going to take care of about 95% of the people. Ninety-five percent of the people who come to me can follow this harmony program and meet their nutritional needs.

The second law is the proper proportion of foods.

THE LAW OF ACID-ALKALINE BALANCE

Now I want you to understand something, and this is very important for you to learn. *The foods we eat should be 80% alkaline and 20% acid*, more on the alkaline side because we need to neutralize so much of the acid wastes produced in the body. The alkaline salts with calcium, potassium and sodium are the main acid neutralizers in the body. The acid-producing foods are the proteins, starches and sugars. When we see that we are going to have 6 vegetables, 2 fruits, 1 starch and 1 protein each day on my **Health and Harmony Food Regimen**, the vegetables and fruits come to 8 out of 10 of the foods we eat. That is 80% alkaline. Proteins, starches and sugars are practically all acid foods. So when we add up the starches and the proteins we have 2 of those compared to 8 of the vegetables and fruits. (We leave out the sugars.) Now if we look at that in a percentage-wise way and in a proportion-wise way, we've got 80% alkaline to 20% acid. And that's the proportion of alkaline-to-acid foods we want.

U.S. government figures show that the average American diet contains only 20% fruit and vegetables and the National Academy of Sciences tells us the average diet has about twice as much fat as it should have. So, at a conservative estimate, I feel the average diet is probably at least 50% to 60% acid-forming foods.

> **No. 3 Law is 80% alkaline and 20% acid foods in your diet.**

With the right foods in the right proportions, you will find that your body makes its improvements from day to day, slowly but definitely, so that at the end of 6 months, you are going to have a better body without going from one diet to another diet. I hope you see this. In the first part of the chapter, we were going over the ideas of natural, whole and pure—the **quality** of our foods. Next we are talking about **quantity**, the proportions of foods we should have.

We don't have to worry about ultimate perfection in this proportion business. If you have your starch at two meals instead of one, you will be all right. If you have your protein at two meals instead of one, I think you'll be fine. On the other hand, you don't have to have a pound-and-a-half of steak just because you're having all your protein at one meal, or two pounds of potatoes because you're having all your starch at one meal. It would be better to take the steak size you usually have, then cut it in half and have it at two meals. The main point is, let's not go to extremes by overdoing the starches and proteins.

By the way, I never have any trouble with people who eat too many vegetables and fruits in their meals. I often have trouble with people who eat too many starches and proteins.

THE SPICE OF LIFE—THE LAW OF VARIETY

> **The fourth food law is variety.**

The next thing we have to consider in our diet is the **law of variety. We have to have the proper variety.** Now what do we mean by variety? My aunt always has vegetables, but it's carrots and peas. She's never had any other vegetables. I mean your body can

16

only work with what you put into it. Some people insist on prunes every breakfast. Every morning they're full of prunes. We find they are restricting their foods so much they are going to make a one-sided body. That's why we have to have variety.

Avocados are wonderful, but not morning, noon and night, week in and week out. You can't have potatoes every day. The variety is important for many reasons. If you get apples from Washington they are entirely different from California apples. We get tomatoes from Mexico, celery from Utah. It comes from different soils.

We have to consider the different soils that these vegetables come from, their different mineral development. For instance, celery grown in New York has 25% less sodium in it than celery grown in the Salt Lake Valley of Utah. So you sometimes find the Utah-type celery advertised, but it is not Utah celery. We find that celery has to grow in a salt soil. And then it is higher in sodium. The soil that grows our Battle Creek celery is very high in sodium. When you grow celery in other parts of the country, it's usually low in sodium. So again, the law of variety is very important.

For example, the average American diet is 54% wheat and milk products and 9% sugar. This violates the **Law of Variety**, because we need fruits, vegetables, whole grains, nuts, seeds and legumes in our diets, and we need variety in our proteins, starches and fats—much greater variety than we are now getting.

When we seek variety, all of our foods should be considered day by day, week by week. What you have today, you shouldn't have tomorrow. You should have different foods from day to day.

One of the most helpful food guides to assist in getting a variety of foods is a little booklet of mine called *Creating A Magic Kitchen*. In it is a chapter titled "Know Your Sevens," which groups many foods in sevens for variety. Why should your salad dressing always be oil, honey and lemon? Why couldn't you have a buttermilk dressing? Why couldn't you have a cheese dressing or an avocado dressing? You don't need to have the same thing every day or even four days a week. That gets into a habit. A short version of "Know Your Sevens" will be presented in another chapter titled "You Deserve the Best."

A good deal of our diet problems come from habits in our eating. The people in England have their tea all the time, and they also have more rheumatism in England than any other part of the world. This is because they add a good deal of sugar to the tea, which aggravates these rheumatic conditions. Sugar robs the body of sodium, which neutralizes rheumatic acids in the body, allowing rheumatism to develop.

Once I visited a little town in South America named Heliconia where the people died at the average age of 29. Their diet was limited to sugar cane and corn. By adding soy powder to their diet as an experiment, the Upjohn Company noticed the average age increased to 39. This increase occurred just from adding a little protein to their diet. You can see what the effect is on people when there is a serious lack of variety in their food regimen.

THE BEST VEGETABLES

You should know that one of the finest vegetables is shredded beet. It's the finest vegetable I can tell you to have in your diet. It's one of the greatest things to get the bile moving through the liver and gallbladder. And, by the way, I never had a patient that didn't have some liver and gallbladder trouble. The liver is your detoxifier in the body. You must have it working at the very best rate of speed so that you can keep well. We find that turnips are wonderful, high in vitamin A and good for catarrhal conditions. I had to take care of all sorts of acidic and catarrhal conditions at the sanitarium, so I was always looking for foods and remedies to take care of that. Turnips are very good for such conditions.

THE LAW OF RAW FOODS

The 5th food law is have 60% of your food raw.

Another important law that I have put together is that **we have to have 60% raw food every day.** Sixty percent raw food. I used to say 50%, but people cheat a little bit—don't take all the raw foods they should—so, I've raised it to 60%. It's in the raw foods that you get the natural enzymes we need in our bodies. We find that cooking and processing destroy these enzymes.

When I treat people who have been on refined foods and overcooked foods for 20 years, I have to make up for it. We make up for it as quickly as we can, and this eating regime will do it. In most cases, it will take a good year to see the changes that will come in your body because of this. If you will follow through, you'll see some lovely things happen.

You often hear that our country has gone bran-crazy. Everybody has gone fiber-crazy now. *Bran is the outside coating of wheat, corn or rice.* Well, why didn't we take care of the fiber problem before? Now you have a remedy for a problem you didn't take care of before. If you knew that fresh fruits, vegetables, whole grains, nuts and seeds were rich in fiber, you wouldn't have to chase the bran wagon. If you ate proper foods, you'd be getting the fiber you need. That's another reason to change over to *my Health and Harmony Food Regimen.*

As I mentioned before, government figures show that the average U.S. diet is about 20% fruits and vegetables, and raw nuts and seeds are not included in the government's statistical tables because they probably amount to much less than 0.1%, and most people eat none at all. Most families have more cooked vegetables than raw vegetables, despite the increasing popularity of salad bars. We need to have at least two large salads a day, each with 5 to 8 raw ingredients. We should be using raw nuts and seeds, seed and nut butters, seed and nut milk drinks much more than milk products. We should be having raw vegetable and fruit juices at least twice a day, and health cocktails with a variety of blenderized ingredients, as described later in this book.

We find also that when you use **60% raw foods,** you tend to have all of the balance from a water standpoint that you should have. Also the greatest thing I can tell you is that everybody needs fiber in the diet, and you get this from chewed-up raw vegetables. You cannot live on soup, soft foods, creamy sauces and expect the intestinal tract to work properly. Raw vegetables and fruit contain a lot of water, vitamins and minerals. This is one of the finest food laws for keeping well. Some people go to the extreme with raw foods, and they are—like they say in London—"going to the edges." Some are going to all raw foods now and we have what we call fruitarians, who live only on fruit. But, let me tell you, I would rather teach you a middle path. Later on, you may want to do things differently. If I wasn't married, I would do things differently. There are times, eating with the family, when you have to compromise with the other person's likes and dislikes. Or the husband may have a physical job needing more protein. We have to make certain, even with individual differences, that we get a balance—*6 vegetables, 2 fruits, 1 starch and 1 protein every day.*

THE LAW OF NATURAL CURE

Law No. 6 is that nature cures, but she must have the opportunity.

Another law is that **nature does the curing, but she must have the opportunity to do it.** Nature cures if we let her. If you don't get enough sleep, you can't be well. If your marriage is not good, you can't be well. If your job disturbs you, irritates you, you can't be well. But I say this— **nutrition is most important.** You can straighten out all these things, but if you don't straighten out nutrition, you find you cannot have good health.

We find that drug therapies, surgery and radiation can stop a disease (or in many cases, drive it deeper into the tissues or cause it to move to some other organ or part of the body), but they cannot bring recovery to tissue. Only food can build tissue. Only food can bring reversal of symptoms, replacing old tissue with new. The only true healing is natural healing, the only kind of healing able to bring full recovery to body tissues.

ABUSING THE BODY—THE LAW OF EXCESS

Now, the next law we will discuss here is law No. 7, the

LAW OF EXCESS

20

When we have an excess, when we have too much of one or two foods, we create imbalance in the body. This law also applies to eating too much food in general, where imbalance results in obesity. Violating the law of excess creates an unnatural body.

An example of violation of the **Law of Excess** is Orson Welles, the famous Hollywood film genius, whose weight reached 400 pounds from overeating before he died on October 10, 1985. Welles was notorious for eating large beef and gravy dinners with lots of rolls and butter, finishing up with generous portions of desserts. Welles knew that his diabetes, heart condition and circulatory problems made overeating dangerous, but once told a friend, "The only thing that makes me happy is eating." According to surveys, over 60% of the American people are overweight, and about 40% are classified as obese. This is due to excess— overeating and imbalanced diets with an excess of only a few foods.

An excess in any of the three major food categories—protein, carbohydrates or fats—causes imbalances in the body and may contribute to obesity.

PROTEIN. Excess protein in the diet overtaxes the stomach, which may not have enough hydrochloric acid to break down the protein for complete digestion and assimilation in the small intestine. This undigested protein causes overgrowth of putrefactive bacteria in the bowel, resulting in many toxic byproducts such as indole, skatole and acidic amines that enter the bloodstream, causing tissue damage and settling in inherently weak organs and tissues. Excess digested and assimilated protein is simply converted to fat and stored in the tissues. Too much protein, then, causes digestive problems, putrefaction and gas in the bowel, undesirable changes in bowel flora and fat.

CARBOHYDRATES. While it is almost impossible to overeat fresh fruits, vegetables and whole grains, most vegetarian diets warn against overeating because overeating *any food can cause overweight.* Refined carbohydrates such as wheat products and white sugar make up 38% of the average American diet, which is an unhealthy excess for two reasons. All refined carbohydrates are quickly broken down into simple sugars by the digestion, and excess sugar puts strain on the pancreatic islands of Langerhans and the adrenal glands and contribute to acidity throughout the body. This may contribute to diabetes, hypoglycemia or arthritis. Secondly, excess sugar is stored in the liver and muscle tissue as glycogen for later use. When all glycogen storage sites are full, the remaining sugar is converted to fat and stored in the body. The experts say that eating too much sugar also increases the rate at which fats in the diet are stored. White sugar, white flour products and all processed carbohydrates are altered in the acid/alkaline ash balance that they had in their natural state. Because of this, they rob the body's reserve of alkaline elements (calcium, sodium and potassium) to neutralize these unnatural acidic foods. If you rob the body of calcium, sodium and potassium, you adversely affect the bones, teeth, joints and all other organs and tissues in the body. Some researchers have pointed out that white bread and many other white flour bakery products contribute to a sluggish bowel and constipation, allowing the assimilation of toxic material through the bowel wall.

FATS. The average American diet contains twice as much fat as the National Academy of Sciences recommends for a healthy diet. Excess fat causes stress on the liver and gallbladder, promotes obesity and contributes to heart disease (arteriosclerosis and atherosclerosis) and cancer. A high-fat diet is also hard on the kidneys.

There are several consequences to violating the *law of excess*. When we have an excess in a few foods, this usually means we are neglecting others and perhaps violating *the law of variety.* So we find that excess of some foods leads to chemical deficiencies due to not eating a balanced diet. Another consequence of excess may be tissue irritation and catarrh. Allergies, colds and catarrhal troubles are more common in those who eat too much of certain foods.

In Chapter 4, "Discovering the Good in Foods," we find that *63% of the average American diet is made up of milk, wheat and sugar. This is far too much! IT SHOULD BE ABOUT 6%.* Another excess in the average diet is meat and potatoes. Government studies have linked diets high in proteins and fats to cancer and heart disease. When we eat too much of the proteins and starches, we are inevitably eating too few of the vegetables and fruits, depriving our bodies of fiber, minerals and vitamins. We need to remember that disease preys on a malnourished body. We cannot upset the chemical balance of the body without serious consequences later on. One of the worst things you can do is overeat. That's abusing the body. And if you overeat, you find that your body has to take care of an excess amount of food. Most of you don't have enough hydrochloric acid to take care of an excess amount of food, especially proteins. We find that we need an excess amount of hydrochloric acid in the stomach to take care of excess food, and if you overeat when the digestion is poor, a lot of that food is not going to be digested well. It is going to cause putrefaction, gas and toxic conditions in the bowel. That can lead to a lot of problems.

Overeating is abuse. If we undereat, it's starvation, another possible form of abuse. So, if you could find out exactly how much you should have, you'd find one of the big secrets of life I believe that is one of the most important secrets of life right there.

If you are already overweight and would have perfectly balanced, perfectly harmonized meals, you should take a third (more or less) of each food on the plate and push it off to the side. *The best way to reduce is on a balanced diet.* If you do a farmer's work, it is all right to have a big farmer's breakfast, because you will work it off. But, it may not be good for a mental-type person who sits at a desk all day. The mental type will gain weight, unless he or she has an unusually fast metabolism.

When you cut back on foods, don't just cut out starches. Don't just cut out proteins. Cut out **part** of the starch, **part** of the protein, **part** of the vegetables, **part** of the fruits. You cut out a little bit of **everything**, but you keep the balance. Eat a "child's portion" more often, especially if you want to reduce. Keep the balance. That's very important.

I once read about a man who lived until he was 108 years of age on just one pint of grape juice a day and 12 ounces of food. He became very thin. The insurance companies tell us that the smaller the waistline, the longer the lifeline.

DEFICIENCY IS LINKED TO DISEASE

Law No. 8 is the law of deficiency.

The **LAW OF DEFICIENCY** is the opposite of the **LAW OF EXCESS**, and it is just as hazardous. What we neglect to eat can affect our health just as much as what we eat. The **Law of Deficiency** applies whether: 1) we are undernourished, malnourished or starving; 2) we are using refined foods lacking vitamins and minerals; 3) we are using foods grown on depleted soils; 4) we are using a diet inadequate to our job demands or daily stress levels; 5) we are using an imbalanced diet or one-sided diet; and 6) we are deficient in one nutrient, vitamin or mineral or many. **EVERY DISEASE HAS A MINERAL AND VITAMIN DEFICIENCY.**

We could give many examples of the **LAW OF DEFICIENCY.** Beriberi is a disease caused by thiamine deficiency (B-1), common among people who use refined white rice. Osteoporosis, a bone-weakening disease, is epidemic in women over 60 in the U.S. possibly due to mineral deficiencies. Kwashiorkor, common in third world countries, is a disease resuting from protein deficiency.

WATER

The next thing that we have to think about is the kind of water we should have. Most urban water supplies are too chemicalized from trying to overcome pollution, and water in many rural areas is contaminated by runoff from agricultural sprays and chemical fertilizers. These substances are of no benefit to the body and many are harmful. So I feel *reverse osmosis* water is the best we can get or, if you have extreme arthritis, distilled water may be best.

During my visit to the Hunza Valley, I saw the old men taking the water right out of the mountainside streams. Pure mountain water is all right. But you can only get it in areas where man has not meddled too much with nature.

COMBINING FOODS

Now another thing we have to take care of is food combinations. I don't put much emphasis on combinations, although I don't want you to combine junk food and fried food. So it is simply a matter of making the natural foods our priority. That's what we put at the top of the list. All of these other considerations we have discussed are more important than combinations. If you aren't sure about what makes good food combinations, it is better to have natural foods of any kind rather than the "foodless" foods available in the stores. Here are a few of the combinations to think about.

Extreme starches and extreme proteins should not be taken together. What is that? That's meat and potatoes. Or, fried potatoes and fried eggs. These are really bad combinations. It is best not to have potatoes at all for breakfast, but I don't object to having protein and whole grain cereals together at that time. If nature doesn't do a perfect job, we will allow you to go with starches and proteins that are not complete or what we might call "compound foods." Most grains and natural proteins are not 100% protein or 100% starch.

We find that melons don't mix well with most of our foods, and should be eaten at a different time. Sweet dried fruit should not be taken with citrus fruit. This is all we need to think about. I don't feel there is any great reason for *always* eating starches and proteins at separate meals, except so we will eat more vegetables instead of filling up on protein and starch before getting to them.

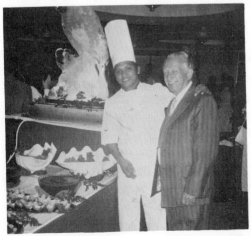

Wherever Dr. Jensen travels, he heads for the kitchen.

SUMMARY OF DR. JENSEN'S FOOD LAWS
If you follow these laws, you will stay healthy.

1. LAW OF NATURAL, WHOLE AND PURE

Our foods should be **natural, whole and pure,** whole foods build a whole body.

2. LAW OF PROPORTIONS

Our foods should be in the proper proportions; each day we should have **6 vegetables, 2 fruits, 1 starch and 1 protein.**

3. LAW OF ACID/AKALINE BALANCE

Our foods should be **80% alkaline foods** and **20% acid foods.** Vegetables and fruits are alkaline. Starches and proteins are acid.

4. LAW OF VARIETY

Our foods should represent proper variety. Different vegetables, different fruits, different starches and proteins every day.

5. LAW OF RAW FOODS

Our foods should be **60% raw.** It is in the natural raw form that we get the most nutritional value (including "live" enzymes) from foods.

6. LAW OF NATURAL CURE

Nature cures, but she must have the **opportunity.** Only when you eat properly is the body supplied with the nutrients needed for tissue repair and replacement, by nature's design.

7. LAW OF EXCESS

We cannot eat one or a few foods to excess without causing deficiencies from lack of variety in our diet.

8. LAW OF DEFICIENCY

A deficiency syndrome in any cell or organ is developed when that tissue has been overworked, burned out from environmental causes or lack of certain necessary foods, vitamins and minerals that are usually assimilated from **natural, pure and whole foods.**

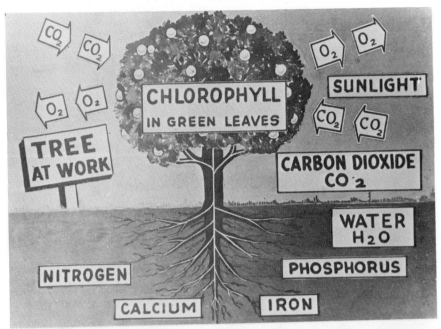

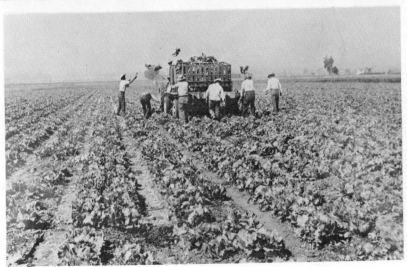

Top: Trees are oxygen factors. Bottom: Harvesting food for the market.

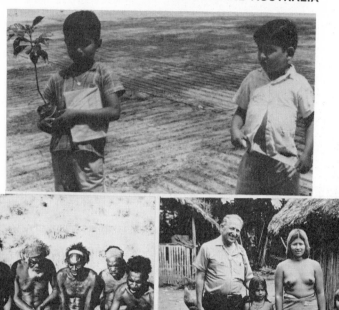

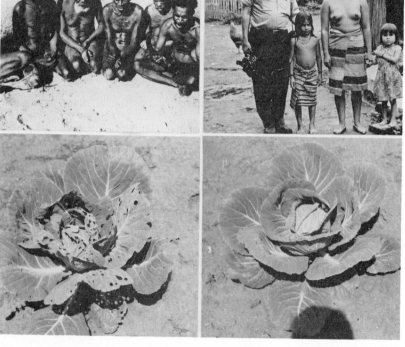

Top: Children planting a tree in South America. Mid Left: Australian Aborigines had little disease until the white man came. Mid Rt: Amazon natives, showing effects of calcium depletion of the soil. Bottom: Insects attack cabbage grown in poor soil but not one grown in rich soil.

3

Where Is Our Farmlife Going?

When I started in my practice of nutrition 50 years ago, the farmer was considered to be our real doctor. We looked to him to produce the food that finally became our bodies.

When farmers were pressured into chemical agriculture, at the instigation of the chemical companies and their agents, human health began to deteriorate. Farmers make up only 6% of the population, raising food for the other 94%. They used to be primarily food producers, but now, due to economic and financial pressures, they have had to become businessmen like manufacturers, retailers and wholesalers.

Farmers now are forced to use artificial fertilizers more than ever to grow foods quickly to reduce their debts, if they can. The balance sheet has become the bottom line.

Agriculture has changed so much that the farmer no longer has to have a green thumb. He is fast losing his natural gift to plant and harvest according to age-old proven principles. He has been sold a bill of goods inducing him to buy a big tractor and other outrageously expensive equipment. In order to pay for it, he has to install headlights in order to work half the night. Farmers no longer have time to be as neighborly as they used to. They must keep their noses glued to the grindstone to keep the sheriff from foreclosing.

The farm of the future, according to a recent congressional report, will be treated financially like any other business—it will have to demonstrate profitability before a bank will finance its operation.

Scientists have become fascinated with changing the genetic pattern of plants. They have created varieties that will grow in frost and snow. But most of these result from hybrids by eliminating the seeds. This destroys the food value for human glands. We thus end up with a full stomach, but we don't have a full nutritional balance in the foods we eat.

For the best nutrition, we should have the smallest fruits, berries and vegetable possible, which have the greatest amount of nutritive values.

Bio-engineering is extremely important in food production. If foods do not have the proper caloric value and a color emanation from a complete spectrum, we cannot expect to get the full value from that food to keep us well. All foods should be measured with a full color background.

The widespread use of agricultural chemicals is very dangerous. In Arizona, for example, several dairies had to be closed because of the spray used on alfalfa. It affected the milk production and eventually the toxins in the spray were found in humans. It affected the human glandular system, as well as the hormone secretions, producing a tremendous buildup of allergies of various kinds.

Because of the enormous use of sprays, Arizona's bee industry was virtually destroyed.

A recent television documentary, "Fields of Fear," showed dramatic consequences of chemical farming in California. Practically the entire state has had its soil infested with overdosages of pesticides and insecticides. The chemical companies long maintained that their products would quickly evaporate and never penetrate the aquifers, but recent tests have shown that approximately two-thirds of the underground water supply has been tainted.

While there are no definitive proofs so far, there have been widespread cases of very young California children dying from leukemia, cancer and heart attacks. One case involved a boy who was born with no arms or legs—similar to the thalidomide horrors of a few years ago.

One segment of the documentary mentioned that out of approximately 50,000 California farmers, only 400 are considered to be practicing organic agriculture. Several scenes showed dramatic examples of how these farmers have solved their infestation problems by using biological controls such as lady bugs and other beneficial insects. They had lowered their costs from $35 to $15 per acre, which goes to prove that large-scale organic farming is not only possible but economically feasible, if the rape of our soil hasn't progressed beyond the point of no return.

In 1985, over one million watermelons had to be destroyed in California because of sprays used which had a dastard effect on the humans who consumed the watermelons.

Allergies are sweeping the country. Many people are being diagnosed with them, no matter what disease they may complain of. In Germany, an allergy was discovered caused by arsenic used on grapes, which even caused cancer. Many of our agricultural sprays contain a carcinogenic agent. Even in processed foods such as muffin and cake mixes, we find suspicious chemicals like EBT and DDT, along with many others that have been proven to be harmful to the human.

Modern technology is going to eventually kill off even more farms. According to the recent congressional study previously mentioned, 60% of North Dakota's wheat farmers, for example, are expected to be out of business within the next five years. Technology is not an unalloyed blessing. It is predicted that by the year 2000 nearly half of the nation's farms will have disappeared.

Chicken ranchers are literally running "factories." They raise chickens packed in cages with lights on all night so they get full egg production 24 hours daily. The chickens get no exercise. Drugs are added to their diets so they put on more fat. Some ranchers fast the chickens so they don't go through the moulting period so much, thus giving extra eggs.

Farmers raising beef cattle often give them stilbestrol, which puts on extra fat, giving a return of $20 to $40 more when the livestock is sold. The same thing happens with dairy cattle. They are bred to produce the maximum amount of milk by mixing chemicals with their feed.

Technology has destroyed most of the bird population which is so necessary for pollination. Chemicals are killing them off. Worms, so vital to proper soil cultivation, now migrate because they can't survive chemical fertilizers.

Computers cannot substitute for the farmer's ancient wisdom of knowing when to plant and harvest, but computers are now being used to tell farmers what kind and proportion of feeds to mix for their chickens or cattle. Old McDonald's farm is not going to be in our future. We may have a plentiful food supply, but of what value will it be to our health?

Could it be possible that a large part of our crime results from poor nutrition? Many nutritional experts believe it is.

There is a large element of our population that is doing even more to raise its own food—a most hopeful sign. But, of course, that isn't possible for millions of city dwellers. However, there are places where city folk are banding together to raise crops cooperatively on vacant lots. It may become necessary, if we are to survive, that more and more of us will be forced to raise our own organic foods.

City children should be taken on regular trips to farms to see how and where their food really comes from. Many of them think milk originates in the carton in the supermarket. I raise goats on my ranch, and believe it or not, some visitors look at them and say, "What wonderful deer you have!"

We must get back to the concept that the farmer is really the doctor in the house. He is the backbone of American agriculture, and if we squeeze him out of his job, we squeeze out our health. And maybe even our food supply.

Another critical factor is that we have less than 10% of natural seeds available. We already have seedless oranges and now they are developing seedless avocados and watermelons. Eliminating seeds genetically wipes out the life and value in food. It has a very harmful effect on the human glandular system.

Vitamin E and lecithin are being eliminated by genetic engineering on our food. This could be responsible for a lot of our sex disturbances today, resulting from glandular malfunction.

Nutritional deficiencies are going to multiply geometrically because of the rape of our agriculture. Farmers must be educated to return to their ancient natural ways, otherwise the rest of us will all end up in hospitals and sanitariums, with not enough knowledgeable doctors to take care of us—or we may end up in a premature grave.

In my humble opinion, the farm problem is the greatest crisis facing America. It is basic and fundamental, and it should have our No. 1 priority for our health's sake. The farmers are really our doctors. The soil nurtures us. Between the farmers and the soil, we have the combination that gives us our well-being for the future.

4

Food—From Soil to Your Kitchen

In some 20 years of practice with diet care, I have found that people are experimenting with themselves through more types of diet and different food combinations than ever before. Before my eyes, many people have improved from all types of disease conditions through correct food science. The food regimen which includes consideration of vitamins and minerals is uppermost in the progressive doctor's mind today. Volumes have been written on how our stomachs are filled with "foodless food," how we are "starving amidst plenty," and on how doctors are looking for a cure. And, truly, our bodies are often suffering from a "hidden hunger."

What follows is a condensation in pictorial form of the many books that are being written these days on experiments and experiences regarding food science and how it affects the human body.

When Dr. McCarrison of Great Britain was appointed Director of Nutrition Research to study the health of the different groups throughout India, he found ethnic groups in Pakistan and Northern India called the Hunzas and Sikhs who were practically free of disease. They were wonderful looking people, having beautiful bodies, properly balanced chemically and long-lived.

Dr. McCarrison fed 1200 rats on the diet of these people, and not a single rat died of a disease. While carrying on the same experiments in Southern India, the same rats—under similar conditions—fed on the diet of these people, died of every disease imaginable from tuberculosis, bronchial disorders, arthritis, rickets, ulcers, etc., and developed bad dispositions and even became ferocious.

33

There is a story in this which applies to our country today. Our food is made up of many chemical elements such as calcium, silicon, sodium, iodine, magnesium, etc., and all these elements are found in good soil to begin with. Through a process of absorption, they are transmuted to plant life where the chemicals of the soil finally become food for man. It is plant life, grown from fertile and chemically-balanced soil, that is necessary for human nutrition. This plant life is transported to the kitchen—and here is where another loss of these vital life-giving chemicals is taking place in America today.

It is possible to starve with a full stomach if the food you eat is grown on depleted soil or is processed or cooked improperly. The water-soluble chemical elements in soil are eventually washed into the ocean, thus robbing it of many of the elements necessary for proper growth and health. We know virgin or chemically well-balanced soil produces the best crops—healthy and fully developed. Depleted soil produces depleted plant life. Much of the fertility and life of the soil in the U.S. has been drained out through constant crop growing so that today we are only getting 20 bushels of corn to an acre on unfertililzed soil, while years ago, when the soil was virgin or chemically well-balanced, production was as high as 50 to 60 bushels an acre. From the chemicals found in plant life, our body structure is built—*what we eat today will walk and talk tomorrow.*

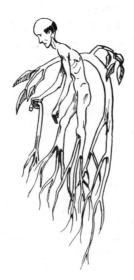

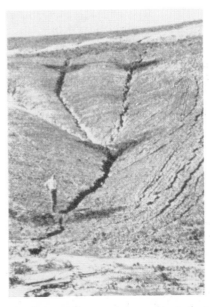

Poor soil cannot grow good plant life for sound bodies.

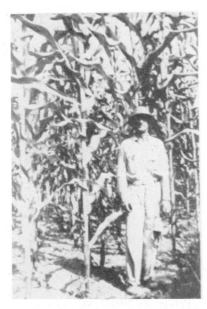

Corn grown as above averaged over 200 bushels to an acre.

Do you know that most of us today are suffering from certain dangerous diet deficiencies which cannot be remedied until the depleted soils are brought into proper mineral balance? The alarming fact is that foods—fruits and vegetables and grains now being raised on millions of acres of land that no longer contains enough of certain needed minerals—are starving us, no matter how much of them we eat!

—U.S. Government Document No. 264

When the soil has been depleted and the soil structure is unbalanced, then we grow plant life which is diseased and undeveloped. By making a more fertile and well-balanced soil, we are able to change these disease conditions. We have to recognize that most of the minerals found in the topsoil of the mountains and valleys are eventually carried away by the rain, are washed into rivers and carried into the ocean. Ocean farming is going to become the dominant thing in the future, because all of our trace minerals are going there.

These illustrations of actual experiments show a healthy plant grown and entwined with an unhealthy diseased plant covered with microorganisms and parasites. Even direct contact failed to transfer disease or parasites from one to the other. The illustration is based on an actual experiment.

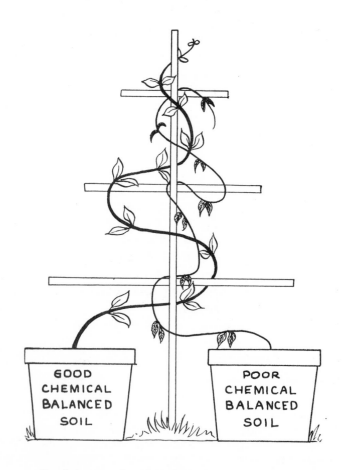

Resistance is developed through proper nourishment.

CHEMICALLY BALANCED SOIL—THE KEY TO GOOD HEALTH

When I studied with Dr. William Albrecht, Chairman of the Department of Soils at the University of Missouri, he taught that *disease preys on an undernourished plant.* When people use foods grown on deficient soils, they, too, become undernourished and subject to disease. The health of food crops depends upon the mineral balance of the soil, and our health depends on our foods.

CALCIUM—A VITAL NEED

In a film titled, *The Other Side of the Fence,* Dr. Albrecht showed how domestic animals fenced in to graze on chemically fertilized ground would reach over the fence to graze on the plants growing in natural soil.

According to Dr. Albrecht, *"Living on soils of the humid region (of the U.S.), our animals, like ourselves, do not get enough calcium regularly to prevent nutritional deficiencies."*

NATURAL COMPOSTING MAKES THE BEST SOIL

As Dr. Albrecht has pointed out, *"Nature uses no concentrated (chemical) salts in building up her soils to an ecological climax, Instead, she uses the decaying organic matter of the past dead generations of exactly the same plant species which she is growing."* Bacteria are constantly at work on decaying organic matter in the soil, breaking the plant life down to its elements again, for use by the next generation of plants. Natural soil is *alive,* constantly replenishing itself. Chemically fertilized soil is *dead*, and the crops it bears lack the vitality and life force of plants grown in natural soils.

PROCESSING AND REFINING FOODS

In the processing, preserving and refining of wheat for example, the vital life elements are destroyed. This leaves only the starchy part of the wheat void of the mineral balance and vitamins needed for healthful body functions such as proper heart function, bowel regularity and many other tissue functions in the body. The degree of health of our bodies depends upon the amount of life in the food we eat.

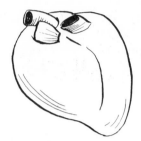

Sound heart tissues develop best from whole natural foods.

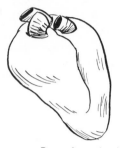

Poor-functioning heart tissues can develop from refined demineralized foods.

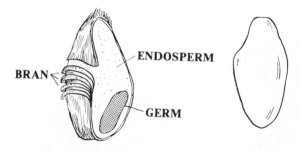

ENDOSPERM

BRAN

GERM

In the whole wheat are the minerals, germ life and bran necessary as food for the body.

Refined and demineralized flour products are void of the proper vitamin and mineral content.

Look at the difference between what polished rice and natural brown rice can do to a pigeon! Within three hours after feeding vitamin B-rich rice polishings, the pigeon was able to stand, and recovery seemed to be complete in 12 hours. (See next page.)

Chemical experiments have been done on rats as shown in the pictures below. Compare the animal which was fed improperly with the larger healthy one which was fed on a chemically well-balanced diet. Rats have been experimented with for many years, and many deficiency diseases have been produced in them that man is heir to. The sad mistake is that these same experiments are going on with human beings daily, only unintentionally.

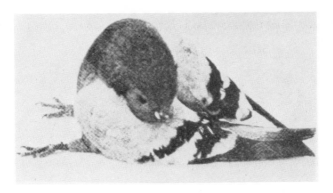

Before

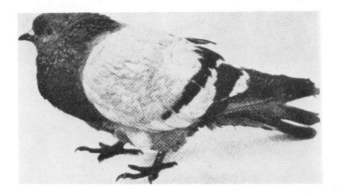

After

The pictures of the chickens shown below indicate what can be done with animals. When fed on diets improperly balanced chemically, the animals are small, scrawny and weak; while those fed on diets properly balanced with the chemical elements necessary for proper growth are strong, well-developed and free from disease.

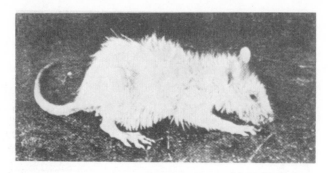

Before

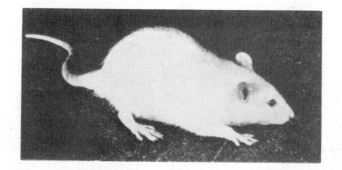

After

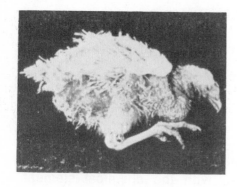

Before

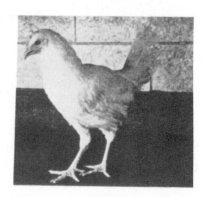

After

40

SOME OF MY OWN CASES

The chemical story is a big story, and does not stop with animals. Actually, humans are being experimented upon today in much the same manner through our refined and preserved foods and through our cooking processes. From my own experience with patients, I have seen arthritis cleared up, spines straightened, and all types of diseases have responded, just by feeding people the proper foods. The following are actual cases taken from my files showing the effect the proper chemicals have on structure and growth of the human body.

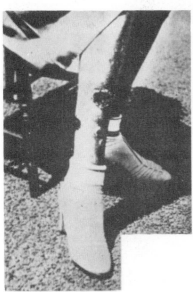
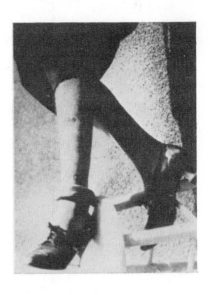

Before   *After*

These leg ulcers defied all types of treatment for years and were healed in a matter of weeks by feeding the proper natural food elements.

We are exaggerating in some of the pictures and examples. This is not intended as a scare tactic but is intended for teaching purposes. You should be aware that these conditions exist.

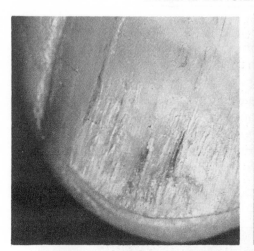
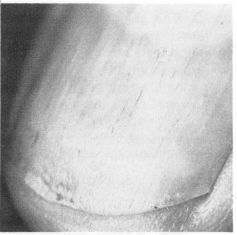
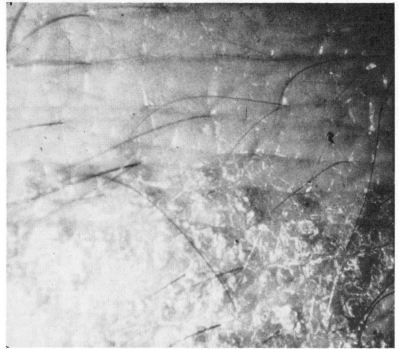

Silicon is one of the vital chemical elements needed by the nails and skin. When the diet is deficient in silicon foods, the nails may become discolored and show irregular ridges or unusual texture. Skin may become dry, scaly, red, crusted and flaky. If the skin and nails are deficient in silicon, then the **whole body is deficient in this mineral.** *This demonstrates new tissue taking place of the old with diet alone.*

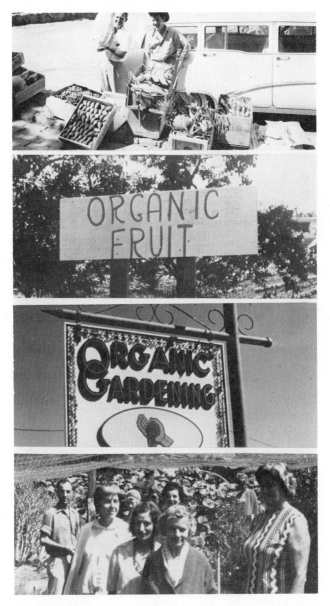

Top: Harvest time! Middle: Signs from a beautiful valley in Canada. Bottom: Tour of the Ranch showing organically-grown produce.

When you are improperly nourished, your posture can become distorted; curvature of the spine can develop; organs can be misplaced and put under undue pressure.

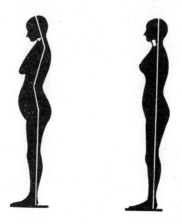

Eight of ten American women have a calcium deficiency and this can begin in girls at 11 years of age.

A dentist sent this 12-year-old boy to me because his teeth decay resulted from a diet lacking the proper chemical balance.

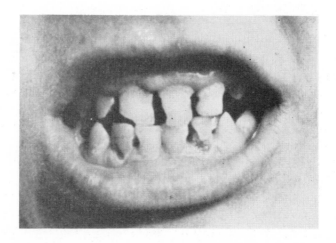

WE NEED A CHANGE IN THE KITCHEN

The responsibility for the health of the entire family rests upon the shoulders of the housewife, mother or cook. Just as a surgeon has the best tools and equipment to save a life, so the housewife, mother or cook should have the best tools and equipment to build and retain a good health-life for her family.

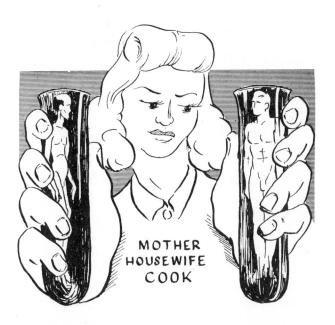

MOTHER
HOUSEWIFE
COOK

One of the greatest mutilations of the chemical elements takes place right in your own cooking utensils. When ordinary cooking methods are used, from 32% to 76% of the essential food values, minerals and vitamins are lost due to oxidation, destruction by heat or being dissolved in water (according to the Bureau of Home Economics, U.S. Dept. of Agriculture). By using waterless cookware and following simple instructions, these important essentials may be retained. Oxidation is practically eliminated, less heat is required and waterless cooking is possible.

Through "vapor sealing," the food values and flavors are retained within the utensil and not lost through evaporation. Immediately after vapor begins to form, it rises to the lid, then travels along the inside surface to the rim where it forms a seal. As a result, vitamins and minerals are preserved—not carried away by escaping steam.

Do you know that some 60% of the potassium content of the potato, for instance, is directly beneath the skin? Through the peeling of vegetables in preparation for cooking, valuable chemical elements are lost.

Three things in the kitchen rob the life from our food, producing a starved mineral condition in our body. These three kitchen robbers are:

1. High temperature
2. Use of water (carrying off minerals)
3. Oxidation (contact with air while cooking).

Keep your mineral values in your kitchen!

Waterless cookware has been designed to cook with only the water on the freshly-rinsed vegetables, to cook below the boiling point and to prevent air from oxidizing food while cooking.

NUTRIENT LOSSES FROM BOILING

Research published in the JOURNAL OF HOME ECONOMICS showed that in cooking foods by boiling, 48% of the iron is lost, 31% of the calcium is destroyed, 46% of the phosphorus is cooked away and 45% of the magnesium is wasted.

Boiling causes a total approximate loss of 50% of the food value of white potatoes, 40% of the value of cabbage and 50% of the nutritional content of an apple.

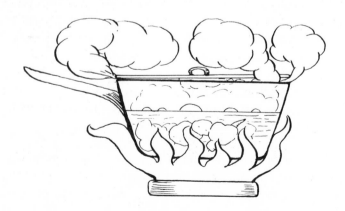

PREPARING OUR FOOD

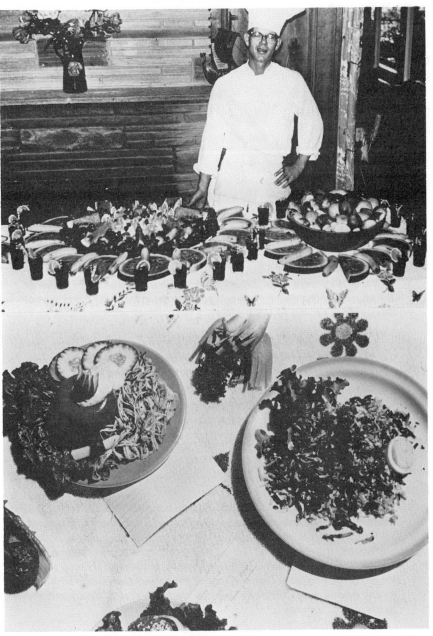

Preparing food is an art, but it should have the practical result of health and long life. This is a table set at our Ranch.

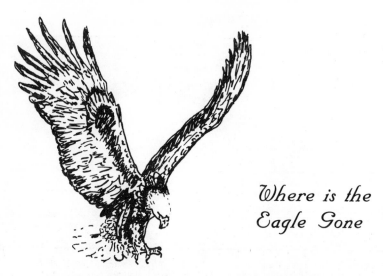

Where is the Eagle Gone

The Great Chief in Washington sends word that he wishes to buy our land. How can you buy or sell the sky—the warmth of the land? The idea is strange to us. Yet we do not own the freshness of the air or the sparkle of the water. How can you buy them from us? Every part of this earth is sacred to my people.

We know that white man does not understand our ways. One portion of the land is the same to him as the next, for he is a stranger who comes in the night and takes from the land whatever he needs. The earth is not his brother but his enemy, and when he has conquered it he moves on. He leaves his fathers' graves and his children's birthright is forgotten.

There is no quiet place in the white man's cities. No place to hear the leaves of spring or the rustle of insects' wings. But perhaps because I am savage and do not understand—the clatter only seems to insult the ears. And what is there to liife if a man cannot hear the lovely cry of the whippoorwill or the argument of the frog around the pond at night.

The whites, too, shall pass—perhaps sooner than other tribes. Continue to contaminate your bed and you will one night suffocate in your own waste. When the buffalo are all slaughtered, the wild horses are tamed, the secret corners of the forest heavy with the scent of many men, and the view of the ripe hills blotted by talking wires. Where is the thickets? Gone. Where is the eagle? Gone. And what is it to say goodbye to the swift and the hunt, the end of living and the beginning of survival.

**—Chief Seattle to President Franklin Pierce
1855**

5

Discovering
the
Good in Foods

I'd like to mention that my years of working in sanitariums have been wonderful experiences for me. People were coming in off Main Street really sick and in wheelchairs. As serious as these conditions were, there is one thing I have learned, which is that the body molds to the nutritional values you take into it. Your body molds to coffee and donuts or it molds to a salad.

The woman I mentioned in the last chapter with the 13 leg ulcers was completely healed in a matter of 3 weeks. Well, the healing resulted because of a shift in tissue to a higher level, the old tissue replaced by the new. Can you see this? We can elevate our health level. We take the body out of the disease level and we bring it to the highest health level possible. And we do this by using the proper nutritional values.

As we take care of different conditions in the body by adding certain nutritional values, the body gets better because the tissue changes. You change the skin; you change the stomach; you change the bones; and this can all be done with nutritious foods. *In fact, only food can repair and rebuild tissue.*

In contrast, we find there is also a tissue shift in the body when we have an excess amount of toxic materials settled there. Tissue deteriorates and becomes less active. Underactivity and toxic materials always go hand in hand. Now, all of us have inherent weaknesses, organs and tissues that are not quite as healthy, strong or disease-resistant as the rest of our body. Toxic materials settle in the inherent weaknesses in the body. To reverse this condition, we have to build up the functional ability. Integrity of all tissue can be improved by taking the nutritional values and chemical elements, as I have explained.

Through my Health and Harmony Food Regimen, I find that toxic materials leave the body, and all tissues function better and more normally. I don't think I've ever had a patient who didn't find that his bowel function was better after utilizing this harmonious way of eating. When elimination is better, you find that the level in every tissue is improved. A chemically well-nourished body will be clean and capable of repairing and rebuilding.

PROPER DIET CAN CHANGE LIVES

The way we think, feel and act is strongly influenced by the foods we eat, as shown by the following news clipping.

LONDON, ENGLAND—"Can Diet Cut Juvenile Delinquency? A survey of 17 maladjusted or delinquent girls between the ages of 11 and 15 in a Salvation Army hostel seems to prove that diet makes good girls from bad ones. Previously the girls lived on the poorest possible types of meals: white bread and margarine, cheap jam, lots of sweetened tea, canned and processed meats. Fish and chips had been one of their most nutritious meals. A year later, their diet was changed to raw fruits, nuts, vegetables, salads, whole wheat bread, dates, prunes, figs, honey, cheese, meat, fish, eggs, oatmeal, crushed wheat. This is what happened. The girls quickly became less aggressive and less quarrelsome, bad habits seemed to disappear, 'problem children' became less of a problem and the bored ones lost their boredom. Physically, they improved almost beyond recognition. A spokesman said, 'It is amazing to see the difference in their complexions, general brightness and poise, but the difference in their behavior is the most significant. The part the diet played in their personalities is undeniable.'"

HOW WE ACCUMULATE TOXIC SETTLEMENTS

Toxic levels in the body always increase as we use the wrong foods, neglect to exercise, don't get enough sleep and deplete **the chemical reserves** in the body. We become tired and imbalanced in our bodies and brain functions and we build up toxic settlements throughout every inherently weak organ in the body. These toxic settlements include drug residues, sprays and chemical additives from foods, chemical pollutants from the air and water supply, and other external sources, but they also include a great deal of catarrh

50

and acidic wastes produced inside the body which are not eliminated. To be overloaded with toxic wastes, we must have had certain habits in our lifestyle, especially our eating habits, that have brought about this situation.

After a time, there is too much toxic material in the body. The elimination organs aren't able to take care of it well enough. So, we have to go back and try to make that damaged, toxic-laden tissue pure, clean and whole again. The only way I know how to do that is through the use of proper nutritional values. You can use bowel cleansing treatments or any other kind of treatments, but if you don't have the nutrition straightened out, you are not going to restore the integrity or chemical balance of toxic-laden poorly-nourished tissue.

When we find excess catarrh or acid wastes in the body, it is always a sign that the body is not working normally. It is slow. We have a lazy colon. We find we don't carry enough of the proper fluids in our body to get rid of the uric acid, carbonic acid and other tissue wastes. We have to lower the level of toxic settlements because we have been adding to that level constantly, and there is a limit to how much we can take. There may come a point of no return, and we develop a degenerative disease. There's no use traveling that path; it is better to prevent it.

A TYPICAL AMERICAN DIET

Many years ago, I had my sanitarium patients write down what they ate every day. You know what I found in everyone's diet? They had salads with iceberg lettuce, which is nutritionally worthless and gas-forming. Everyone had orange juice, to get their vitamin C. They had bacon and eggs, ham and eggs, sausage and eggs—always fried. And everyone had bread. It was hard for me to believe all the bread they were eating. They were building their meals around bread and other baked wheat products. Everyone had milk or at least a lot of milk products—butter, cottage cheese, buttermilk, processed cheese, cream, ice cream, whipped cream. I began *to see that all their younger years had been built mainly on wheat and milk!* Also, everyone was having meat and potatoes. Can you see this? Can you see how people get in the habit of using the same few foods cooked the same way, day after day?

WE CAN DO BETTER

To start living by the food laws mentioned in Chapter 2, we could change to Romaine lettuce, bib lettuce, a red leaf lettuce, Boston leaf lettuce or the different greens such as endive and watercress in our salads. We need variety and more nourishing greens. We need two green vegetables a day. But, we do not need iceberg lettuce. It furnishes no nourishment, and it is gas forming. It also contains a chemical substance that slows down the digestion. You find most people's digestion is already too slow.

I wondered why they used orange juice every day, and the people said, "We take it for the vitamin C. We have a lot of catarrh and we'd like to get rid of it." If they'd been eating right, they wouldn't have been producing catarrh and they wouldn't have needed extra vitamin C! Where is our law of variety if we are only going to have orange juice every day? They didn't seem to realize that we need to eat the orange pulp too. *The calcium balance is in the pectin of the pulp which also provides bulk for the bowel.* The problem here is that we neglect having a variety of juices from day to day. I don't tell people to eat the skins of oranges or bananas, but we do need to remember to eat as much of the whole fruit as possible. *We should have foods that are whole, pure and natural.*

Now, I live in a citrus belt and they pick the citrus 6 weeks too early, in most cases. Most of you are getting green citric acid in your oranges and juice, which can stir up more acids than the kidneys can carry off. The sodium in citrus is only fully developed when the sun shines on the fruit until it is completely mature.

This is one reason I don't believe in a fruitarian diet, *because the average person can't get ripe fruit.* I once read that no Bostonian had ever tasted a vine-ripened blackberry, because it was all shipped in. We wouldn't deliberately eat either a green apricot or an overripe rotten one. We want that apricot right on the button, perfectly ripened by the sun.

The sun is a sodium star, and we find that is what ripens fruit. Because the citrus fruit we find in the store is picked early, I don't believe in using it or the juice. Citrus stirs up acids and puts an extra load on the kidneys, two of the most important eliminative organs. There are many other fruits beside citrus, and they should be used for variety. Oranges should be organically grown, tree ripened, peeled and eaten in sections. We should use citrus only occasionally.

If we lived closer to the Equator, we could eat more fruits because we could get it ripe and because—since we perspire more in a warmer climate—we would eliminate enough acids through the skin so the kidneys would not be overloaded.

VEGETABLES ARE A DIFFERENT STORY

In contrast to fruit, vegetables, in most cases, don't have a critical maturity date. You can have young beets or old beets, young squash or old squash. Vegetables can be picked and used almost any time. That's another reason why I put 6 vegetables and only 2 fruits in my food regimen. This is 3 times as many vegetables as fruit. In the summertime, when you're perspiring a lot, you can take extra fruit because the extra sodium helps to replace what is lost in perspiration. If you've ever tasted perspiration, you know it is very salty. We need more sodium in the summertime.

I would like to emphasize that vegetables carry off the acids, while fruits stir them up, and citrus stirs them up more than all other fruits. This is something to stop and think about.

Two foods I advise against using are rhubarb and cranberries. These are two of the highest foods in oxalic acid and can cause disturbances with the joints, even after they are cooked.

The next thing is the fried eggs and bacon, ham or sausage for breakfast. Frying and high heat (over 212 degrees), in general, destroy the lecithin in eggs or any food, which is meant to balance and take care of the cholesterol. This is one reason we find an imbalance of cholesterol in so many people today. The fatty meats such as bacon, ham and sausage overload the system with overheated fats and leaves the cholesterol without the balancing element of lecithin or unsaturated fatty acids. This is just too much fat and cholesterol for the normal system to handle. *High heat makes chemical changes in the nutritional balance and ingredients of foods.*

It is all right to have eggs twice, three or even four times a week, but they should be boiled or poached. High heat should not be used in cooking eggs, as in baking or frying. And, **we should be taking the whole grain cereals cooked under low heat,** otherwise lecithin is not there as a balancing agent.

WHEAT LOGGED—BEGINNING OF CATARRH

When I had everyone write out their diets, I noticed they all made their meals around bread. They had toast, French toast or muffins for breakfast, then they had sandwiches for lunch. How many sandwiches did they have? Goodness me! I had patients who said they had 5 or 6 sandwiches for lunch! At the evening meal, they had bread on the table again. This is a lot of wheat. Then I asked what kind of cereals they had. Most always they had wheat cereals. And how many different varieties are there? Something for everyone's palate and taste. So I began to look at wheat in the same way I looked at the overloading of toxic material in the body.

When I found out how much bread and wheat were being used, I wondered what they were doing to the body. I found that bread can be very constipating because the lecithin, vitamin E and natural oils are altered and ruined because of high heat used for baking. All our breakfast cereals are anything but **natural**, and many are cooked with added white sugar. I found out that you can never heat lecithin above 212 degrees, the temperature of boiling water, otherwise you destroy this wonderful brain and nerve food. Lecithin is a brain and nerve fat. They cannot keep these oils in foods naturally because oxygenation sets in, and they get rancid. Bread is baked at very high temperatures and sometimes for over an hour. I include pies, cakes and pastries (all of which I like) when I talk about bread, because they are usually all wheat products. We have to consider this for a moment because, in addition to wheat, I began to look at milk, dairy products and white sugar.

WE'RE MILK LOGGED

I found government tests that told how the average American diet was running 29% wheat products and 25% milk products. This violates the **Law of Excess.**

WE ARE WHEAT LOGGED AND MILK LOGGED.

When we add it all up, that is 54% of the total average diet! I feel this is far too much of these two foods! I believe this amount should be no more than 6%.

Think of this—don't let this escape your mind. When are you going to have leaf lettuce? Watercress? When are you going to have asparagus? When are you going to have beets? When are you going to have these lovely foods? You have squeezed them out by the amount of wheat and milk you have in your daily eating tht makes the average person *WHEAT LOGGED AND MILK LOGGED.* This has been accumulated. You have gone through your childhood and early adult years troubled with all the catarrh problems that affect growing children.

WHY MY EARLY PATIENTS WERE NOT GETTING WELL

When I first started out in health work, I didn't understand why some of my patients were not getting better. Then, over the years, I began to see that the people who were having the greatest problems were the ones who were having the same foods over and over, and I began to see there was a problem with tolerance. The body is not designed to take too much of the same foods day after day. We have to consider that possibly we have overloaded our bodies; we have put in the wrong proportions of certain foods; and, we are suffering from the fact that we cannot tolerate any more of them.

The foods causing the greatest reactions were milk, wheat and sugar. I had always felt that milk and wheat were good foods, but when I began to understand how much of them people were using, I had to stop and think about it. Many times I have asked my lecture audiences how many were raised on wheat products and every time 90% or more raised their hands. I asked how many were raised on milk and, again, 90% raised their hands. Many of them had also used a good deal of sugar.

According to published reports, Americans use 29% wheat, 25% milk and 9% sugar in the average diet—63% of the total food intake. Finnish medical researchers found that problems with gluten in a considerable number of children were connected with problems assimilating sugar, and published their findings in *Acta Pediatrica Scandinavia* in 1970. A 1962 article by D.C. Heiner in the *Journal of Pediatrics* linked gluten intolerance with milk intolerance. Problems with wheat (gluten), milk and sugar seem to appear fairly often together. Excessive use often leads to intolerance, and intolerance of one food may lead to intolerance of others.

Several Scandinavian studies linking wheat intolerance with milk intolerance were published in the 1960s, while a 1970 study by Dr. O. D. Kowlessar indicated that children intolerant of wheat should have both wheat and cow's milk removed from their diets. Other studies in Canada and Belgium have shown that sugar intolerance in diabetes is often associated with wheat intolerance, especially refined wheat products. There is a great deal of published research, in fact, which supports what I found out on my own in my sanitarium work.

It is the most common foods that seem to cause a good deal of the trouble, so we're going to have to get to the place where we use *other* foods to get the right percentage balance in our bodies. In other words, we eliminate the wheat, milk and sugar—the most common foods in the diet—and we look for substitute foods. We restore chemical balance by bringing in more variety in our food program, by getting into those foods we haven't had a lot of in our lives. If we will do this, *I am sure the body will balance of its own accord.*

WHAT I FOUND IN OTHER COUNTRIES

I have traveled around the world, searching for the keys to health and long life, and I have found different foods emphasized in other cultures. We can look to these foods as substitutes for the foods we tend to use in excess in our culture.

What can we use as a substitute for wheat? In Latin America, I found yellow cornmeal used more than any other grain. In India and the Far East, rice and millet were the most commonly used. The Turkish people use a great deal of sesame seeds. These cultures don't have the same health problems, the same chronic diseases we have. In fact, the greatest health I have seen was in the Hunzas of Pakistan, who use a great deal of millet in their diet. Corn, rice and millet are apparently the least fattening cereal grains and cause the least problems, even in gluten-intolerant people according to a study by J. H. van deKamer published in a 1959 issue of *Acta Pediatrica*. I found the same thing over 30 years ago.

Instead of milk and milk products, we can use the seed milk drinks and the nut milk drinks, as well as the seed and nut butters, to get the calcium and fats we need. Soy milk powder mixed with water and a little honey makes another good drink. In many cases, raw goat milk is tolerated much better than cow's milk, in part, because the fat particles are much smaller in goat's milk. I have also found that many of the older people in the world use a little yogurt or kefir, a **predigested** form of milk which is more easily taken in by the body without creating disturbances. These foods are discussed elsewhere in other chapters at greater length. Instead of sugar, we can use a little honey, maple syrup or carob, now and then, but I feel we should be careful with concentrated sweets of any kind. It is better to use fruits as sweeteners, and this can be done very nicely with raisins, dried apricots, dates, figs, pineapple and other sweet fruits.

WHAT WILL YOU DO WHEN YOU EAT OUT?

We have to decide in advance what we are going to do when we go on picnics, to banquets and barbecues, out to dinner, either at friends' homes or at restaurants. What is available may not be the best for us, so we have to be a little bit choosy, a little bit selective about what we take. Many of the foods available on these occasions are the cheapest foods possible, especially at picnics, barbecues and banquets. Any time a large number of people is going to be served, cheapness is usually one of the main concerns. So we have to make sure we are not building our body on just what others give us to eat. We can't afford to use foods that will cause problems, foods that will not nourish us properly.

Think of foods this way: *You deserve the best!* Food is fuel, a

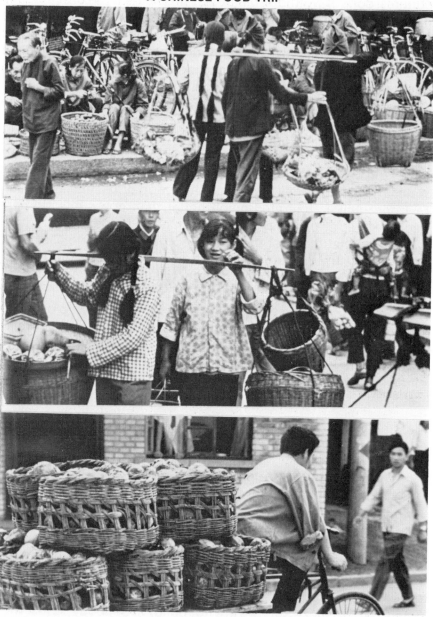

In China, fuel is expensive and manpower is cheap, so food is often transported in baskets by people.

replenisher, a rejuvenator of tissue, and we need the best foods to build the best health and the best body. It is said, "God can only do *for* you what He can do *through* you," but you have to have the vital energies in your body for good things to come through your life. If you have no ovaries, you can't expect God to help you conceive a child. If you have toxic-laden, underactive ovaries, what are your chances of having a healthy baby? This is something to stop and think about. We have to have the proper foods, rich in the vitamins and minerals our bodies need, to have healthy bodies and to give the next generation the best possible start in life.

DISEASE PROBLEMS OR FOOD PROBLEMS?

What we have to realize in so many of our health problems is that many symptoms and disturbances come from poor food habits, malnutrition that breeds imbalances, intolerances and deficiencies in the body. "Disease preys on a malnourished body," as Dr. William Albrecht of the University of Missouri has pointed out. If we take care of our diet by eating the proper amounts of *natural, whole, pure* foods and by following the *Law of Variety,* the *Law of Proportions* and the *Law of Excess,* then we are preventing disease by creating a body that disease cannot touch.

We tend to build bodies based on the food culture of the country in which we live, and when the food culture is in the hands of commercial interests and not health-minded interests, it is easy to see where problems can arise. The profit principle is not often harmonized with the principles of healthy living.

FOOD INTOLERANCE CREATES PROBLEMS

As I said before, I once thought that wheat and milk were healthy foods, and I couldn't understand why my patients were not getting well on them. Then in 1950, the research of a Dutch doctor, W. H. Dicke, showed that gluten—the protein in wheat—can cause such a severe reaction of the wall in the small bowel that nutrients can't be absorbed through the villi, the tiny finger-like projections that take in the digested food particles. With regard to milk, intolerance may be due to a deficiency or absence of lactase, the enzyme needed to digest milk sugar or to a milk allergy, according to Dr. Jean Monro. Intolerance of sugar may be due to insufficient insulin secretion from the Islands of Langerhans of the pancreas. Insulin is needed for the cells to absorb sugar from the blood. These "islands" of the pancreas not only make insulin, they regulate very carefully the amount being released, and if they are not functioning properly, a blood-sugar imbalance results. Wheat, milk and sugar cause intolerance in different ways, but we need to realize that these causes are well established by researchers. Intolerance of these foods is more common than we think in the United States.

Taber's Cyclopedic Medical Dictionary says that *celiac disease is intestinal malabsorption caused by a substance in gluten and characterized by diarrhea, malnutrition, bleeding tendency and hypoglycemia. Treatment is a gluten-free diet perhaps continued indefinitely.*

The gluten causes inflammation and damage to the bowel, leading to extreme malnutrition, starvation and chemical depletion. Extreme losses in celiac patients of iron, calcium, magnesium and vitamins A, D and E have been noted in the research of Drs. J. F. Phillips, G. L. D. Bensen, J. A. Balint and S. Goldman. One British researcher found that fingerprints were missing on many celiac patients, which caused considerable concern on the part of the police for awhile. Celiac disease may appear at any time during a person's life, and the only effective treatment yet found is a gluten-free diet, removal of all wheat (also oats, rye and barley, which contain some gluten) from the diet.

Celiacs react strongly even to small amounts of gluten in food. An article by Dr. L. S. Reed in a 1970 issue of *The New York State Journal of Medicine* described how celiac children and adults, symptom-free for some time on a no-gluten diet, would immediately go into severe shock if they ate any wheat or other gluten grains or products—even a small amount. I found out about celiac disease during a visit to England over 30 years ago, but have seen problems with wheat intolerance in my sanitarium work for over 50 years.

Milk intolerance is the most extreme in Orientals and Negroes who lack the milk-sugar digesting enzyme, lactase. Bloating, gas and diarrhea result soon after taking milk or milk products such as cheese, butter, whipped cream and so forth. There are also milk allergies and reactions in which a great deal of catarrh and mucus develops, showing tissue irritation in response to the milk.

Extreme sugar intolerance is found in diabetes mellitus. Diabetics lack enough insulin for proper regulation of blood sugar. If untreated, this type of diabetes leads to nausea, dizziness, coma and death.

Wheat, milk and sugar all have produced extreme reactions that are well-known to doctors, but I feel what most doctors don't realize is that intolerance often develops from *using too much* of these foods and that the intolerance reaction *can exist in degrees.* At lower levels of use, wheat, milk and sugar may produce catarrh. At a little higher level, we find allergic reactions to wheat and milk, and increasing disturbances of sugar metabolism. At even higher levels of use, these three foods produce conditions in the body that may invite any of a variety of chronic diseases.

BETTER HEALTH WITH BETTER DIET

When I began putting my sanitarium patients on a noncatarrhal diet, which is basically a gluten-free diet with a few more restrictions, improvement and recoveries became quicker and more numerous. A patient with a severe case of psoriasis who also developed arthritis and diabetes was greatly helped by diet. I have had wonderful results with hundreds of arthritis patients by putting them on a noncatarrhal diet. Many diabetics have been helped by diet to the point where they can reduce their insulin or stop taking it altogether. Dr. R. Shatin of Melbourne, Australia, has suggested that multiple sclerosis may be linked to gluten intolerance, and that poor absorption in the small intestine is sometimes linked to rheumatoid arthritis. Other studies have linked eczema with gluten foods.

I have found that any catarrhal condition, any catarrhal discharge, will generally improve if we cut out wheat, milk and sugar, while using a balanced regimen of whole, pure, natural

SWEETER IS NOT HEALTHIER

According to food researchers, the average American uses about 130 pounds of sugar a year, five times the average consumption in 1900. Since the total average food intake per person in the U.S. was 1,402 pounds in 1980 (USDA), simple division shows that over 9% of the average American diet is refined white sugar!

**REFINED SUGAR USED IN FOOD PRODUCTS (PER PERSON, PER YEAR)
INCLUDING ALL REFINED SWEETENERS: CANE SUGAR,
BEET SUGAR, CORN SYRUP, ETC.**

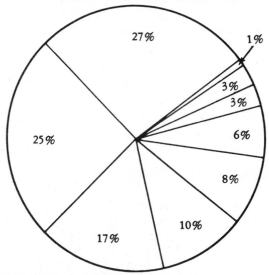

27% =	34.56 pounds:	Beverages (largely soft drinks)
25% =	32.00 pounds:	Added to foods at home
17% =	21.76 pounds:	Commercial bakery and cereal products
10% =	12.80 pounds:	Commercial candy
8% =	10.24 pounds:	Commercial canned and frozen fruits and vegetables, jellies and preserves
6% =	7.60 pounds:	Commercial dairy products
3% =	3.40 pounds:	Other processed foods
3% =	3.40 pounds:	Restaurants
1% =	1.28 pounds:	Institutions
100% =	128.00 pounds	pounds per capita

(From USDA SUGAR & SWEETENER REPORT 5 (7): 35; 1980.)

foods. Most people can tolerate a little wheat, milk or sugar once in a while, but a person with extreme intolerance cannot. Such people must remain on a very exacting diet.

USE MORE FOODS FROM NATURE'S GARDEN

There is a great variety of foods in nature's garden, and we need to use *more* of them to give our bodies the *variety* of nutrients the various organs and tissues need. Wheat, milk and sugar probably make up a small portion of nature's bounty, yet they provide a greater percentage of the average American diet. I feel very strongly there would be far fewer health problems in the U.S. if we limited our intake of wheat, milk and sugar.

Wheat, milk and sugar are so common in our packaged, canned, refined and baked products that it can be difficult to find any prepared food that doesn't have one or more of the three in it. Wheat flour may be used as a thickener in commerical gravies, puddings and soups. Powdered milk or "milk solids" are added to processed meats and other refined meat and protein products as a cheap method of boosting protein content. Sugar is added to thousands of packaged foods these days. Wheat, milk and sugar products are among the most heavily advertised products we see these days, but we must be careful. We are creating deficiencies by lack of variety and proportion in our foods and by inadequate nutrition. This is not the pathway to *health*, but the pathway to *disease.*

In the United States, a great deal of high pressure media advertising is centered on getting the consumer to buy more wheat, milk and sugar products. I sincerely believe that Americans would eat much less of these foods if magazines, newspapers, billboards and television were not saturated with ads promoting milk products, cake mixes, pastries, pancakes, waffles, muffins, bread, sugar-loaded breakfast cereals, snack foods, desserts, chocolate, cookies, syrups, jam, jelly, soft drinks, high-sugar fruit-flavored punches and candies; each brand competing against all the others to prove it has more eye appeal, taste appeal and sales appeal.

There is seldom any mention of nutritional value in any of

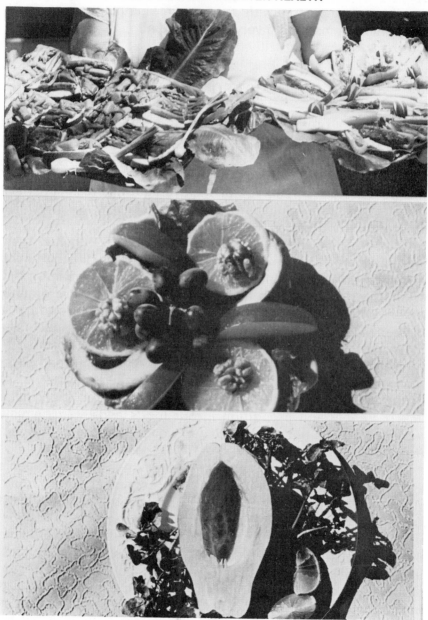

Foods properly prepared and artistically arranged contribute to better nutrition, attitude, appetite, digestion, assimilation and healthful living.

these commercials for the very good reason that most of these so-called foods are nutritionally worthless, foodless foods, without an ounce of good in them, harmful to the body in the amounts eaten by the average person, fattening, hard on the digestion and bowel contributing to an imbalance in the blood chemistry and glandular functions. Advertising like this is promoting what we call the "dollar foods," foods whose main purpose is to make as much money as possible.

We must realize that advertising is not interested in your health or well-being, it is interested in your pocketbook. The newspapers tell us that Philip Morris attempted to take over General Foods in 1985. Do you think a cigarette manufacturing company would be the slightest bit interested in producing healthy foods for your family? We need to understand these things and wake up, or else we will be raising our children to become doctor bills.

It is not always what we eat that counts, but what we digest and assimilate. The small intestine is where most digestion and assimilation takes place, but if the intestinal wall is inflamed and coated with wheat gluten and irritated by undigested milk particles, digestion and assimilation may be greatly hindered, even if the best foods are eaten. But, when we see how much refined, chemicalized, preserved, devitalized foodless junk foods the average person eats, we can begin to see what we are doing to our bodies.

This is where we get all our catarrhal inflammations such as gastritis, stomatitis, diphtheritis, rhinitis, bronchitis, pulmonitis, conjunctivitis, otitis, meningitis, enteritis, colitis, appendicitis, hepatitis, pancreatitis, nephritis, vaginitis, metritis, ovaritis, cystitis, prostatitis, arthritis, phebitis, pericarditis and endocarditis. But we don't need to take care of these things if we use a proper diet to prevent them and if we avoid those foods our bodies most easily develop intolerances toward. I feel proper percentage balance in foods is the key to better health and a longer life.

ALLERGIES FROM TOO MUCH MILK AND WHEAT

One of the best known allergy specialists in this country sent a number of allergy patients to me for counseling. One boy who came to my Ranch had an estimated 3000 eye ulcers. At home, he would break out in eye ulcers after every meal, but not at the Ranch. Because we didn't use any of the artificial fertilizers or pesticide sprays on the food we grew, he had no eye ulcers. So the ulcers he brought from home would disappear after a few days. After he left the Ranch, the eye ulcers came right back as soon as he ate food at restaurants or at home. Now on his own place he grows his own food without sprays and chemicals, and he no longer has the eye ulcers.

I learned something very important from this allergy specialist who used to refer some of his patients to me. He said his patients were allergic to two foods more than any others. *And what do you think they were? Wheat and milk.* The boy with the eye ulcers and many other allergy patients became wheat logged and milk logged before they developed allergies to so many other things. Too much wheat and milk can trigger allergy reactions to other food and substances.

According to Ronald Deutch in *Realities of Nutrition,* "...There is no substance so toxic that the body cannot manage some tiny amount of it harmlessly; and there is none so safe that a great enough excess will not do injury."

Today, allergies are one of the biggest health problems in the U.S. I had many patients with serious allergy problems who were taking shots and drugs for their conditions, but we find that suppression of symptoms is not the solution. I believe that excessive use of certain foods triggers allergies in our body. Many people in this country are *MILK LOGGED AND WHEAT LOGGED.* That is the main problem. It is to your advantage to understand this.

We find that researchers at the University of Chicago have discovered a link between the food we eat, the moods we have and fluctuations in the body's immune system. Dr. John Crayton, the psychiatrist in charge of the study said, "We're not talking about traditional food allergies...but marked changes in mood and behavior. Food induced mood changes studies in 35 volunteers, included irritability, anxiety and depression." We realize how important it is to have a balanced diet, especially in view of the fact that Americans eat such large amounts of wheat, milk and sugar, totaling 63% of the average annual diet. Dr. Crayton's study proves that foods can disturb the emotions, and this could be either through an effect on the glandular system on the brain, but they also apparently disturb the immune system, which has a direct relation to our health level. This is something to stop and think about.

The Pakistani government supplies to its needy people daily rations of a little over a pound of wheat, an ounce of edible oil, an ounce of dried skim milk, under an ounce of sugar and a little tea. While this is hardly more than a survival diet, we find that wheat makes up over 86% of it, pointing to the future probability of great wheat-sensitivity reactions in the Pakistani people. A Japanese newspaper commented, "We Japanese, living as we do amid a superabundance of material goods, cannot imagine what it means to live on 500 grams of wheat a day."

I am convinced we can make a change. I am convinced that every organ can be changed. It may take a couple of years to get rid of all the wheat and milk that you've stored up in your right shoulder, hips, legs, bones, muscles and other tissue. The body has its reserves of minerals, balancing materials, materials for neutralizing acids and so forth, but can bring itself back to normal if the proper foods are used. It's going to possibly take a year, two years, cutting out all the wheat and milk products. Eventually when we realize what it is to take only 6% of wheat and milk in our diet and not more, then we will keep the proper balance in the body and not develop catarrhal discharges. Some people are constantly treating the catarrh, they are constantly treating the discharges and they are treating them with suppressive methods, driving this discharge back into the body until symptoms appear. Have a look at the list of symptoms Chapter 23, with one thing in common—catarrh.

The secret in this whole matter of getting rid of these allergies and heavy catarrhal conditions which are working together in so many people throughout the United States, is to find a variety of substitutes for wheat and milk. How many years have we been doing this? Far too many! Yes, far too many, and now we have developed consequences. In my practice I have definitely reduced

67

the discharges of every one of those catarrhal symptoms listed by cutting down the wheat and milk taken into the body. You must balance the systems of the body—elimination, glandular, respiratory, circulatory—in order to keep this catarrh on the move with the proper nutritional program. This body molds to coffee and donuts. It molds to pancakes and cereals, to the various kinds of devitalized wheat products, manhandled and developed wheat products to such an extent that they're constantly in need of a move and thus we have this discharge. We need to know that wheat is a fattening grain, and if it has produced fat in you, you will lose it when you cut out wheat. Can you understand? How many people are taught how to avoid these catarrhal discharges and manifestations while growing up?

Abnormal and unbalanced foods have settled in and made up the various organs and tissues in the body. But there is a nice thing about this body, and that is, it constantly changes. You build new skin on the palm of your hand every 24 hours. You can make a new stomach. You can make a new shoulder. But you must have the proper chemical elements to do it. If you have been milk logged in the past, wheat logged in the past, you can wash them out. The body molds to the foods you eat and the amount you eat. That's the lovely thing about the body.

I tell my patients they can't be well unless they give nature an opportunity. Here is a chance for you to give nature the opportunity. Wheat and milk are two of the most heavily advertised foods on the market today. How long will it take to get your body balanced enough not to need the discharge state of catarrh? We find the body has its own clock, its own inherent weaknesses, its own mineral balance and its own pattern of habits, especially food habits and enervating habits of tiredness and fatigue to compensate for what is not working well at the proper time. It is possible that we should listen more to our food laws and less to the advertisements.

THE LAW OF EXCESS

When we eat so much of a few foods, we are violating the law of excess, which leads to imbalance in the body and creates an unnatural body.

When we feed the cells and tissues with over 50% wheat and milk, this is an excess. This excess forces a shortage or imbalance of other foods we should have been eating. Milk-logged and wheat-logged people produce an excess of catarrh, phlegm and mucus, which, in time, will develop into discharges. *These discharges are signs of chemical excess or deficiency—a chemical imbalance in the body.* When we realize we are violating the law of excess, it is important to change to a balanced eating regimen. When I found out that people were *wheat logged and milk logged*, I began to look for alternatives. I cut out wheat in the average patient. I couldn't tell they were wheat logged—outside of noticing allergies, excessive catarrhal conditions and so forth—but I knew I had to have something to replace the wheat.

WHAT DO WE ORDER FOR BREAKFAST?

According to the"Nation's Restaurant News," restaurant breakfast customers increased nearly 57% between 1977 and 1984, and what they ordered for breakfast gives us a very interesting picture of U.S. food patterns. The following figures represent the percentage of customers ordering each particular item. Keep in mind that a single customer may order several items from the list.

*Bread	32%
Bacon, sausage	23%
Juice	19%
*Breakfast sandwiches	18%
Potatoes	18%
*French toast, waffles, pancakes	16%
*Donuts, sweet rolls	15%
*Cereal	1%

*Notice that all items marked * contain wheat, which accounts for 5 out of 8 food items listed. This amounts to 63% wheat-containing foods in the average breakfast, when people eat out.*

Six percent of the American people eat breakfast out, amounting to $9.1 billion each year out of $141.6 billion total in commercial restaurant sales.

You may think I'm exaggerating, but a simple diet formula has turned out to be one of the greatest things I have found in my work to clear up original catarrhal discharges. As an idealist trying to balance the different foods needed in the body, I came up with the formula: *6 vegetables, 2 fruits, 1 protein and 1 starch daily.* This is as close as we can get, I feel, to the place where we develop a nondischarging, noncatarrhal body. This is an ideal. Get as close to it as you can. Without ideals we get sick; without ideals we die.

WHAT CAN WE USE INSTEAD OF WHEAT?

When I visited the Hunza Valley, I discovered that they use a good deal of millet, and these people are among the healthiest in the world. *In Northern China, they use a lot of millet. It is claimed that these people are much hardier than those who live in the South and don't use millet.*

MILLET—THE TOP CEREAL GRAIN

You know, I didn't know much about millet. The average person doesn't know much about it either. I found that Pythagoras used millet and recommended it to all his students. Hippocrates used millet with his patients. I checked further and found out about experiments with millet at Yale University by Dr. Osborn and Dr. Mendel. They discovered that a diet of millet alone gave dogs a glossy coat, a pink tongue and high vitality. No other grain or single food kept them as healthy. So I began to recommend millet. Millet is not fattening in the way wheat is. Many people don't like it, but it is one of the best cereal grains we can eat.

RYE BUILDS MUSCLE

I went a little further and spent time in Finland. The greatest runners in the world, such as Nurmi, come from Finland. They use rye grain. I noticed the wonderful muscular bodies the Finns had, and they were using rye. We have found that wheat puts on fat. Rye puts on muscle. *Like millet, rye is a fine substitute for wheat.*

BROWN RICE—THE LEAST FATTENING GRAIN

A third nutritious grain is whole grain brown rice. Did you ever see a fat Chinese? No, you don't see fat Chinese. You don't get fat with rice. And, of course, I'm talking about whole rice now. The polishings are very important because the silicon they contain feeds the nerves and glands, and prevents catarrh formation in the body when put in proper combination with other foods. Rice doesn't have gluten in it. The grains highest in gluten are wheat and oats, and these are the grains most people are eating. There is very little gluten in millet, yellow cornmeal, rye and rice.

CORN—THE AMERICAN CEREAL GRAIN

During trips to Central and South America, I found one of the main foods was corn. Yellow cornmeal is a very good cereal food. If you go down to Mexico, Guatemala, Costa Rica or many of the South American countries, these people use yellow cornmeal and have no constipation.

The American Indians considered corn the most important food in their gardens. They had black corn and colored speckled corn and they found it to be very wonderful. The different colored corn does have a different chemical balance in it and I am sure they varied the chemistry of their diet a good deal by having the variety of corn that they especially ate, that they especially lived on.

In Mexico, we studied the Mayan Indians. Their sculpture and pottery often showed man with corn in his hands. They considered corn the most important food they could get. In fact, they considered it the staff of life. Corn could almost be considered a complete life-giving food, especially the yellow cornmeal.

You should use corn and the other grains I have mentioned here until you get the excess wheat washed out of your body. By taking these wheat substitutes and having a different one each day, you will balance out and reduce the amount of wheat stored in various organs and systems of the body and, finally, the heavy catarrhal conditions that most people are having treated today will get less and less.

CEREAL GRAINS: THE STAFF OF LIFE FOR MAN

Cereal grains are the seeds of cereal grasses that go back in history as far as man knows. As seeds, they carry the life force, genetic material and nutrients to give life to the next generation of cereal grasses, and it is this wonderful combination of life-giving factors that makes whole cereal grains such an excellent food for man. When grown on rich soils, grains provide man with the materials to help give the next human generation the life force, genetic material and nutrients for the healthiest possible start.

Wheat is one of the finest grains I know of, used more than any other grains, except in Asian, African and some Latin American countries. The problem is that we have used too much of it, and many people in the Western nations have developed sensitivities, allergic reactions or even complete intolerance to wheat, gluten or both. Wheat has been historically important in Egypt, Palestine and even among some prehistoric cave dwellers in Europe as early as 7,000 B.C. The U.S., Russia and Canada are the main producers and consumers today. I am sure that much of the problem with wheat comes from using refined, bleached white flour and the products made with it, which tend to irritate and slow the bowel, according to research studies. There may also be problems with the hybrid wheat types, as developed by man instead of nature.

WHEAT FACTS

- *One acre of wheat yields 2,686 one-pounds loaves of bread.*
- *A modern combine machine harvests 1,000 bushels of wheat per hour, which represents 73,000 loaves of bread.*
- *Today, it takes 10 man-hours to produce 100 bushels of wheat, as compared to 373 man-hours in 1880.*
- *One bushel of wheat contains about one million kernels.*
- *The U.S. uses over 3 million bushels of wheat per day.*

■ *There are over 400 varieties of wheat estimated to be grown in the U.S.*
■ *Archeologists have found evidence to show that wheat has been a food grown by man since about 2,000 B.C.*
From the National Association of Wheat Growers.

Rye is a grain that will grow in climates too harsh and cold for wheat, such as northern Russia, the Sandinavian countries and northern Germany. Rye is less fattening and more muscle building than wheat, and has more of the chemical elements. Rye crackers are a good alternative to wheat, but should be used along with a variety of other cereal grains and grain products.

It has been said that barley may have been the first grain crop cultivated by man. Barley cakes are mentioned in the Bible, and barley is still widely used in Israel, according to published reports, where it is used as a breakfast cereal and also made into a pudding. "Pot" barley has had its outer husk removed; Scotch barley is the husked grain crudely ground; and pearled barley is the polished grain with outer and inner husks removed. Barley is used in bread making in Europe, but in most countries, it is used mainly in soups. Barley and green kale soup is one of the richest sources of calcium we can use. Barley gruel is soothing to stomach disturbances.

Corn (or maize) is said to have originated in the tropical areas of North, Central and South America, where it was used by the Indians for centuries before Columbus, and spread to tribes far from the tropics. Europeans quickly adopted corn as a food, and in North America, steamed corn on the cob, fresh cooked sweet corn kernels, cornbread, grits, mush and other forms became widely used. In Latin America, the corn tortilla and tamale are popular foods, and a good deal of corn is used in Africa, especially South Africa. In the U.S. and other heavy meat-eating countries, corn is often also used to fatten cattle and hogs and is mixed with chicken feed.

Millet is the name for a number of small-seeded cereals that form the chief cereal grain crop in parts of India, Pakistan, China and other countries. It is one of the grains highest in potassium and silicon, when grown in good soil, and some varieties grown in Hungary produce more bushels per acre of land than wheat. Millet was the predominant cereal grain in the Hunza Valley where I visited some of the healthiest, long-lived people in the world. It is becoming increasingly popular in Western countries and can be added to bread, steamed as a breakfast cereal, used in soups or cooked slowly over low heat as a side dish for any meal.

Rice is one of the few cereal grains which can be grown continuously for several decades without depleting the soil. First grown about 3,500 B.C., rice now feeds a third of the world's population. It is a staple in Asia, the most densely populated area of the world. Rice needs a hot, humid climate with plenty of water; it is high in minerals, B vitamins, vitamins E and K. Brown rice is the unhusked whole grain rice, considered the most nutritious; white rice is milled and less nutritious. A steam-pressure treatment of unhusked rice is used to drive nutrients into the grain before milling and polishing, which results in a nutritious rice that can still be stored for long periods (whole grain rice does not keep long). Rice is threshed, screened, shaken and passed through pneumatic and vibrating machines to remove sand and foreign matter. Milled and polished, the rice is separated from broken grains, which are packed. Byproducts of rice processing include animal feed, bran, starch, oil, straw, groats, rice flour, rice wine and rice polishings.

While we recognize that some grains spoil quickly if the germ and hull are not removed, we must also recognize that the term is where the "life material" for the next generation is stored, along with substantial quantities of vitamins and minerals. Milled grains are not whole grains, not natural grains. The "next generation" material has been removed, *but we need this material* to preserve our health, our genetic integrity, our ability to bring forth a new and healthy generation. By using milled grains, we will find that our health and genetic structure slowly deteriorate. For these reasons, it is important to use whole, unprocessed cereal grains as much as possible.

THE CHEMICAL ELEMENTS IN UNCOOKED GRAINS (mg/100 gm)

	Whole Wheat	Rye	Yellow Cornmeal	Barley (Pearled)	Brown Rice	Millet
Calcium	40	54	20	34	35	20
Iron	3	5	2	3	2	7
Magnesium	113	115	106	36	96	162
Phosphorus	372	536	223	290	235	311
Potassium	370	860	248	296	234	429
Sodium	3	1	1	-	10	-
Silicon	43	30	-	-	40	160

In a grain of wheat, the following percentages of nutrients are in the germ and bran (lost by milling) and the rest are in the refined kernel.

NUTRIENT LOSSES IN MILLING WHEAT

	Germ (3% of wheat)	Bran (14% of wheat)	Milled Kernel (83%)
Thiamin	64%	33%	3% (97% loss)
Riboflavin	26%	42%	32% (68% loss)
Pyridoxine	21%	73%	6% (94% loss)
Pantothenic acid	7%	50%	43% (57% loss)
Niacin	2%	86%	12% (88% loss)
Protein	8%	19%	73% (27% loss)

WHAT CAN WE USE IN PLACE OF MILK?

What can we use in place of milk? When we have taken such a high intake of milk into the body over the years, especially while we have been growing up and forming the different systems in our body, *it is necessary we realize that having 25% milk in our diet is crowding out the other lovely foods we should be having. It is equally important that we find a substitute for milk,* and I have found a wonderful substitute in the seed and nut milk drinks.

Children and adults with serious catarrhal problems do

extremely well, and a noticeable improvement in catarrhal conditions can be be seen in a matter of weeks by giving up wheat and milk and by using these alternative drinks made from seed butters, sesame seeds especially, and also almond nut butter. Sunflower seeds make very good butters also. *THESE DRINKS CANNOT MAKE CATARRH.* They make wonderful milk substitutes. *You do not have to worry about the balance of chemical elements. All the calcium and growth elements are there that are necessary for a child to build a good body.*

MILK SUBSTITUTE DRINKS (NONCATARRH FORMING)

Seeds and sprouts are going to be the foods of the future. Today we have found that many of the seeds have the hormone values of male and female glands. Seeds carry the life force for many years, as long as they are enclosed by the hull. Seeds found in tombs, and known to have been there for thousands of years—when planted—have grown. To get these seeds into our body in the form of a drink gives us the finest form of nutrition.

Sesame Seed Milk. Use 1/4 cup sesame seeds to 2 cups of water, raw milk or goat milk. Place in blender and blend 1-1/2 minutes. Strain through a fine wire strainer or 2 to 4 layers of cheesecloth. This is to remove the hulls. Add 1 tablespoon carob powder and 6 to 8 dates. For flavor and added nutritional value, any one of the following may be added to this drink: banana, stewed raisins, apple or cherry concentrate, date powder or grape sugar. Your own imagination or taste may dictate other combinations of fruits or juices. Whenever adding anything, run in blender again to mix. This milk may also be used as the basis for salad dressings.

I believe that sesame seed milk is one of our best drinks. It is a wonderful drink for gaining weight, for lubricating the intestinal tract and its nutritional value is beyond compare, as it is high in protein and minerals. This is the seed used in the making of tahini, a sesame seed oil dressing. This is the seed used so much in Arabia and is used as a basic food in East India.

Other uses for sesame seeds: Salad dressing, add to vegetable broth, add to fruits, mix with nut butter of any kind, for after-school snacks, use on cereals for breakfast, add to whey drinks to adjust intestinal sluggishness, drink twice daily with banana to gain weight, add supplements such as flaxseed meal or rice polishings.

Almond Nut Milk. Use blanched or unblanched almonds. Other nuts may also be used. Soak nuts overnight in apple or pineapple juice or honey water. This softens the nut meats. Then put 3 ounces of soaked nuts in 5 ounces of water and blend for 2 to 2-1/2 minutes. Flavor with honey, any kind of fruit, concentrates of apple or cherry juices, strawberry juice, carob powder, dates or bananas. This can also be used with any vegetable juice.

Almond nut milk can also be used with soups and vegetarian roasts as a flavoring. Use over cereals too.

Almond milk makes a very alkaline drink, high in protein and easy to assimilate.

Pumpkin Seed or Sunflower Seed Milk. (The vegetarian's best protein—sunflower seeds.) The same principles as previously described can be employed to make sunflower or pumpkin seed milk, i.e., soaking overnight, liquefying and flavoring with fruits and juices. Use in the diet the same as almond nut milk. It is best to use whole sunflower or pumpkin seeds and blend them yourself. However, if you do not have a liquefier, the seed meal can be used. Add other seeds and/or nuts. (Do *not* add peanuts! They are legumes—not nuts.)

Soy Milk. Soy milk powder is found in health food stores and is another alternative to cow's milk. Add 4 tablespoons soy milk powder to 1 pint of water. Sweeten with raw sugar, honey or molasses and add a pinch of vegetable salt. For flavor, you can add any kind of fruit, apple or cherry concentrate, carob powder, dates and bananas. You can add any other natural sweetener.

Keep in refrigerator. Use this milk in any recipe as you would regular cow's milk. It closely resembles the taste and composition of cow's milk and will sour just as quickly. Therefore, it should not be made in too large quantities or too far ahead of time.

I would have nothing to say against milk or wheat if we had no more than 6% of them in our daily diet, which amount we should really have. But since these two foods make up 54% of the entire diet, they are overwhelming for the body to take care of. Because we cannot use such an excess in the body, it eventually has to slip into an elimination of catarrh, acidity and discharges which we may fight most of our childhood. It affects adults also, running into cysts, growths, etc. It may take 2 years, but I am not going to starve you doing this. You're going to have good carbohydrates; you're going to have things you didn't have before, and it's only balancing this out that's going to keep you from being logged on one or two foods, a problem facing the entire nation.

When I look at this percentage of 54% milk and wheat, I think it should be about 6%, as I mentioned. This would bring wheat and milk more into balance with other foods.

THE CANDIDA ALBICANS PROBLEM   (A VITAL PROBLEM)

When we find so many American families building their meals around bread, it is not so surprising that some researchers claim 80% of the people in the U.S. have a problem with the yeast called candida albicans.

Candida albicans is a yeast spore normally lodged in small colonies in the intestinal tract of man. Why do we find the candida getting out of control in so many people in the U.S. today? Candida multiplies most rapidly when it has plenty of yeast foods to consume. Nearly all wheat flour bread and bakery products are made with yeast, and these products make up 29% of the average American diet. Milk and sugar, respectively, 25% and 9% of the average diet, also feed candida. *Yes, this is something to stop and think about!*

Candida albicans is a vital problem in America today. When we look at the pies, cakes, pastries, and the amount of wheat and milk and sugar we have had, I am convinced that you will find that at the basis of candida albicans the problem lies right in the wheat, milk and sugar excess. We have been doing this for so many years now that this has crept up like a thief in the night, causing intestinal disturbances that have been very difficult to handle.

The candida problem will change when the right changes are made in the diet. In other words, I believe in letting nature do this work from day to day without pushing the candida too fast, as they do with drugs.

78

MORE GOOD CEREALS AND STARCHES

A good cereal you can have is buckwheat. Buckwheat is not really a type of wheat, but it is a good cereal, high in rutin which they extract from the grain to put in supplements that help fragile veins. It is high in silicon, which is also a great catarrhal eliminator.

Wild rice is actually a grass seed rather than a true grain, but it is very nourishing, with twice the protein of brown rice and almost three times the amount of iron. An ounce of wild rice has 99 calories, 4 grams of protein, 21 grams of starch and almost no fat. It has 2 mg sodium, 64 mg potassium, 5 mg calcium, 95 mg phosphorous, 36 mg magnesium, 1.2 mg iron and 2.8 micrograms of fluoride. It has several B vitamins and a trace of vitamin E.

NUTRITIONAL VALUE OF WILD RICE

	Wild Rice	Raw Brown Rice	Raw White Rice
Food energy (calories	1601	1633	1647
Protein (gm)	64.0	34.0	30.4
Fat (gm)	3.2	8.6	1.8
Carbohydrate (gm)	341.6	351.1	364.7
Calcium (mg)	86	145	109
Phosphorus (mg)	1538	1002	426
Iron (mg)	19.1	7.3	3.6
Sodium (mg)	32	41	23
Potassium (mg)	998	971	417
Thiamine B-1 (mg)	2.2	1.52	0.32
Riboflavin B-2 (mg)	2.87	0.24	0.12
Niacin B-3 (mg)	27.9	21.4	7.2
Magnesium raw (mg)	585	-	127

The above is from: Composition of Foods, USDA Agricultural Handbook Number 8.

Other starches can be used occasionally but even these starches mentioned have been used in excess in the past. And for us to decrease it a bit is going to help our whole body, especially the allergies and catarrhal conditions that are running rampant throughout the U.S.

You can use oats once in a while, but keep in mind they are high in gluten.

Baked potato is a good starch to have occasionally, but not every day. I don't care if you are Irish, you don't need potatoes every day. I don't care if you are German, you don't need potato pancakes every day. I don't care if you are Russian, you don't need potato soup every day. I'm not picking on the Irish, Germans or Russians, but we must have **variety.** Every country has its imbalances, but God made stomachs the same, no matter what country we come from. I should know. I was raised on Danish pastry and 12 cups of coffee a day. Wow! Even today I hear people talk about coffee substitutes. Listen, there's no substitute for coffee. Coffee is the real thing! I only tell you this because I was raised on it, and I like it. But I had to make changes because it almost destroyed me. A shot from a gun brings instant death, but imbalanced, improper foods bring slow death.

What I know I have given you, and I know it works because I have used it for years at my sanitariums. *One of the greatest discoveries I feel I have made is how to straighten out your diet.*

Many varieties of wheat are hybrids, while barley is an original grain, and I don't want to get into this subject too deeply, but hybrids are getting people into trouble. They are not a "natural" food as God created them, but new food biologically crossbred with another. There are over 250 varieties of soybeans, but only one original—the mungbean. There are soybeans bred to grow in cold weather, soybeans bred to grow in hot weather, soybeans bred to make the best Ford steering wheel. They grow almost anywhere in almost any kind of climate, but they are genetically changed and are **not always good foods.** We need to get back to the original grains. Hybridization weakens the gene life and the original life force that is in our foods. It is well to realize that the more hybridization our foods go through, the less seed power we have to develop a good, strong glandular system. *The seeds contain the hormones for developing a good glandular system.*

The orange used to be a tiny berry filled with hundreds of seeds, but man has developed it into a large fruit with few or no seeds. Removing the seeds—which are the "glands" of the fruit—

has changed the orange into a "sexless' food. It is seeds that give our glands building factors, our hormone-producing factors. Remove the seeds from a food, and it will not build the glands, as in the case of oranges. We live in a "seedless" generation right now, because man has interfered with nature's way and created unnatural "seedless' foods.

Hybrids are not natural or whole, so they violate one of the greatest food laws, *that our food must be natural, whole and pure.* We should stay with nature's original foods. Most original foods had many seeds, which are the most vital part of those foods. Man is making many hybrids today, and I feel he is really getting us into trouble for the future. Our original foods were made for man. Try to get them at every opportunity.

THE BEGINNING OF THE REVERSAL PROCESS

The secret of getting well is through the elimination of catarrh, balancing the body, having a greater nourishing value in our foods so that we may replenish the chemical elements for a stronger elimination and rejuvenation that can take place in the reversal process.

With so many Americans wheat and milk logged and not having a chemically-balanced diet, you need to realize that this condition can't be taken care of overnight or in a week or even in a month. I have to wait until you get cleaned out. I have to wait until you get well. I have to wait until the chemical deficiencies in your body are fed and balanced before you can take the next step on the health path.

We have to consider elimination of the toxic settlements in your body that build toward chronic disease over the years. When you realize that you are cleaning out or eliminating what has been put into your bodies for many years, you can see that we are *reversing* what has taken place in the past. I want you to see that cleansing the body is the beginning of *reversal,* reversal of direction from the pathway to disease toward health instead. By nutritionally balancing the chemical elements in your body and

81

presenting foods in the proper proportions, I am able to start the reversal process and get you out of the chronic disease direction you may be taking.

We have to consider also that when we throw off catarrh, phlegm and mucus it might not just come from the foods you are eating today. As you get stronger, you start eliminating a greater amount of catarrh and actually liquefy it, bringing it to a running stage. You can stay in a catarrhal elimination stage for a period of a year before you actually see a lot of good changes taking place, and a lessening of the discharges.

A HARMONY WAY OF LIVING

One of the biggest problems in this country today is overweight, and I am convinced it is because a lot of the allergies, catarrh, phlegm, mucus have settled in the body. As you follow this Harmony Way of Living, you will see this all change for the better.

We should all seek a balanced, harmony way of living. With all the "dos" and "don'ts," there are still many nice menus you can follow. There are many nice menus you can make from the foods we have discussed, and we will be getting back to them in later chapters. If you will use these ideas as the basis for food planning in your home, I think it will fit the whole family, including the children. If you want to reduce, you can go on a reducing diet such as outlined in my book *Slender Me Naturally.* But come back to the family food plan we are giving here.

BIBLIOGRAPHY

For those interested in further study of health problems due to wheat, milk and sugar, here are some of the sources I have used.

Diabetes, Coronary Thrombosis and the Saccharine Disease by Dr. T. L. Cleave and Dr. G. D. Campbell, John Wright and Sons, Bristol, England, 1966. (The dangers of refined carbohydrates.)

Beckwith, A. C., *et al., Archives of Biochemistry and Biophysics, 117* (1966), pp. 239-249. (Describes the toxic substance to which gluten-intolerant persons react.)

Anderson, D. H., *et al., Pediatrics,* Vol. II, **3** (1953), p. 207. (Extreme gluten intolerance, celiac disease and what it does.)

Reed, L. S., *New York State Journal of Medicine,* Vol. 70, **16** (1970), p. 15.6. (Recovery from symptoms by using a gluten-free diet.)

Bayless, T. M., *et al., Journal of Clinical Investigation, 41* (1964), p. 1344. (Shock effect when gluten-intolerant people have been on a gluten-free diet for some time then ingest a little gluten.)

Creamer, B., *Transactions of the Medical Society,* London, Vol. 85 (1968). (Gluten-intolerant persons may never become tolerant of gluten.)

Ebbs, J. H., *American Journal of Disabled Children, 79* (1950), p. 930. (Gluten intolerance may be inherited.) See also Thompson, M. W., *American Journal of Human Genetics,* Vol. 3, No. 2, June 1951; Carter, R. C., *et al., Annals of Human Genetics,* Vol. 23, Part 3 (July 1956), p. 266; Boyer, P. H., *et al., American Journal of Disabled Children, 91* (2), 1957, p. 131; and Sheldon, W., *Pediatric Journal of the American Academy of Pediatrics,* Vol. 23, Jan. 1959.

Frazer, A. C., *Journal of Pediatrics, 57,* 2 (Aug. 1960). (Gluten intolerance due to enzyme deficiency, possible link with intestinal parasites.)

Challacombe, P. N., *et al., Archives of the Diseases of Children, 46,* April 1971. (Gluten intolerance and missing enzymes.)

DiSant Agnese, P. A., *et al., Journal of the American Medical Association, 180* (1962), p. 308. (Discussion of causes of gluten intolerance.) See also Collins, J. R., *American Journal of Digestive Disturbances* (July 1966), p. 564.

McWhinney, H., *et al.*, *Lancet, 2,* 17.7 (1971), pp. 121-124. (The immune system and gluten intolerance.) See also Reed, L., *New York State Journal of Medicine,* Vol. 71, **16** (1970), 15.8.

Thompson, M. W., *American Journal of Human Genetics,* Vol. 3, No. **2** (1951). (High incidence of diabetes in celiacs.) See also Hooft, C., *et al.*, *Lancet, 2,* (1969), 19.11, p. 1192.

Wells, G. C., *Modern Trends in Gastroenterology,4* (1970), pp. 328-348. (Skin problems and gluten intolerance.) See also Van Tongeren, J. H., *Metabolic Dermatology, 140* (1970), p. 231; Seah, P. P., *et al.*, *Lancet, 1* (1971), pp. 834-836.

Heiner, D. C., *et al.*, *Journal of Pediatrics, 61* (1962), p. 813. (Milk intolerance linked to gluten intolerance.) See also Pock-Steen, O. C., *et al.*, *British Journal of Dermatology, 83* (Dec. 1970), pp. 614-619; Lipshitz-Fima, M.D., *et al.*, *American Journal of Digestive Disorders* (May 1966); Visakorpi, J. J., *et al.*, *Acta Pediatrica Scandanavia, 56* (1967), pp. 49-56.

MILK INTOLERANCE

Cuatrecasas, P., *et al.*, *Lancet, 1,* 14 (1965). (Milk intolerance in a family of Mexicans with 13 children, 4 of them gluten intolerant.) See also Lipshitz-Fima, M.D., *et al.*, *American Journal of Digestive Disorders,* May 1966.

Visakorpi, J. K., *et al.*, *Acta Pediatrica Scandanavia, 56* (1967), pp. 49-56. (Forty children intolerant of milk, gluten or both.)

Chung, M. H., *et al.*, *Gastroenterology, 54* (1968), p. 225. (Milk sugar intolerance in adults.) See also Dawson, A. M., *Modern Trends in Gastroenterology, 4,* Butterworths (1970).

Freier, S., *et al.*, *Clinical Pediatrics, 8* (Aug. 1970), pp. 449-454. (Intolerance of milk protein.)

Dean, R. F. S., *Recent Advances in Pediatrics,* London, 1963. (Milk sugar intolerance in Buganda infants.)

Cook, G. C., *et al.*, *British Medical Journal, 1* (1967), p. 527. (Lower activity of milk-digesting enzyme in Bantu natives in Africa.)

Brock, J. F., and Hansen, J. D. L., *Clinical Nutrition,* Harper Brothers, 1962. (Impaired absorption of milk sugar in children acutely ill with protein deficiency.) See also Kowlessar, O. D., *et al.*, *Medical Clinicians of North America, 54,* 3 (May 1970).

MULTIPLE SCLEROSIS AND GLUTEN-FREE DIET

Kuland, L. K., *American Journal of Medicine, 12* (1952), p. 561. (Relation of dietary habits and M.S.) See also Swank, R. L., *New England Journal of Medicine, 246* (1952), p. 721.

Shatin, R., *Neurology, 14* (1964), pp. 338-341. (Multiple sclerosis may be caused by gluten intolerance.)

SCHIZOPHRENIA AND GLUTEN-FREE DIET

Dohan, F. C., *Acta Pediatrica Scandanavia,* Vol. 42, **2,** (1966). *British Journal of Psychiatry, 115* (1969), pp. 595-596. *Mental Hygiene, 53,* 9.10 (1969), p. 9525. (Effects of gluten-free diet on schizophrenics.)

Lancaster-Smith, *et al., Lancet, 21,* 11 (1970). (Factors in common between schizophrenia and gluten intolerance.)

Dohan, F. C., *Lancet, 25.4* (1970), pp. 897-899. (How gluten intolerance and schizophrenia occur in the same person or family more frequently than by chance.)

RHEUMATOID ARTHRITIS

Shatin, R., *Lancet, 499,* 2.3 (1963). *Medical Journal of Australia, 2,* (1964), p. 169. *Rhumatologie, 17* (1965), p. 69. *Rheumatism* (1966), pp. 48-51. (Use of a gluten-free, high-protein diet with supplements to treat arthritics.)

REGIONAL ENTERITIS (LOWER BOWEL INFLAMMATION) AND AUTISM

Rudman, D., *et al., Journal of Clinical Nutrition* (1971), pp. 1068-73. (Patients with enteritis put on a gluten-free diet for 12 days had gluten-intolerant reactions when gluten was added to diet again.)

Goodwin, M. S., *Journal of Autism and Childhood Schizophrenia, 1,* 1 (1971), pp. 48-62. (Found abnormal responses to the toxic factor in gluten among autistic children.)

COMMON NUTRIENT DEFICIENCIES
IN GLUTEN-INTOLERANT PEOPLE

Phillips, F., *New York State Journal of Medicine, 70,* 11 (1970). (Lack of essential fatty acids and fat-soluble vitamins in gluten intolerance.)

Bayeli, P. F., *et al., Minerva Medica, 19* (1961), p. 25. (Folic acid deficiency.)

Herbert, V., *American Journal of Clinical Nutrition, 12* (1963), p. 17. (Soaking and boiling vegetables destroys vitamins and minerals.)

Olson, O. E., *et al., Journal of the American Dietetic Association, 23* (1947), p. 200. (Nutrient losses due to canning.)

Bensen, G. L. D., *et al., Medicine, 43* (1964), p. 1. (Iron deficiency.)

Balint, J. A., *et al., New England Journal of Medicine, 265* (1961), pp. 631-633. (Calcium deficiency.)

Goldman, S., *et al., Pediatrics, 19* (1962), pp. 448-452. (Magnesium loss is four times more than intake.)

Kowlessar, F., *et al., Medical Clinicians of North America, 54,* 3 (May 1970). (Gluten-free diet should be rich in protein, especially the amino acid tryptophan.)

Monro, Jean, *British Medical Journal, 14.11* (1962). (Those on gluten-free diet not responding as well as they should may need pantothenic acid as a supplement.)

COOKBOOKS

Wheatless Cooking (including gluten-free recipes) by Lynette Coffey (1984), Greenhouse Publications, 385-387 Bridge Road, Richmond, Victoria, Australia. (Written by a housewife and mother of a boy severely allergic to milk and wheat.)

6

How Much and What Kind of Protein Should We Have?

I am not attempting, in this chapter, to change either vegetarians or nonvegetarians, but to show that a proper balance of foods, according to our food laws, requires a certain amount of protein. One of our food laws says **we need 6 vegetables, 2 fruits, 1 starch and 1 protein every day.** That protein is very important—not only for the building and repairing of tissue—but for the proper maintenance of the 20% acid/80% alkaline ratio of nutrients in the bloodstream, which comes from another of our food laws. Whether you are vegetarian or not, nutritional balance must be part of your food program.

I read an article about the "caveman diet," based on research by two Emory University scientists, that showed how our ancestors ate about 251 grams of protein daily (nearly 5 times the amount now recommended), about 333 grams of carbohydrates, and about 98 grams of fats (half of the amount in the average daily U.S. diet). Their diet contained almost the same amount of cholesterol as eaten by the average American, several times the amount of fiber and much more than the amount of vitamin C in the average diet today. This high cholesterol, high protein diet, was partly balanced by the great amount of work these people had to do to find their food. None of the foods were refined, contaminated by toxins, compromised by chemical additives or grown in soil fertilized by manufactured chemical fertilizers. We need to realize that after thousands of years of "natural foods," the change within the past century to more and more refined foods, sugar, white flour and fatty foods is not something the human body can easily adjust to. We can learn one great lesson from our cavemen ancestors: eat natural foods and exercise every day.

Before we get into the proteins, I want to point out that vegetarianism is the cleanest way of life, but it is a mental way of life as well as a physical way of life, and we have to be prepared mentally before we can go into it. It isn't just a matter of removing meat, fish and poultry from your food program. The mental and the physical must be harmonized and prepared to go the vegetarian way. A nonvegetarian considering the vegetarian way might find coming into it by degrees the best way.

THE HIGHEST PROTEIN FOOD

When we talk about proteins, I have to tell you *meat is the highest protein food available.* I am not saying you should have it but simply stating a fact. *Meat is also the most stimulating of the proteins,* and some who are sensitive to it find they must take it for breakfast or lunch, because they don't sleep well if they have it at the evening meal.

Many people have meat two and three times a day, which is too much, but since so few are willing to make such a big change in their food habits all at once, I recommend initially cutting meat down to two or three times a week and substituting more chicken and fish for red meat. I don't tell anyone they have to cut it out completely. Experience has shown that I have to help people through a learning period until they are ready for the next step. *Every path is taken one step at a time.*

If you are going to eat meat, it should be lean meat, no fat, no pork. Lamb is one of the better meats. Meat should be baked, broiled or roasted; never fried.

THE BEST PROTEIN FROM THE SEA

The second-best protein is fish. Use white fish that has fins and scales. That is clean fish. Shell fish are scavengers. The white fish with fins and scales are clean and that includes salmon. In spite of the fact that it is not white, salmon is a fish that takes care of itself and swims as much as 3000 miles, under fasting conditions, to go back and spawn in the same place where it was born, to make sure the next generation is taken care of. Fasting makes this fish clean. They follow a healthy way of life, and that's why I say the salmon belong with the white fish as the best.

THE MOST PERFECT LAND PROTEIN

After fish, I consider eggs the perfect protein. Many people say they are high in cholesterol, which can cause hardening in the arteries, hardened fat settlements. Now, eggs are high in cholesterol, but what food contains the highest amount of lecithin? Egg yolk. We find that God put the lecithin right next to the cholesterol because it is lecithin that breaks down and dissolves cholesterol to balance it in the bloodstream.

COOKING TEMPERATURES OVER 212 DEGREES F. DESTROY LECITHIN

If you fry eggs, you ruin the lecithin, and all you've got left is cholesterol. If you fry or bake anything with oil or fats, you ruin the lecithin, leaving cholesterol-forming food. This is why we have to cook all foods with oils or fats in them at low temperatures, temperatures below the boiling point of water. There are experiments with prisoners who had 15 eggs a day for a solid year without raising their cholesterol. In Egypt, a man over a hundred years of age averaged 13 eggs a day for 30 years, and didn't have a cholesterol problem. Without lecithin, the fats in eggs will form a hardened fat in the body and will be attracted to the arteries and settle there. This applies to all foods that have oils and fats in them. The high cholesterol is from that lack of lecithin destroyed with high heat. I'm talking about all eggs, fertile or otherwise.

The best eggs to use are fertile eggs from chickens free to walk around and forage. We should have what we call "earth eggs." This is very important.

I consider eggs the most perfect of all foods, in part because Professor Alexis Carrel was able to keep a chicken heart alive for 29 years feeding it egg yolk. That, to me, is a very, very wonderful experiment. You can't name another experiment concerning foods as valuable as that. Another reason I consider eggs the perfect protein is that they have all eight essential amino acids in the amounts needed by the human body.

Now, we go still further, and this is something to think about. They claim that eight essential amino acids are necessary for our nervous system and especially for the brain. Some of these are found in foods with lecithin, which is also needed by the nerves and brain. There is very little lecithin in vegetarian foods. You can find some in all the oils and fats, and you find it in soybeans. In fact, lecithin in the concentrated form often comes from soybeans. Most of us using lecithin are burning it out of our system through overworking the brain and nerves. And we find it is hard, from a vegetarian diet, to restore lecithin and the essential amino acids once they have been depleted in the body.

While we have very little of these essential amino acids in the vegetarian foods, the egg yolk has all eight essential amino acids and lecithin. Now, of course, there are a lot of cults, a lot of religions, there are a lot of people and doctors who do not believe in the egg yolk, but I lived in Sri Aurobindo's ashram in India, where at the beginning, they never believed in using eggs or milk. But now, they have the largest herd of cows in all of India today. They have the largest egg ranch in all of India also. All the Olympic records won by India came from young people who lived in Sri Aurobindo's ashram. Vegetarianism without eggs or milk is extremely difficult for nutritional reasons and because the lifestyle of the vegetarian is different from those who eat more stimulating foods.

Another reason we need proteins, fats and lecithin is because they build and maintain the glands, and they tell you, you're as young as your glands. That doesn't mean you should have proteins for sexual purposes only. You find if you have good glands, you're not going to develop wrinkles; you're not going to develop flabbiness under the arms.

There's a lot that you can find in studying the different religions and ways of life associated with each one. If you want to go that transmutation way, it's perfectly all right. And it is a way of life, isn't it?

Most of the people who come to me are living a life that needs extreme changes, so I have to take them through these changes by degrees. It is often a slow process. Those of you a little farther along may be able to take larger, faster steps on the path to this kind of knowledge.

Laucks
Testing Laboratories, Inc.
1008 Western Avenue. Seattle. Washington 98104 (206)622-0727

Chemistry. Microbiology. and Technical Services

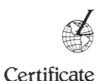

Certificate

CLIENT Briar Hills Dairies
279 S.W. 9th
Chehalis, WA 98532

LABORATORY NO. 73419

DATE June 19, 1981

REPORT ON GOAT MILK WHEY

SAMPLE INDENTIFICATION Marked: 1) Whex Dehydrated Goat Milk Whey
Net. wt. 6 oz.

TESTS PERFORMED AND RESULTS.

Ash, %   9.3

SEMI-QUANTITATIVE SPECTROGRAPHIC ANALYSIS
(on ash)

Potassium	41.%
Sodium	4.0
Phosphorus	3.1
Calcium	1.1
Magnesium	0.79
Silicon	0.58
Boron	0.012
Aluminum	0.037
Manganese	0.0043
Lead	0.015
Iron	0.068
Tin	Less/0.0031
Lithium	0.0043
Copper	0.0054
Titanium	0.0076
Silver	0.00035
Strontium	0.0054
Chromium	0.0054
Other elements	nil

Respectfully submitted,

J. M. Owens

JMO:ks

This is an analysis of a concentrated goat whey called Whex. I use this a lot with my patients.

USING MILK AND MILK PRODUCTS

After the egg, milk is close to the most perfect protein, but you don't have to have it as most people drink it today. You should prepare it in another way, such as clabbered milk or yogurt. Most of us have been overdoing this, haven't we? We don't usually have anything but pasteurized milk, and far too much of it. That's where we're getting into trouble. We don't need the milk if we use the seed milk drinks.

I recommend that vegetarians find out the best animal-protein substitutes, but try to follow my Health and Harmony Food Regimen as much as possible.

GOAT MILK

The best milk is inspected and certified raw milk, and if you can get raw goat's milk, that is the best of all. (All dairy products should be from clean, healthy animals.)

Next, we come to cheese, and we should use raw goat milk cheese if you can possibly get it. You can send for some at Mt. Capra Cheese, 279 S.W. 9th Street, Chehalis, Washington 98532. This is the best source I have found and we send for our cheese. They have raw goat cheese they call the Olympic-type cheese or Cascade cheese, and this is what the Olympic champions used to eat during training in years past.

I don't believe in using milk as it comes in the regular form, with the exception for young children. There are better ways to have it. The scientist Mechnikoff brought out the fact that in Romania and Armenia, the people who lived longest had the finest intestinal flora, and it was because of the way they took their milk. We call it yogurt or clabbered milk. Some call it "spoon milk." And you find this form of milk contains the natural bacteria to keep the intestinal tract saturated with the acidophilus bacteria.

92

YOGURT AND CLABBERED MILK ARE EASY TO DIGEST

In Russia, clabbered milk is called "matzoni." In Turkey, they call it "kumiss." In a great many countries they call it yogurt, and it is used especially by old people who have more difficulty digesting their foods.

When we make clabbered milk, the liquid whey separates from the curd in about three days. I want to tell you something. Whey, a high natural sodium food which the stomach needs for good digesting, is the old man's drink. The old men took the whey from the clabbered milk. I never found one with arthritis or joint troubles, as food sodium keeps us from having stiff joints. They were doing something right and didn't know it. Yogurt, clabbered milk and whey are all easy on the stomach, easily digested.

Many people who have difficulty with digestion take digestion aids to support the acid, enzyme and bile activity of the stomach, pancreas, liver and small bowel. At any health food store there is usually at least one good vegetarian digestive substance available which has no animal products in it.

LACK OF HYDROCHLORIC ACID IN THE ELDERLY

In hospitals, they have discovered that after the age of 50, about 85% have insufficient hydrochloric acid. It happens to many long before that, too. When you have enough hydrochloric acid and you put milk into the stomach, what happens to the milk? It curdles. You clabber it. But, when it is already clabbered, older people or people with poor digestion don't need as much hydrochloric acid. The first stage of digestion was taken care of *before* they put it into the stomach. So with the lower amount of hydrochloric acid they could still have the calcium from the milk they needed for strength and long life.

HOW TO MAKE YOGURT

Milk is the highest food in calcium and you find that most of these people from Russia, Armenia and Romania are calcium types. They have square shoulders, large bones and when they shake hands with you, you're shaken! Calcium is that long life element in milk. You don't die young when you have that long life element. That's the reason I believe in yogurt, and it should be raw if you can possibly get it.

You can make yogurt or clabbered milk in shallow pans, two inches high or so. Use raw milk and put in a teaspoon of raw yogurt for a starter or use a little rennet. You can also use a little pineapple juice or lime juice. Whichever way you start, let it curdle with cloth over the top for a couple of days. That's a nice quick raw way of making it. People from some other countries who make yogurt use a "starter" from the last batch to start fermentation in the new batch. Yogurt and clabbered milk go on to develop and bring a food to the friendly bacteria in the bowel, the acidophilus bacteria.

SESAME SEEDS—ONE OF OUR BEST PROTEINS

Many seeds are high in protein, and we find the quality of this protein is very good. We find that the sesame seed is the champion of all seeds. Sunflower seeds are very good, indeed, but the smaller the seeds, the better they are for you—the more powerful. powerful.

If you have ever spent time in Turkey, you find they use so much of the sesame seed. The strongest men in the world are in Turkey. I saw a 75-year-old man there carry a piano on his back for nine blocks. Did you know that the champion wrestler in Turkey is 75 years old? A man very much enamored by the food value of sesame seeds made a sesame candy. He showed it to the football team at one of the big universities in Arizona and made a bet with those big athletes that even at his age of 50, he could outdo anyone on the football team in loading a truck with sand. He won over every member of the football team. Sesame seeds were quite popular with the team members after that.

The sesame seed is one of the finest glandular foods you can have. When my patients are lacking in glandular material, what is it I do? I advise all my patients to take a tablespoon of sesame seed butter every day.

There are other seeds you can use, too, such as pumpkin seeds and sunflower seeds. Some doctors recommend taking pumpkin seeds for prostate trouble. Sunflower seeds are an especially good vegetarian protein.

ALMONDS—KING OF THE NUTS

The almond is the king of all nuts. You should use almonds often, but I want you to realize that few people chew nuts adequately. Most people seem to just breathe them in. Nuts must be chewed very fine to be digested. I've given colonics to many people who eat seeds and nuts, and they come out the same way they are chewed. They are not digested and broken down.

If you will break down these nuts and seeds and have them only in nut butter and seed butter form, you will get the most good from them. I do not approve of them in any other way (except the seed or nut milk drinks), because you're eating them and you're not getting any food value out of them. You don't chew them well.

You can do better by soaking them in apple juice or honey overnight and they'll be nice and mushy the next morning. Put them in a liquefier, and you'll find in this form they are easily digested. Otherwise, if you eat these seeds, they will leave the stomach in less than 2 hours, in much the same way they went in. It takes 10 hours to properly soak dry nuts or seeds. The hydrochloric acid in the stomach works best on finely broken up particles of any "hard" protein such as seeds and nuts. These have to be almost in a milk form, finely ground, for the stomach to digest properly. I don't think you'd have to liquefy it if you would chew it well or "fletcherize" it, but most people don't do that. It can take hours to soak up nuts so that man can get the protein values out of it, but in making nut milk and seed milk drinks, it gives the body the easiest protein and one of the finest proteins.

Too many people are in a hurry. They want to get eating over with, get it down, because they think they have more important things to do. Play and work are considered more important. We don't take enough time to eat properly. That's what our whole country is based on today—fast-food situations.

LENTILS—KING OF THE LEGUMES

After the nuts, *the best protein we have is the legumes.* The king of all the legumes is the lentil. It is a small bean, the smaller the bean, the higher the food value. The reason the bean causes gas in the body is not because it is part starch and part protein, but because of the hull. It is the hull on the lima bean, the hull on the soybean, that causes gas. Legume hulls are very irritable to the bowel.

So, there you have the protein values for the body. This has been a very condensed lesson, but a good lesson.

OILS, FATS AND HEART DISEASE

Because eggs are high in cholesterol, many say they could cause heart disease. But when cholesterol is balanced with lecithin, the hard fat deposits can't develop in the arteries. When we have the proper amount of lecithin, we don't have to worry about cholesterol, but we find that high heat destroys lecithin. Oils and fats in foods such as eggs, nuts, seeds, milk, cream, butter and cheese are held by the lecithin, which is destroyed when we heat it above 212 degrees. This means that lecithin in whole grain cereals and flours is also destroyed when we bake bread, pies, cakes and pastries of all kinds. It is destroyed whenever we heat cooking oils or fry any food above the boiling point of water.

Now, if you're going to control cholesterol, you can't do it if you fry your eggs, scramble them or use them in baking. Cooking at higher heat changes the lecithin, and makes it inactive so it can no longer dissolve the cholesterol. Then the cholesterol can take over and manifest itself in hardening of the arteries, in arthritis and other conditions in the body. Often, it leads to coronary disturbances and is one of the leading causes for heart disease, the number one killer in the country. This principle of not using high heat applies to any foods that have oils or fats in them. This is the reason that we should not roast almonds, peanuts or any nuts or seeds. This is why we cannot have foods cooked at high temperatures with milk or cream. If you want to have a creamed soup or dish, put the cream in at the table. If you want a nice protein broth or soup, add a teaspoon of almond butter or sesame butter at the table, not while it is cooking. Never fry or cook with oils at high heat, and don't use concentrated fats or oils on or in foods while they are cooking. Instead, add cream or butter to foods such as soups or casseroles after they have been cooked.

If you will have your eggs raw, soft-boiled or poached, you will not destroy the lecithin. This is the important thing to know.

I might also mention the egg white does not have to be used. An excess amount of the raw egg white is hard for the kidneys to take care of.

EGGS ARE A WHOLE FOOD

I might just mention that the egg yolk is a whole food. Having whole foods means that all the vitamins and minerals needed to build a whole body should be in that food.

The egg yolk is the seed that produces the whole chicken. We need the chemical elements from the egg yolk to build the skin, nerves, glands, brain tissue, eye tissue, spinal cord and so forth, so we use the egg yolk more. I think the average person could have 2 egg yolks a day. If taken raw, boiled or poached, it would seldom produce cholesterol problems in the body. It is when we are preparing the egg yolk at high heat that we get into trouble.

We have mentioned that the egg yolk is probably the most perfect of all proteins, but there is no use mutilating a perfect protein and robbing it of its nutritional balance by destroying lecithin.

Many people will give up the egg yolk because it is very high in fat, but the liver and gallbladder can take care of fatty foods if they receive the proper nutritional support and cleansing. If you will use dandelion tea, if you will use the liquid chlorophyll drink you will help the gallbladder and the liver, it will be better able to take care of the fats. Black cherry juice is one of the best foods in taking care of the liver. This, blended with a raw egg yolk, would be an easy food for the liver to take care of.

Having whole foods means that all the vitamins and minerals needed to build a whole body should be in that food. In other words, we must keep those 6 vegetables, 2 fruits, 1 starch, 1 protein combination going during the day.

We consider the egg yolk a whole food because it builds the whole body. There are many supplements a person can take, but a doctor's counseling is needed to take care of the specific organ problems. There are foods that feed one organ better than another. In general, my Health and Harmony Food Regimen will help build the whole body and provide all the elements to rebuild the individual organs. However, when you are working with my food program, you should follow the food laws in Chapter 2 to get the proper balance in your foods and to get the good out of them.

VEGETABLE COMBINATIONS

When we advise taking vegetables, you should always have underground vegetables such as carrots or beets when you are having above-ground vegetables such as lettuce or broccoli. When you have beets, you should have the beet greens. When you have turnips, you should have the turnip greens. And, you'll find that you will have much better health if you will have a couple of greens a day in your diet.

We should consider that nuts and seeds are whole foods. To make the seeds easier to digest, it is best to get them in sprout form, and sprouts will add bulk and fiber for better colon health.

GETTING CLOSER TO VEGETARIAN LIVING

There is much that could be said about raw goat milk, especially for those looking to the vegetarian way of living. The balance of food factors in my Health and Harmony Food Regimen applies also to the vegetarian way of living, particularly in keeping a balance of 6 vegetables, 2 fruits, 1 starch and 1 protein daily.

I feel that the average vegetarian starves because he doesn't have a good protein in his diet. A good vegetarian should know about raw goat milk.

Raw goat milk, first of all, is said to resemble the chemical makeup of mother's milk more closely than cow's milk does.

Raw goat milk comes from an animal that acts a good deal like the human. The goat is active, intelligent, quick and does not have heavy horns, hooves and hide like the cow. The bones are very large in the cow, which is a huge animal compared to a human. The goat is lithe, nimble in its activities, and we find that the milk from that type of animal is better for the human being. We can go still further. If you look at the temperament of the goat, you will find that it has feelings. Goats are social and like to have friends around. They appreciate peace and harmony, and they respond to good music by increased milk production even more than cows. If the goat is not being milked by someone she likes, she will drop from 1 to 2 pints a day in the amount given. Goats are like pets, and they need to be shown kindness and care.

We find that 65% of the world today is still living on goat milk. In the Good Book when the "land of milk and honey" is mentioned, the milk is goat's milk. In many places, a goat is the family dairy. However, this is not the case in the Western industrial nations. As we consider the milk from this type of animal, we find there are many reasons for the vegetarian or anyone else to consider it a valuable source of protein for his diet.

GOAT MILK COMPARED WITH COW MILK

It is better to take goat milk than cow milk. Many people don't want cow milk because it has a certain feeling that goes with it. If you have such a feeling, then you should go to goat milk.

Another thing we should consider is that fat globules in the goat milk are 6 times smaller than those in the cow's milk. We find it is naturally homogenized, *much easier for the liver to take care of than cow's milk, with its large fat globules.* The goat is really a higher-evolved animal. It is a browser, not a grazer. It is not earthy like the cow, and you find it likes to have fine foods. They are much cleaner than cows.

THE GOAT IS A FEELING ANIMAL

And talk about the feelings, if a human takes a bite of its food or if the food isn't clean and right, the goat won't eat it. It's very particular. This is the kind of milk we should use if we are particular and want to have the best for our bodies.

GOAT MILK FOR BETTER HEALTH

Most people don't realize that goat milk is usually used by people for health reasons. Perhaps the man of the house has an ulcer or the mother has tuberculosis or the child has tonsil troubles. Goat milk helps them all.

Goat milk is very high in fluorine—the chemical element that helps keep germ life from developing in the body. Fluorine is a natural antiseptic. There is 10 to 100 times as much fluorine in goat milk as there is in cow's milk. So it is good for sick people. It is good for people who want to keep well, and in this day and age, where it is so difficult to keep well and to keep free of germ life, it may be well to consider the possibilities of getting raw goat milk if you are not in the best of health.

EGGS AND THE VEGETARIAN WAY

The egg, especially the yolk, is a wonderful protein food for everyone, including the vegetarian. We find that many who have tried to go the "pure" vegetarian way have encountered problems with dizziness or dizzy spells, periods of weakness, difficulty in thinking and so forth. When milk, eggs or both were added to the diet, these problems cleared up. Nuts and seeds are fine supplemental proteins, but it is very hard to get by with them as the main protein source. The same is true of the grains and legumes. Some people can digest these cold proteins better than others, but it is difficult for many people to handle them. It takes a fairly healthy person with good digestion to take care of cold proteins.

If a man wants to become celibate and give up sex entirely, he doesn't need much of the cholesterol for the glands or lecithin for semen. But for those who are sexually active, you must pay back to the body what you use up, and the glands need proteins, fats and lecithin to stay healthy. You should know that the egg yolk carries all eight of the essential amino acids and a good balance of fats and lecithin. The brain and nerves use the same foods as the glands.

Other sources of lecithin are the nuts, seeds, grains and especially soybeans. We can get concentrated lecithin from soybeans at most health food stores in capsule form.

I am not trying to make a vegetarian out of anyone, but if you want to go the cleanest way in foods, the vegetarian way is it. What I am trying to show is that even the vegetarian must go by the food laws in my Health and Harmony Food Regimen to meet all the chemical needs of a healthy body.

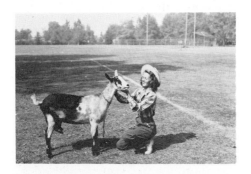

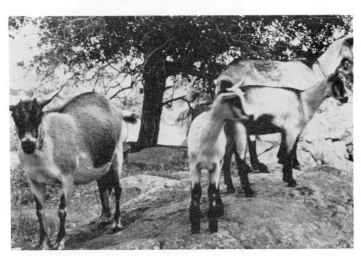

Top: Goat's milk is the best you can get. Bottom: Dr. Jensen's prize-winning goats.

101

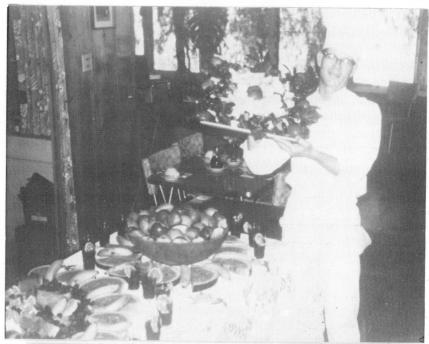

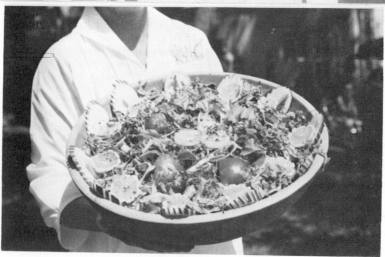

Food prepared to look lovely whets the appetite, stirs the digestive juices into action and makes mealtime a nice experience.

7

The Four Survival Foods

I consider four foods so important to the survival of man that we need to know about these foods more than any of the others. We live in a world with so many toxic substances, unnatural and "foodless" foods, high-stress jobs, emotional upsets and so forth that survival is now an issue for the average person to take seriously.

The four survival foods are chlorophyll, seeds, sprouts and black berries. Before getting into a discussion of each of these foods, I want to say that nobody should try to live on these foods alone. When I call them "survival" foods, I mean they are important to **man's survival** not that man should try to survive on these four foods without using others.

CHLOROPHYLL

Among the four survival foods, Number One is chlorophyll. The person who wants to get well will be helped more by adding chlorophyll to his diet than anything else. Chlorophyll is the great cleansing and detoxifying food, supportive of the liver activity and sweetening to the bowel.

There are many foods that have some chlorophyll, but the green, leafy vegetables are highest. Any time you take greens, it's going to help make the greatest change in your body.

If you are going to have sandwiches, it's perfectly all right, but they should be "Dagwood" sandwiches with fillings of green, leafy vegetables and other vegetables, with snacks of crisp vegetables on the side, such as celery and carrot sticks. Make the vegetable filling the greatest part of the sandwich.

Never eat bread unless you eat vegetables with it. Bread will dry out in the intestinal tract, but the proper amount of vegetables will carry enough water to keep the bread from being constipating and causing a dry stool. We need to remember this when we send our children to school with sandwiches, so they will not become constipated.

When one of my sons was young, we always sent him to school with a nice sack lunch. With his sandwiches, we always included snacks of celery stuffed with fillings such as chopped dates and nut butter. The sandwich itself always had leaf lettuce in it and sometimes sprouts, cucumber slices and other vegetables. So there were vegetable fillings in the sandwich and vegetable snacks to eat along with it, such as bell pepper slices, carrots and celery sticks.

Once I asked my son, "How are you getting along with your lunches?" He said, "All right, but they call me a rabbit at school, because I take so many vegetables." And I said, "Well, what do you say back to them?" He said, "I tell them at least I'm not a constipated rabbit!"

START EARLY IN HELPING CHILDREN
TO HAVE GOOD ELIMINATION HABITS

It is always best to establish regular, natural elimination habits in our children as early as we can. In nature, the digestion of food in the stomach starts the peristaltic motion in the bowel, so it is ***natural to have a bowel movement after each meal.***

If we don't answer nature's call, bowel contents become more compacted, and we weaken the bowel tissue. It takes fiber and bulk in our foods to give the bowel something to "push" against to move bowel wastes along as fast as they should. When bowel wastes are held too long, toxins move through the bowel wall into the bloodstream. Any benefits we are getting from good nutrition can be spoiled unless we learn to follow nature's call when it comes. Constipation and gas work against what we have accomplished.

Over the past 50 years, I would say about 80% of my patients have had rectal problems due to the lack of proper bowel activity and management. Prolapsus, hemorrhoids, pressure on the prostate and pelvic organs—all these and other bowel disturbances can develop when we have undue strain in forcing a

104

bowel movement.

To correct bowel problems, the first thing to think about is nutrition, then bowel exercises. In addition to following my Health and Harmony Food Regimen, I recommend that my patients with rectal problems (especially hemorrhoids) take 1 chlorophyll capsule, 1 garlic oil capsule and 1 vitamin A capsule as rectal suppositories every night for a month to help heal the rectal area while problems are being corrected throughout the body. Every organ and tissue in the body is affected by bowel conditions, so we have to take care of the whole body as we take care of the bowel. Exercises such as the slant board exercises, as shown on pp. 82-83 in my book *TISSUE CLEANSING THROUGH BOWEL MANAGEMENT*, should be used by those who are well enough to take them. If you have high blood pressure, ulcers or any condition which may contra-indicate the use of the slant board, **DO NOT USE THE SLANT BOARD WITHOUT CONSULTING A PHYSICIAN FIRST.**

We find that the toilet is probably man's worst invention as far as bowel health is concerned. Primitive people all over the world have seldom had bowel problems, generally because they get plenty of bulk in the diet and because they squat to eliminate. Squatting is man's most natural position for bowel elimination. There is no strain in squatting.

When I was staying in the palace of the Mir of Hunza, the "toilet" was a hole in the floor, and squatting was the only way to use it. At my sanitarium, I taught my patients to hold their hands above their heads when using the toilet. There was a rope to hold onto above the head, and when the arms are raised, there is no strain on the bowel.

Chlorophyll, chlorophyll-rich vegetables and chlorophyll-rich algae such as chlorella help detoxify the bowel and feed the beneficial bowel bacteria. Chlorophyll assists in the detoxification of the bloodstream, the liver and all other tissues and organs of the body. Our carbohydrates are made by solar energy acting on chlorophyll in plant leaves, and I feel that chlorophyll can be considered a form of concentrated sunlight, with similar antiseptic and cleansing powers as sunlight.

Chlorella tablets are very high in chlorophyll and in a growth factor and in other nutrients that are wonderful for taking care of digestive disturbances and bowel troubles. According to published medical reports from Japan, chlorella speeds the healing of stomach and duodenal ulcers, takes care of gas and bloating, and restores regularity in most cases of bowel underactivity and constipation. In four published cases from Japan, normal bowel activity was restored in patients paralyzed due to spinal injuries. From my own experience, I know what a wonderful healing agent chlorophyll is, and we find that chlorella is the highest known plant source of chlorophyll—3% to 7%. Chlorophyll helps cleanse and deodorize the bowel, helps feed the friendly bacteria in the colon and helps cleanse and build the bloodstream.

Care of the bowel is explained fully in my book *TISSUE CLEANSING THROUGH BOWEL MANAGEMENT*, which I strongly recommend.

SEEDS

Seeds are Number Two in the survival foods.

The most active vital principles we can put in our bodies come from seeds. The smaller the seed, the more vital it is, the more powerful in its energies.

The seeds are the glands in our plant foods and they contain the vital principles that nourish the glandular system, the nervous system and the brain.

The Cavalda Date Company has found that the date seed is one of the highest in the male hormone. Citrus seeds are very high in the female hormone. I don't know if you knew that we make our hormones from the fats and life factors in seeds, but when we have been using white flour, white rice, refined cornmeal, and other refined grain products, the vitamin E and the germ with the life factors in them have been taken out. The life factors that support your glands are found in the seeds. And now we've got a seedless generation to take care of, a generation that has lost its natural sex and replaced it with abnormal substitute activities.

THE SEEDLESS GENERATION

If you are a reader or TV watcher, you find out that child molestation, pornography, rape, sexually explicit films and TV shows on these subjects are common these days. The people responsible for these things are the "seedless" people. These are people who don't have the proper hormones. These people are hungry for natural sex, but because the body chemistry is abnormal, the sexual expression is abnormal. They are starving in the mental sex area because they are deficient in the seed factors that build their sex hormones. Can I be that definite?

Consider that the same nutrients that build the sex glands also build the brain. The "seedless generation" is not only deficient in the factors that normalize sex life but also deficient in the factors that normalize brain function and mental life. How can we expect those lacking the proper glandular, nerve and brain foods to think or act properly?

SEEDS FOR THE CHANGE OF LIFE

I believe seeds are the greatest thing you can have in your diet. When you ladies go through the change of life, you haven't been building the glands for proper hormones. We develop all kinds of change of life symptoms and it has occurred because we did not have the proper glandular foods such as vitamin E and lecithin from our seeds, nut butters, etc. And then what do you take? You take artificial hormone substances in the form of drugs, some of it made from the urine of pregnant mares! Did you know that? Why don't you get the hormone substance from seeds? You may have to chew them. You may have to grind them into fine meal or make seed milk drinks from them, but you should be using these seeds. It's something to think about, isn't it? You men should know that pumpkin seeds are the greatest thing for the prostate gland.

One of the things I tell my patients is to take a tablespoon of sesame seed butter every day. I personally believe this helps to keep up or restore the glandular activity in those who have neglected taking seeds and other glandular foods.

SPROUTS

Number Three of our best survival foods is sprouts.

Sprouts are whole, pure and natural. There is no excuse for not using sprouts because if you can't buy them you can easily make them. The sprout is the new babe or new generation coming from the seeds. We find that after a certain number of days the sprout develops leaves which bring in the chlorophyll. That's the time it is supposed to be eaten or planted in soil, and it's one of the finest things because it has all the vitamins and minerals you can use for the body. The sprout is still part of mother, the mother seed. Sprouts are among the most nourishing foods we can have. In a wide-mouthed jar (a quart preserving jar), place the seeds. Put cheesecloth over the top of the jar and secure with a rubber band. Soak the seeds for 10 hours; drain off the water; and place in a cool dark area. Rinse three times daily to freshen the grain. In three days, they're ready to eat.

BLACK BERRIES

The fourth survival food is black berries.

This does not mean just blackberries, but all berries that are black. It means blueberries, huckleberries, loganberries, black raspberries and others. This includes black cherries. All of these are particularly high in iron. You'll never have enough oxygen in your body without enough iron.

The first thing the doctor takes care of when a woman is pregnant is to make sure she has enough iron in her body. The first thing a good athlete needs is plenty of iron. I'm going to tell you that iron attracts oxygen out of the air. Iron and oxygen are the two frisky horses that give you energy to run, work, play and the energy to repair and rebuild your body. The iron is found in black berries.

Living in Los Angeles or other large cities with smog and carbon monoxide gas, you find it is much more difficult to get enough oxygen from the polluted air. Getting plenty of iron from berries helps you survive and be healthy, sometimes in conditions that are not the best.

Other survival foods are beans, honey, raw goat milk and nuts with hard shells.

We have to be willing to make changes, and I am giving you things to think about. If you feel eating is everything or you can't have a meal without a glass of beer or a sweet dessert, maybe I can't help you. Maybe you haven't gotten sick enough yet. Some people have to wait until they are sick of being sick. Then they decide they can give up the old ways. Then they are willing to change. But I tell you, if you want to be well, you can start on a new path and establish a higher level of well-being.

S.O.S.—SAVE OUR SEEDS

Few Americans are aware that increasing use of hybrids has led us to the peculiar place where we are in danger of losing original seeds for thousands of varieties of perfectly useful fruits and vegetables. We find that all the vegetable varieties available at the turn of the century, perhaps fewer than 20% have survived to this point.

In 1975, Kent Whealy started the Seed Savers Exchange when an elderly gardener gave him seeds from three treasured varieties his family had brought over from Bavaria five generations ago—cabbage, pole beans and a purple morning glory with a red star at its center. By 1980, the Seed Savers Exchange had expanded to 328 members in the basic network, which, in the previous 5 years, had offered about 3,000 vegetable varieties, many of them unusual or possibly unique, to over 9,000 gardeners. There is a government storage facility for seeds in Fort Collins, Colorado, but the government can't do everything and may not have the funds to continue this project indefinitely.

All of our present-day fruits and vegetables are said to have evolved from herbs at some point in the past, and many of the originals provided smaller fruits, berries and vegetables than we find today, with the same nutritional value in a "smaller package." Today, large corporations are buying up the seed companies and dropping many regional or unprofitable varieties from their catalogs, leaving more and more hybrids, which I feel have far less nutritional value than seeds from true natural stock.

We have to realize that seeds are the glands of plants, the source of many of the hormone factors needed by man. When we eat seeds from berries and fruits and varieties like sesame, sunflower and pumpkin seeds, we are building our glands. Hybrids do not provide the glandular factors people need. If use of hybrid foods continues to increase, we may be building a "seedless" generation of people in the future.

One of the greatest dangers today is that the variety of original seeds which kept such diversity of plant life on the face of this planet is being slowly and persistently diminished until we are becoming in danger of losing the hardiness and adaptability of plant stock in the face of changing environmental conditions. In other words, I feel if our seed supply drops too low, some temporary imbalance of nature could wipe out most of our food supply and blight the seeds, leaving us facing a bleak, seedless future with no reserves, no stock of alternative seeds to use to try to replenish the earth.

The Creator left man a wonderful garden as an inheritance, but unless we learn to take better care of it, we will never know what a wonderful place this earth was meant to be. This is something to stop and think about, isn't it?

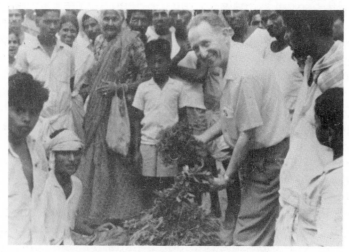

In an Indian market—herbs and greens are parts of most of their meals.

8

My
Daily Health and Harmony
Food Program

Many people don't realize that they wouldn't have to turn to diets if they had a right way of living. By applying my Health and Harmony Food Regimen every day, you will be on the way to better health. You won't have to think so much about vitamins, minerals and calories. For the average person, this regimen will supply a good balance of the chemical elements.

A club, which I started in New Zealand, called *Dr. Jensen's 729 Clubs*, are made up of people who want to live correctly so they can avoid doctor bills. There was one doctor there to every 729 people, so these clubs throughout the South Seas, New Zealand and Australia became active in teaching other peope how to live correctly, and this is the food program they taught. This club took on a proposition one time to change the diets of 250 school children to see what healthier food would do for them as compared with the average diet prepared at school cafeterias and eaten on the school grounds. The children were watched quite carefully.

It was difficult to get the cooperation of the parents, teachers and so forth, to have the children's diets changed as they considered it meddling in their personal affairs. But they finally agreed. Refined foods were replaced with whole meal breads and plenty of fresh fruits and vegetables were served. *To the surprise of the mothers and teachers, there was quite a change—especially in reduced tardiness and colds.* Many of the mothers reported that their children didn't have the *constipation* with which they had been troubled. Their *bowels became regular. They did not have the fevers and many of the childhood diseases that usually prevailed.*

Eating right will make a great deal of difference in your family

111

life. Carefully read the following rules and food laws and think about them. While these rules are ideal goals for the average person and may vary a little with the individual, start out by following them closely.

RULES OF EATING

1. ***Do not fry foods or use heated oils in cooking.*** Frying lowers nutritional value, destroys lecithin needed to balance fats and makes food harder to digest. The temperature at which foods are fried or cooked in oil alters food chemistry, which is not a safe practice. This can be one of the greatest contributing factors to cholesterol formation and hardening of the arteries and heart disease.

2. ***If not entirely comfortable in mind and body, do not eat.*** We don't digest food well when we are upset or when we are not comfortable. It's better to wait. A little waiting period from food will allow us to digest our food properly.

3. ***Do not eat until you have a keen desire for the plainest food.*** Too often, we eat simply because it is mealtime, not because we are hungry. Break this undesirable habit. To have the best possible digestion, eat when you are hungry.

4. ***Do not eat beyond your needs.*** Overeating is not good for the health.

5. ***Be sure to thoroughly masticate your food.*** Chewing well increases the efficiency of digestion. You get more food value for the money you spend on food.

6. ***Miss meals if in pain, emotionally upset, not hungry, chilled, overheated or ill.*** Each of these conditions is a signal that we need rest, warmth, calmness or something other than food which, if eaten, ties up considerable energy and blood in the gastrointestinal tract. Often, rest is the thing most needed. Food takes energy to digest and involves work by several organs, and it may take hours before food energy is available.

RULES FOR GETTING WELL

1. Learn to accept whatever decision is made. Do your best to keep your peace of mind. Peace is a healer.

2. Let the other person make a mistake and learn. This is so

much better than standing over people and supervising every move. Learn to give the person the opportunity to grow and grow up. We are bound to make mistakes. Let's not gloat over them and live in remorse about them.

3. Learn to forgive and forget. Many studies have now shown that forgiving enhances health and helps prevent chemical changes in the body that may lead to disease.

4. Be thankful and bless people. These are two of the main secrets to a healthy life.

5. Live in harmony—even if it is good for you.

6. Don't talk about your misfortunes or illnesses. It doesn't do any good for you or the person you tell, and it presents an opportunity for them to do the same to you. Save it for your doctor. He's paid to listen to your troubles.

7. Don't gossip. Gossip that comes through the grapevine is usually sour grapes.

8. Spend 10 minutes a day meditating on how you can become a better person. Replace negative thoughts with positive ones.

9. Exercise daily. Keep your spine and joints limber, develop your abdominal muscles, expand your lungs—with specific exercises on a regular schedule.

10. Walk 10 minutes barefoot in the dewy grass or sand the first thing in the morning to stimulate the blood circulation.

11. No smoking or drinking of alcohol. Both nicotine and alcohol are depressant drugs. Both require energy to detoxify the body which is needed for more useful life processes.

12. Go to bed by 9 pm at the latest, when you can. If you are tired during the day, rest more. Rest allows the body to give its full attention and energy to healing and rebuilding tissues. Write down your problems at the end of the day and go over them first thing in the morning when you are refreshed, so you can look at them with a fresh mind and body.

TOTAL HEALING LAWS

Food is for building health. You need to have foods that will meet the needs of a vital, active life and the following laws are designed to do exactly that. These are physical laws to be carried out. Try to understand what it means to get your diet program working out according to these laws.

1. Food should be natural, whole and pure.

Reason: *The closer food is to its natural, God-created state, the higher its nutritional value.* Some foods, such as meat, potatoes, yams and grains must be cooked. Whole foods are more nutritious than refined, bleached or peeled foods. I'm not telling you to eat banana skins and avocado seeds, I'm just giving you a practical guideline. Pure foods are much better for us than foods with preservatives, artificial colors or flavors or chemical additives of any kind. Many chemicals now added to commercial food products were never meant to be in the human body. Our bodies were designed for natural, whole, pure foods and that's what keeps us in the best condition. We have learned our greatest lesson with experiments on animals using denatured, peeled, polished foods. They have become sick because of the chemicals that have been deleted and they are no longer whole, as God designed for us.

2. We should have 60% of our foods raw.

Reason: *I am not advising a raw diet because I like the taste, I'm saying it is better for us.* Raw foods provide more vitamins, minerals, enzymes, fiber and bulk, because they are "live" foods at the peak of nutritional value, if properly selected. Raw foods help the digestive system and bowel. I mean fruits, berries, vegetables, sprouts, nuts and seeds. We have to cook cereal grains, lima beans, artichokes and other foods, but there are many we can take raw.

3. We should have 6 vegetables, 2 fruits, 1 starch and 1 protein every day.

Reason: *Vegetables are high in fiber and minerals. Fruits are high in natural complex sugars and vitamins.* Starch is for energy and protein is for cell repairing and rebuilding, especially the brain and nerves. *This is a balanced combination of foods.*

4. Our foods should be 80% alkaline and 20% acid.

Reason: *We find that 80% of the nutrients carried in the blood are alkaline and 20% are acid. To keep the blood the way it should be, 6 vegetables and 2 fruits make up that 80% alkaline foods we need, while 1 protein and 1 starch make up the 20% of acid foods.* To keep the blood balanced, we should eat 2 fruits, 6 vegetables, 1 starch and 1 protein daily. Proteins and many starches are acid-forming and nearly all of the metabolic wastes of the body are acids. We need alkaline-forming foods such as fruit and vegetables so their alkaline salts will neutralize the acid wastes. I believe that we should recognize that to keep the proper alkaline-acid balance in the body we must have 6 vegetables, 2 fruits, 1 starch and 1 protein daily. There is no reason why we should add too heavily to the acid conditions in our body by adding heavy acid foods such as we find in the proteins and starches. In my experience, acid wastes not properly disposed of are the cause of many disturbances, health problems and chronic diseases.

5. Variety: Vary proteins, starches, vegetables and fruits from meal to meal and day to day.

Reason: *Every organ of our body needs one chemical element more than others to keep healthy.* The thyroid needs iodine, the stomach needs sodium, the blood needs iron and so on. We also need variety in vitamins. The best way to take care of this is to have variety in vitamins. The best way to take care of this is to have variety in our foods. Foods, in a way, are matched to our body organs in that each food is usually highest in one or two minerals and vitamins. But every food is different and even the same foods grown in different localities, different soils, have different nutrients. As we take in a variety of foods, we must realize that we are made from the dust of the earth. To get calcium foods, we need grains and different kinds of grains. Some grains have more calcium than other grains. It is necessary to realize that in our variety, especially our salads, they must be made up of different colors. Each color has its own activity in the body, because each color carries a chemical element particular to that color. All red foods are stimulating foods. All yellow are of a laxative nature in the natural food routine. All green foods repair, rebuild and are high in iron and potassium. For example, a rainbow salad will have all the chemical elements we need in the various colors of vegetables. The same applies to the main dish. If you can follow this reasoning and go into it deeper and see how each chemical element has its own vibration, each color found in the foods has its own vibration. We are eating the life force, the sun-giving force from these fruits and vegetables in the color that was placed there by nature. This is one of the greatest laws to follow.

6. Eat moderately.

Reason: *The healthiest people I have met in my world travels were the same weight later in life as when they were in their 20s, and some of them were over 120 years old!* In the U.S., 60% of the people are overweight, which leads to many health problems. Leave that extra food on the plate. Eating at home is more desirable. *The bigger the waistline, the shorter the lifeline.*

7. Combinations: Separate starches and proteins.

Reason: *Have your proteins and starches at different meals, not because they don't digest well together but so you will be able to eat more fruits and vegetables each meal.* People tend to fill up on protein and starch, then neglect their vegetables. I want you to have a lot of vegetables with each meal for your health's sake, and when you are hungry, they taste wonderful. There are poor combinations, and I'll mention a few. Dried fruits do not go well with fresh fruits. Unless dried fruits have been reconstituted and brought back to their natural state, it is best not to eat them. It is best not to have grapefruit and dates together. Dried fruits must be reconstituted by putting the dried fruit in cold water at night and bring them to a boil, let the water boil for about 3 minutes, then turn off the flame; let stand overnight. Melon should always be eaten at least half an hour apart from any other foods.

Don't have ice-cold drinks with meals because they interfere with digestion. Herb teas can be taken with meals and so can vegetable or fruit juices, since they are foods. There is a lot of discussion about having liquids with meals. It is best to have your fruit at breakfast and 3 pm.

8. Be careful about your drinking water.

Reason: *Most public water systems are now highly chemicalized because ground water sources are increasingly polluted.* The fruit and vegetables in my Health and Harmony Food Regimen supply much of the water your body needs. If you use broths, juices, soups and herbal teas, they will take care of any remaining thirst during the day. If you are still thirsty, try cutting down or eliminating salt on your foods. Salt creates a thirst. Use vegetable or broth seasonings instead. I advise distilled water for those who have arthritis but we don't really need much drinking water on my Health and Harmony Food Regimen. Reverse osmosis water purification units provide the best water for household consumption.

9. Use low-heat, waterless cookware; cook with little or no water and do not overcook.

Reason: *High heat, boiling in water and exposure to air are the three greatest robbers of nutrients.* Low-heat stainless steel pots with lids that form a water seal are the most efficient means of cooking foods in such a way as to preserve the greatest nutritional value. For oven cooking, glass casserole dishes with lids are fine. I approve of crockpot cooking, because it offers another low-heat method.

10. If you use meat, poultry and fish, bake, broil or roast it—but have it no more than 3 times a week.

Reason: *Baking, broiling and roasting—while far from perfect cooking methods—are at least more acceptable in terms of preserving more nutritional value. Cook at lower heats for longer times to retain the most nutritional value.* Avoid pork and fatty meats and use only white fish with fins and scales. Salmon is permitted, even though it isn't a white meat. Fatty meats lead to obesity, heart trouble and so on. Beef is very stimulating to the heart and I do not recommend using it. Eating meat more than three times a week can produce excess uric acid and other irritating by-products causing an unnecessary burden on the body. While I do not believe that the meat will cause heart trouble, I believe when we live a fast, hard lifestyle that includes having a heavy amount of meat, it can lead to heart troubles. Those who study the positive and negative effects of food will find that meat is positive, starches are negative. Starches feed the left side of the body, and that is the side where the heart is. Proteins feed the right side of the body.

11. Avoid having an excess of one or a few foods in the diet.

Reason: *An excess of one or a few foods may provide too much of certain food chemicals for the body to handle, causing irritation, inflammation or possible allergies.* Celiac disease is caused by gluten from wheat and other gluten grains damage the wall of the small bowel. An excess of one or a few foods also means that other foods are not used in sufficient variety in the diet, which causes chemical deficiencies.

12. Don't neglect important foods.

Reason: *Our health is determined as much by what we don't eat as well as by what we eat, which can cause nutritional deficiencies that lead to a future disease.* If we neglect most vegetables, for example, we prevent our bodies from receiving needed chemical elements and enzymes. Lack of sufficient proteins, carbohydrates and fats—any or all—can cause disturbances in the body, as can lack of vitamins, minerals, lecithin, enzymes and trace elements.

DAILY EATING REGIMEN

Organize your meals to use the food laws and instructions properly. Here is an outline of what your daily food regimen should be like, and this will take care of the food laws—the law of variety, the law of proportions, the law of acid/alkaline balance, the law of 60% raw food and so forth.

You can have half your daily allowance of protein at breakfast and half at dinner; half of your starch at breakfast and half at lunch. Starches and proteins together help keep you from snacking and experiencing hunger between meals, but you shouldn't have so much that you don't have room for vegetables.

Breakfast
1/2 starch
1/2 protein
Health drink
10 am—Vegetable juice or broth
Lunch
3 vegetables (cooked, raw or salad)
1/2 starch (see list of starches)
Health drink
3 pm—Fruit or fruit juice
Dinner
3 vegetables (cooked, raw or salad)
1/2 protein
Health drink

BEFORE BREAKFAST

It is best to have a couple glasses of water or a drink of some kind before breakfast. This cleanses the bladder and kidneys. I have found the practice of taking a teaspoon of liquid chlorophyll in a glass of water is one of the best things to start off the day. I avoid citrus juices in the morning, as they stir up acids. Remember citrus stirs up acids, while vegetable juices carry them off. Other juices you might have could be a glass of natural, unsweetened fruit juice—grape, pineapple, prune, fig, apple or black cherry.

BREAKFAST

Fruit, one starch and a health drink (broth, soup, coffee substitute, buttermilk, raw milk, oat straw tea, alfa-mint tea, huckleberry tea, papaya tea, etc.) Dried, unsulphured fruits should be reconstituted. Fresh fruit such as melon, grapes, apricots, figs, pears, berries, apple slices (or baked apple) may be sprinkled with ground nuts, seeds or nut butter. Ground sesame seeds, flax seeds, sunflower seeds and almonds are good. Try to use fruit in season. If you have a cooked whole grain cereal, sprinkle ground nuts and seeds on top, add chopped dates, raisins, prunes, figs or other dried fruit for sweetening or use a little honey or maple syrup. A handful of steamed raisins in any cereal has been a favorite with our family. We can use Swiss muesli any time. There is a formula for making it in our menus. Avoid citrus or citrus juices with breakfast, except an occasional ripe orange, sliced in sections.

LUNCH

Raw Salad: Tomatoes, lettuce (no head lettuce), celery, cucumber, spinach leaves, sprouts (bean, alfalfa, radish, etc.), green pepper, avocado, parsley, watercress, endive, onion, garlic, cabbage, cauliflower, broccoli, etc., in any combination. Top with grated carrot, beet, parsnip, turnip—in any combination. Sprinkle with ground nuts and seeds. Add a little grated cheese, if you like. One or two starches may be used, plus a health drink.

DINNER

Protein, vegetable or fruit salad, one or two cooked vegetables (such as squash, artichoke, cauliflower, spinach, chard, Brussels sprouts, broccoli, etc.) and a health drink. If you had a large salad for lunch, have a small one for dinner and *vice versa*.

DESSERTS

I do not believe in desserts, however, we find occasionally many people have to have it, so here are some suggestions. We can have a sliced apple, a raw fruit salad, a mixture of cut-up apples and steamed raisins with maple syrup. Mix gelatin with cherry juice and put a little whipped cream on it. Or why not have a banana, apple, pear or apricot? There are homemade candies, and one is made with nut butter and dried fruits, rolled in coconut.

SUGGESTIONS FOR PREPARING
BREAKFAST, LUNCH AND DINNER

BREAKFAST. In many countries, breakfast is considered the main meal because most people believe a good breakfast is necessary to get them going. They believe they have to have something in their bodies to get every organ stimulated and working. They think that in that stimulated condition they are ready for work. However, the strength and power to work with is in the tissues. The strength we have in the morning comes from our meal at noon the day before. After eating food, it takes some 18 hours before it gets to the tissues to give strength to our bodies. Once the "response" part of the body—the nervous system—is fed and repaired, we have the strength to work. The food we eat at noon today will give us our energy tomorrow afternoon. But what we eat for breakfast will be reacting tonight, when we go to bed. This is not the time when we should be stimulated. This is one reason why we should have a light breakfast. We don't want to be ready to go to work at night when it is bedtime. We should have our heavy meal at noon. The strength derived from that comes just in time to start our day right the following morning.

Preparing whole grain cereals. The best way is to use a wide-mouth thermos. Put the cereal grain into the bottle, cover with boiling water and let soak overnight. Make sure there is room for the cereal to expand without breaking the thermos. Exception: Cornmeal must always be added to cold water and brought to a boil in a pan first or it lumps. When it has boiled, pour the mixture into a thermos and leave overnight. Cereal can also be cooked in a double boiler.

Ground nuts and seeds. You can grind several types of nuts and seeds in advance and keep them in small jars or plastic containers in the refrigerator. Bring them out at mealtimes. You can sprinkle these on fruits, vegetables, salads, cereals, baked potato—almost any food.

Other supplements. You can add psyllium husks, wheat bran, wheat germ, oat bran, flax seed meal, dulse or broth powder seasoning on many foods to add fiber, flavor and nutritional value. Herbs are a fine addition.

Now I know that we can have our German pancakes for breakfast, and I know that the German people like a big breakfast. They claim they cannot put in a full day's work without it. There have been many plans brought forth: A no-breakfast plan, a fruit-breakfast plan, an Oslo-breakfast—it is difficult to set a program that is going to fit each and every person. However, the main thing we are trying to bring out in all our diet work is *what is right* for a person and not *who* is right. We find there must be some regular or definite program which fits most people. We believe there are exceptions to all rules. However, "breakfast" comes from the root "break fast." Whenever we fast or go without food; for instance, all night long digestive juices flow slower, our whole body is working slower; therefore, when we wake, we should break the fast with a fruit juice or a light nourishing drink of some kind. Then we should have a fruit breakfast. Fruit is the proper thing to break a fast. If we like, a little protein is a good combination with fruit and it may be allowed. We can also have dried fruits and carbohydrates together for the breakfast. The idea of having fried foods, a lot of muffins, bread or French toast, and all the other heavy foods for breakfast is not right. It is not a matter of trying to see how much we can eat.

LUNCH

If you want energy for the next morning, eat a good lunch. That "washed-out" feeling with which so many housewives start the day is probably due to the fact that they can't always be bothered to fix a nourishing meal for themselves at midday. They may fix a sandwich with white bread and a filling with no nutritional value, and a cup of coffee.

We will follow along with the starch idea at noon because most people are in the habit of having sandwiches or bread for this meal. Make sure your sandwiches are made of thinly sliced whole-grain breads, and stuffed heartily with good fillings and plenty of vegetables to aid the digestion. Avocado, grated carrot, celery and nuts, cottage cheese and alfalfa sprouts, olives and lettuce, nuts and dates, sunflower seed meal and honey are a few suggestions. Use a spoonful of health mayonnaise, cream or mashed banana to stick them together. Flavor with vegetable seasoning and dulse. Along with your sandwiches, take extra salad ingredients such as green leaves, carrot and celery sticks, green peppers, cucumbers or tomatoes. A health cookie is permissible, but wouldn't a bag of nuts, sunflower or squash seeds, raisins, dates or figs be more pleasing?

Did you know you could make sandwiches without bread? Bread is not the only starch, in fact, it is one of the least desirable and even if you pack a lunch, other starches are easily possible. Slice an apple horizontally and wedge cheese between the slices for instance. Raw baby zucchini slices make a nice "bread" to stuff with nut butter; some people use raw eggplant sliced thin and filled with a tasty mayonnaise spread. Even lettuce leaves will sandwich together many lovely fillings.

Salads: See Chapter 19, Food Tips, Recipes and Menus for a lot of good ideas.

Starches: Yellow cornmeal, baked potato, ripe or baked banana, yam, sweet potato, barley, rye, millet, brown rice, wild rice (actually this is a seed), buckwheat, squash such as banana, acorn or spaghetti. A couple of dead ripe bananas can become the hub of your lunch. Never forget variety. These can quite easily be put in a thermos if you have to carry your lunch. A thermos has many uses. It can hold your cold fruit or vegetable cocktail in summer, your hot broth or herb tea in winter. It can also hold a cool fruit whip or soy or nut milk beverages.

Lunch time is salad time. You will be on the move again shortly, and it takes exercise to handle raw food. Have your big green, raw salad at noon, using as many vegetables as possible. It is amazing the number we can use raw such as summer squash, asparagus, Jerusalem artichokes, okra, cauliflower and turnips, to mention just a few of the more unusual. These can be extremely tasty grated and occasionally dressed with a tangy mayonnaise. For eye appeal, sometimes stuff a green pepper, tomato or celery sticks. (These can even be carried to work in a jar. So can salads, although they lose value if cut up too long. It is best to take vegetables along whole.)

Have a cooked, low-starch-type vegetable with your meal, too, if you like. When serving a root vegetable, always make sure you have a "top" vegetable with it—not necessarily the matching top or green. On colder days, a nourishing soup is welcome. And why not try a cool raw soup in summer?

Finish your meal with a health drink: herb tea, dandelion coffee, buttermilk, raw milk, whey or any good health beverage.

It really doesn't take so very long to prepare a lunch such as we have suggested, and the lift it will give your vitality and good humor will be well worth it.

DINNER

If you value your health, eat at home! No one suffers more from malnutrition than the clergyman's wife, who is always out to supper at Mrs. Brown's, attending a church luncheon or supervising the Sunday school.

Dinner should be a family affair, a happy get-together at the end of the day when news can be exchanged convivially at the family dinner table. Here, children can learn by example the rules of healthy eating, a happy attitude, quiet enjoyment, manners, cultivation of a desire for plain food, eating slowly and masticating, and most important, knowing when to stop eating.

Use the evening meal to balance your day nutritionally. If you skimped on your salad at noon, have a bigger one at dinner or begin the meal with a raw vegetable cocktail. Did you get your

123

quota of two fruits today? Have a fruit dessert or Waldorf salad for dinner. A mixed vegetable broth is an excellent way to bring up your vegetable intake for the day—there are very good recipes for raw soups, too.

Plan your dinner around this basic formula: A small raw salad, 2 cooked vegetables, 1 protein and a health drink. If you are not a vegetarian, have meat two or three times a week, but make sure it is lean meat and cooked by broiling or roasting without fat. Fish once a week is a good protein high in iodine and phosphorus. Choose fish with fins and scales and steam, grill or bake it. Two nights a week serve a cheese dish. You'll find a popular summer supper is plain cheeses with fruit. Cheese which breaks or cottage cheese and a variety of fruit make a complete meal. An egg dish, such as a souffle or omelet, plain, poached or scrambled eggs on spinach or other greens can complete the week's dinners. There are all the vegetable proteins to bring in the changes. Nuts are one of our high-protein foods. The almond is king. Always soak nuts for several hours in fruit juice, tea or honey water for better digestion. Nuts are best eaten raw. A good form is as a nut butter. Beans baked or in roasts, lentils, split peas and sunflower seeds can also be used. An excellent vegetarian protein made from the soybean is tofu or soy cheese. Occasionally, the soy substitute meats are permissible.

With your protein dish, serve a small raw salad. Vary this from day to day. It is good to have a sulphur vegetable (cabbage or onion family) along with proteins to help drive the nerve fats to the brain. The two cooked vegetables can be of any of the non-starchy type. Remember the value of greens and eat plenty of them.

Your beverage may be a broth or soup. also vary beverages with all the different herb teas, whey, raw milk or buttermilk.

It is permissible to have a health dessert at this protein meal, although the idea is not highly recommended. If you feel the need for something sweet to finish off your meal, fresh raw fruit is best. Fruit desserts such as gelatin molds, fruit whips and sherbets, yogurt and fruit concentrates are far superior to the usual puddings, pies and ice creams. (Keep the starchy dessert idea for an occasional lunch treat after a healthful salad.)

You may exchange your noon meal for the evening meal, but follow the same regime. This is sometimes a good idea, especially if you have trouble getting to sleep. Starches predispose one to sleep more than proteins which are more stimulating.

No matter how wonderful the dinner, remember if you are emotionally upset, chilled, overheated, ill or lacking the keenest desire for plain food, miss the meal! That will do you more good.

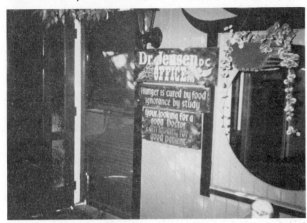

The door is open to those who are ready.

INSTRUCTIONS TO THE KITCHEN STAFF

Here are the instructions my kitchen staff at the Ranch has followed for many years in meal planning and preparation.

BREAKFAST

Fruit. One fresh fruit and one dried fruit. Also, prunes every morning with juice or water.

Drinks. Milk, if desired. Whey. Tea: Three different teas should be served during each day. Five different kinds should be kept on hand in the kitchen.

Cereal. Yellow cornmeal (twice a week). Muesli (twice a week). Rye. Oatmeal. Millet. Always serve five different ones during the week.

Eggs. Soft and hard boiled.

Sunday Mornings. O.K. to serve cornmeal hotcakes.

Bread and Butter. Toaster in working order.

Supplements. Wheat germ. Rice polishings. Flaxseed meal. Sesame seed meal.

Coffee Substitutes. If desired, Pero, Sano-Caf or Postum.

LUNCH

Salad Bar: Dish of olives. Waldorf salad (peel apples) once or twice a week. Gelatin mold (shredded carrot and pineapple) once or twice a week. Stuffed celery (almond or cashew butter) twice a week. Stuffed dates (almond or cashew butter) once a week. Carrot and cashew salad (on Champion juicer) once a week. Carrot and pea salad (cheese) once a week. Cole slaw once a week.

Always Serve: Finely shredded carrots, beets, turnips; carrot sticks; celery sticks; sliced tomatoes; sliced cucumbers; sliced green peppers.

Anything else in season, used raw: Jicama, zucchini, summer squash, onions (small), parsley, watercress, endive.

Serve alfalfa sprouts daily, and other sprouts occasionally.

Salad Dressings: Avocado; cheese and yogurt; nut butter; cottage cheese with blue cheese and yogurt; oil, vinegar and honey.

Vegetables: Two (cooked): Use one vegetable from under the ground and one vegetable from above the ground. One *bland* vegetable must be served, such as: beets, squash (yellow neck, banana, winter, etc.), zucchini, peas, carrots, string beans, wax beans, spinach, asparagus. Other vegetables *may* be a *sulphur* one (but doesn't have to be). These are: cabbage, cauliflower, Brussels sprouts, onions, broccoli, turnips, kohlrabi. Steamed onions may be served (creamed with parsley) once a week as a separate dish. *Do not put onions in soups, loaves, etc.*

Starch: Brown rice (twice a week); baked potato (twice a week); lima beans; cornbread; yams.

Drinks: Milk, whey, buttermilk, tea. Nut milk drink (once a week). Doctor's drink (once a week).

DINNER

Protein: *Meat* (lean, no fat, no pork) use: Chicken, turkey, beef, beef roast, meatloaf, lamb roast. A meat meal is to be served no more than three times a week.

Fish (baked) served on Friday. Ocean white fish, halibut, bass, trout, salmon loaf.

Nut loaf for vegetarians.

Other nights, instead of meat or fish use: Cheese souffle, cottage cheese loaf, spinach loaf, eggplant and cheese loaf.

Two cooked vegetables and salad, as for Lunch.

Two Nights A Week: Fruit and cheese.

Assorted cheeses: Swiss, Jack, Cheddar, Cottage Cheese. Yogurt.

Assorted fresh fruit. Three kinds, such as melons, apples, persimmons, pears, cherries, berries, oranges, apricots, peaches.

Nuts and Dates

Crackers: Ry-Krisp, Ak-Mak or Sesame.

Desserts: Natural desserts allowed 3 times/week—but not recommended.

Juices. People can have a juice in place of any meal. If a person is on a juice diet, they usually have some every three hours: 8 am: Fruit juice; 11 am: carrot juice; 2 pm: carrot juice; 5 pm: fruit juice. Sometimes they will have an extra juice to take with them at 5 pm. Fruit juice may be: apple, grape, papaya or liquid chlorophyll (1-1/2 teaspoon to a glass of water). Liquid chlorophyll may be used at 8 pm as a juice drink.

Breaking The Fast. Always break with juices: one, two or three days, as directed by doctor.

First Day of Solid Food. Two oranges (sliced) or dish of shredded carrots (slightly steamed: cook for 2 minutes to just wilt). Fresh, soft peaches or apricots may be used. Juices (any kind) given with these solid foods at 10 am and 3 pm.

Desserts. Always on Sunday and two times during week. Gelatin mold (twice a week). For example: homemade ice cream (frozen fruit, whey and honey); carrot cake; custard; gelatin mold (cherry, grape, raspberry); Apple Betty; or, as requested.

SUGGESTED BREAKFAST MENUS

Reconstituted dried apricots
Muesli with bananas and dates
Oatstraw tea
Add eggs, if desired or sliced peaches w/cottage cheese
Herb tea

Fresh figs
Cornmeal cereal
Shavegrass tea
Add eggs or nut butter or raw applesauce & blackberries

Reconstituted dried peaches
Millet cereal
Alfa-mint tea
Add eggs, cheese or nut butter or
Sliced nectarines and apple
Yogurt

Prunes or any reconstituted dried fruit
Brown rice with cinnamon and honey
Or reconstituted raisins
oatstraw tea
Grapefruit and kumquats
Poached eggs

Slices of fresh pineapple with shredded coconut
Buckwheat cereal
Peppermint tea
Or baked apple, persimmons
Chopped raw almonds
Acidophilus milk

Cornmeal cereal
Reconstituted dried fruit
Dandelion coffee or herb tea

Cooked applesauce with raisins
Rye grits
Shavegrass tea
Or cantaloupe and strawberries
Cottage cheese

SUGGESTED LUNCH MENUS

Vegetable salad
Baby lima beans
Baked potato
Spearmint tea

Vegetable salad (with health mayonnaise)
Steamed asparagus
Very ripe bananas or steamed unpolished rice
Vegetable broth or herb tea

Raw salad plate w/sour cream dressing
Cooked green beans
Cornbread or baked hubbard squash
Sassafras tea

Salad w/French dressing
Baked zucchini and okra
Corn on the cob
Ry-Krisp crackers
Buttermilk or herb tea

Salad
Baked green pepper stuffed with eggplant and tomatoes
Baked potato and/or bran muffin
Carrot soup or herb tea

Salad
Steamed turnips and turnip greens
Baked yam
Catnip tea

Salad w/lemon and olive oil dressing
Steamed whole barley
Cream of celery soup
Steamed chard
Herb tea

SUGGESTED DINNER MENUS

Salad
Diced celery and carrots
Steamed spinach, waterless cooked
Puffy omelet, vegetable broth
Herb tea

Salad
Cooked beet tops
Meat or fish
Tomato sauce
Cauliflower
Comfrey tea

Cottage cheese, cheese stix
Apples, peaches, grapes, nuts
Apple concentrate cocktail

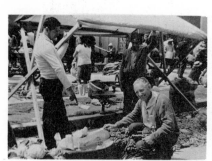
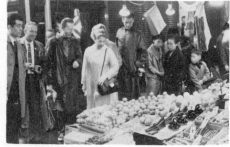

Left: Japanese marketplace. Right: Mexican street market.

Salad
Steamed chard, baked eggplant
Poached fresh salmon
Persimmon whip (optional)
Alfa-mint tea

Salad
Yogurt and lemon dressing
Steamed mixed greens, beets
Tofu with soy sauce
Leek soup, herb tea

Salad
Cooked string beans, baked summer squash
Carrot and cheese loaf
Cream of lentil soup or lemongrass tea
Fresh peach gelatin w/almond-nut cream

Salad
Diced carrots and peas, steamed
Tomato aspic
Roast leg of lamb w/mint sauce
Herb tea

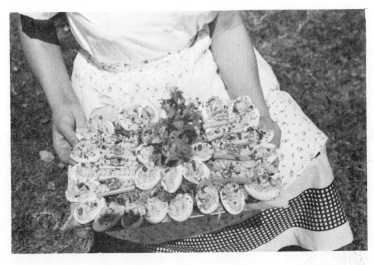

Stuffed hard-boiled eggs make a wonderful protein food.

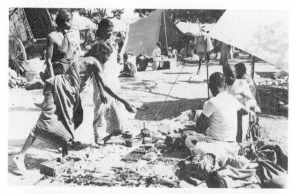

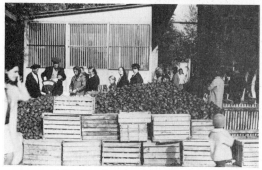

Top: Herb store in India. Bottom: Get your potatoes—they really have plenty in Russia.

TO GAIN OR LOSE WEIGHT

My **Health and Harmony Food Regimen** is designed to be **half building and half eliminating,** which will tend to reduce the **weight of overweight persons and increase the weight of underweight persons.** However, if you overeat or undereat in the same way you did before, you will remain in much the same body form. So, here are some tips for you.

To lose weight, eat zucchini, yellow crookneck or summer squash instead of other starches at lunch and dinner. It is all right to eat millet, cornmeal, brown rice and rye, but not wheat or oats, for the time being. Cut the use of butter, oil and nut butters to an absolute minimum. Use salad dressings that have a minimum of oils and fats, since these have 9 calories per gram as compared to 4 calories per gram for carbohydrates and proteins. For dressings, you can use apple cider vinegar and oil, nut butter, homemade

French dressing, lemon and honey; use only a tablespoon on your salad. Avocado, buttermilk, mayonnaise, roquefort and bleu cheese dressings can be thinned with low-fat or skim milk.

Fill up on salad and vegetables as much as possible before eating your protein. Take 5 chlorella tablets before eating; be sure to crack them before swallowing. Eggs are a fine protein but contain a good deal of fats, so eat them as directed in the past chapter. Nuts are high in fats. Surprisingly, dried fruits, sweet fruits and fruit juices, because of the concentration of fruit sugars, are high calories, so cut down on them or thin them down by diluting with water. Snack on vegetables and drink more vegetable juices.

At any meal, avoid eating to satiety. One good way to accomplish this is to push one-third of every food on your plate aside and stop eating when you finish the other two-thirds. Even healthy desserts can be high in calories. Reduce desserts to one a week—maybe two and make them natural.

Exercising for half an hour every morning raises the metabolic level and burns off fat faster than usual for up to 15 hours afterward. Exercise to music to make it more fun. If you are over 40 or 15 pounds overweight, or if you have any chronic disease or debilitating condition, consult your doctor before starting any reducing diet and exercise program. **See my book SLENDER ME NATURALLY for a safe effective reducing program.**

To increase weight: building weight, interestingly enough, also is helped by exercise, and we all need it unless our job requires physical labor with considerable muscular effort. If it does, however, I doubt that you would be underweight.

For increasing weight, here are a few key ideas. You may increase your protein intake—meat, eggs, fish, milk products, cereals, etc.—but don't cut down on your vegetables. You can have proteins twice a day instead of once. Between meals, have protein drinks as described in my chapter on **Raw Juices, Broths, Soups and Tonics.** Be sure to add an egg yolk or two to your drink, and add nut or seed butter or meal if the recipe doesn't already specify it.

Try to arrange your exercise period so that you can have a protein drink or meal afterward. You'll need plenty of rest—at least 8 hours of sleep, a nap during the day—10 minutes at 3 o'clock (if possible), and a sitting-down rest period of at least 10-15 minutes after your exercise. Weight lifting or exercise machines are helpful.

If you have any trouble digesting your food, take an intestinal digestive aid tablet with each meal for relief of gas, dry stool, slow bowel transit time, and as something temporary until the body can carry on without it. A teaspoon of wheat germ oil every morning will also help you put on weight. Chew your food slowly and thoroughly to get the most good out of it.

Whether you are trying to lose weight or gain, don't "fight" your body. Learn to love yourself now and be prepared to love the way you are going to look and feel when you take off or put on more pounds. Be success oriented. Imagine how you want to look several times a day. Give your inner mind a visual goal to shoot for.

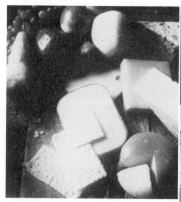
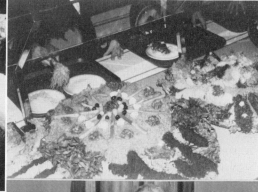
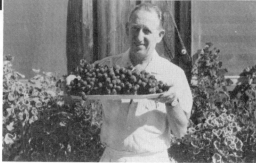

We served cheese of many kinds; cakes made of natural ingredients and home-grown grapes for snacks.

9

Feeding Children

The foods you start your children out with will strongly influence their health and food patterns later in life, so it is important to follow the path of wisdom. First, keep fatty foods to a minimum. Studies have shown that most kids overweight in the first grade are also overweight when they reach high school. Avoid giving salty snacks to young children, because it develops into a craving for salty foods very soon, increasing their chances of high blood pressure later. Fruits, vegetable sticks, unsalted raw nuts and seeds are much better as snacks. Don't reward children for eating well at mealtimes by giving them a sweet dessert. Use fruits for dessert instead, helping them develop a taste for healthier foods. Encourage children to help in the kitchen so they can see for themselves how healthy meals are prepared—and encourage them to exercise with you to show them you value exercise.

TEENS AND NUTRITIONAL DEFICIENCIES

Many teen diets these days are heavily slanted toward fast foods, soft drinks and snacks, lacking in fresh fruits, vegetables, whole grains and other foods needed to provide a balanced diet. A recent USDA survey, taken together with the previous Ten-State Nutrition Survey and the Health and Nutrition Examination Survey showed that most teens are seriously deficient in calcium (11-29%) and iron (21-30%), moderately deficient in vitamins A and B-1 (1-20%) and mildly deficient in vitamins B-1 and B-2. Because the teen years are such rapid growth years, diet is extremely important at this time. One of the best ways to supplement teen diets is to make "empty calorie" foods unavailable in the house for snacks

135

while having plenty of easily available snack foods such as cheese, yogurt, raw nuts and seeds, sprouts, carrot and celery sticks, raisins, dates, figs, fresh fruit and fruit and vegetable juices. If breakfast can be prepared for the teenager, he or she is less likely to rush out for a quick donut-and-coffee brakfast, which I consider the worst breakfast habit in the U.S. School lunch sandwiches should always contain some vegetable fillings—lettuce, sprouts, zucchini slices, tomatoes and so forth. It is always best for the family to share meals together as often as possible, but on busy days, sometimes dinner may be the only shared family meal. In that case, always try to have high calcium foods with the meal (or, if necessary, calcium supplements for the teenagers, such as bone meal), and high iron foods such as meat, green vegetables, raisins, dark berries and so forth. I feel that the key factor, however, is in what snacks are left around for teenagers, for several reasons. If healthy snacks are left near the TV, they are likely to be eaten while favorite teen TV programs are on, simply because they are convenient. Secondly, if they are encouraged to snack on healthy foods at home, they will be less likely to buy junk away from home simply because they aren't hungry. The one thing I strongly advise avoiding is "nutritional lectures" or nagging. Teens tend to rebel against both. So stick to positive approaches, consistent effort and frequent encouragement.

WEANING THE BABY

The first thought in taking care of the baby is to take care of the mother. See that the mother has as perfect a body as possible. See that her milk comes from a perfect body. When she is not able to give enough milk, add greens to her diet. The tops of vegetables furnish what the baby needs. Add two to three pints of raw vegetable juices a day to the mother's diet.

There are times when the mother does not give much milk and probably there is a definite reason. Probably the baby shouldn't have very much. The baby and mother are one; as the mother is, so is the baby, even some little time after he is born. If you want to add a formula along with the mother's milk, you may.

SUGGESTED FORMULA TO USE ALONG
WITH MOTHER'S MILK OR IN WEANING CHILD

1 oz goat milk or certified raw milk
3 oz distilled water
1/2 oz pure cream
1 tsp sugar of milk

You may make changes by lessening the certified milk and substituting soybean powder that has been mixed with water to the consistency of milk. This formula may be used in weaning the baby. When that time arrives, it is best to start adding a little barley gruel and gradually, raw vegetable juices.

After the baby is three or four weeks old, make sure he has orange juice every day. When weaning the baby you may add a little broth made of carrots, onion and parsley, finely cut. This is to be strained and only the broth given. A little prune juice or fig juice can be made from unsulphured dried fruits and used very well.

THINGS TO KNOW ABOUT MOTHER'S MILK

1. Breast milk is not always adequate in vitamin content and the mother's body cannot produce vitamins unless they are contained in her own diet.

2. The baby's body cannot store a proper amount of vitamins if those vitamins were lacking in the mother's diet during pregnancy.

3. Vitamin C is not stored in the mother's body and the amount in her milk is small, varying according to the amounts received in her diet. So begin early to supplement baby's diet with orange and tomato juice, whether breast or artificially fed.

4. Be sure the infant gets all he needs of vitamin C as this vitamin is so essential in his early development of teeth.

5. The mother is conferring a real favor on her baby if she takes sun baths during the nursing period as vitamin D is produced in the mother's milk as a result. This is the best known way of getting this vitamin.

SUPPLEMENTARY FEEDINGS FOR THE
ABOUT-TO-BE WEANED BABY

1. Orange juice strained, with some pulp, diluted with distilled water.

2. Fresh tomato juice.

3. Figs and prunes, raisins and dates, which have been soaked for about 12 hours and pureed or mashed.

4. Any fresh, uncooked fruit, pureed, mashed or cut up in small quantities at first to accustom the child to the taste of each new food.

5. Any whole grain cereal, including brown rice and cornmeal, which has been steamed or double-boiled over a long period of time and left to stand overnight. Stress steel-cut oats and be sure to cook long enough.

6. Any fresh vegetable in season, steamed, mashed or cut up, preferably no more than two kinds at one sitting. Use small quantities at first.

7. Supplement goat milk for the breast milk gradually so that the break is a normal and natural one.

8. Do not flavor baby's food. The natural flavor of the food itself should be sufficient. If the baby shows a dislike for any cereal, flavor with a little pure honey or dried fruit sweetening. *Do not use salt.*

BABY'S MENU AT WEANING TIME

6 o'clock: Milk formula
8 o'clock: Fruit or fruit juice
10 o'clock: Cereal and milk formula
2 o'clock: Milk and cooked vegetables or puree
4 o'clock: Broth or celery and onion soup
6 o'clock: Cereal and formula
8 o'clock: Fruit or fruit juice
10 o'clock: Milk or formula

Interchange vegetables and fruits so that baby gets used to variety. Celery and onion soup, with a little finely-cut parsley, should be strained.

As the baby begins to grow, add a little bit of hard food to the diet to help keep the teeth strong. Fresh goat's milk is the finest milk to feed growing children. Steel-cut oatmeal, cooked for 2 or 3 hours in a double boiler and allowed to stand overnight before eating, is marvelous for building a strong body.

Never use sugar for children. To sweeten, use fruits. For instance, mix a few raisins, prunes, figs, dates into the oats before serving. It is best not to give children meat. Let them get their protein from milk until they reach the age of seven.

Greens are best for building strength and bones. Orange, grapefruit and pineapple juices are also marvelous for supplying the necessary vitamins for the child's body. Children should have at least two glasses of fruit or vegetable juice daily.

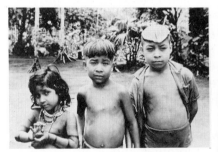
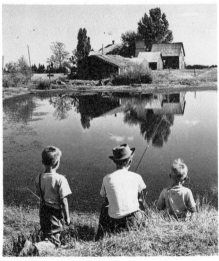

Left: Pigeon chests and pronated ankles result from calcium deficiency. Photo taken on the bank of the Amazon River, South America. Right: Nutritious food from balanced soil builds healthy bodies and sound minds. Start your child out right, otherwise you are raising doctor bills.

CHILD FEEDING

Do not be afraid to fast the children or skip a meal or two. Children seem to know when it is best to eat or not. Do not force them to eat fruit. Do not allow them to eat between meals, except fruit or fruit juice. When they do not grow properly or have abnormal growths on their bodies, are cold blooded, have eye trouble, throat ailments or running sores, it may be a sign they are lacking silicon. Add steel-cut oatmeal to the diet or oat straw tea.

Find out what the best natural foods are for keeping the body in good health. Start your children on natural foods and they will want only natural foods during their lives. They will be opposed to anything that is too sweet or too salty. A natural body wants natural food. Children raised on natural food will not care to smoke, drink or indulge in any of the abnormal habits that young people have today. The average child should have a nap every afternoon and go to bed at sundown.

For further information, it is best to consult a doctor who understands child feeding and child care. As a word to mothers, remember that *There is an unspoken word between mother and child. There is nothing purer than the source.*

Milk. Milk is a good food for children and should be taken in plentiful amounts up to 7 years of age. After that age, cut down the milk to one glass a day. Use raw goat milk, and when you cannot get it, use raw, first-grade certified cow's milk. It is best to use milk with fruit or vegetables or in between meals.

Butter. Butter may be used on vegetables and dry toast, but be certain you are using unsalted (sweet) butter.

Cottage Cheese. Cottage cheese is not as good for children as the whole milk. However, occasionally it may be used.

Eggs. Eggs should be in the child's daily diet. They may be slightly cooked, soft boiled, poached or coddled.

Meat. Meat is not a necessity in the child's diet, if you are using plenty of milk, eggs and nuts.

Vegetables. Vegetables should be steamed or baked, but never boiled. Give the child plenty of salads. A carrot chewed raw or some other hard vegetable helps the jaws to develop normally.

Cereals. Cereals may be given once a day and if they are cooked, cook them well. Sweeten by adding cut-up sweet fruits as raisins, dates, figs or prunes. Use only natural, unrefined cereal such as those you buy in health food stores. Dry cereals are best.

Sugar. Sugar should never be used as it will leach out the calcium of the body, interfering with proper body construction. Bad teeth are caused mostly from artificial sweets and refined grain products.

Broths and Soups. Broths and soups should be as natural as possible, like our Vital Broth. Never make heavy soups by adding too much thickening such as milk or cream.

Bread. Stale bread and dry toast are best for children. Make them chew their foods by giving them hard foods.

Rich Desserts. Rich desserts should never be indulged in. Use natural sweet fruits. Dried fruits should be soaked first.

School Lunches. Lunches should be eaten at home, if possible. If not, let them take their lunches to school. Do not allow them to have hot dogs, hamburgers and cheap, sickening lunches that are served on the school grounds.

Vegetable Juices and Fruit Juices. These may be drunk between meals.

Oat Straw Tea. Oat straw tea is exceptionally good for children.

Appetite. The appetite is generally good in a child. Do not force them to eat.

TRY THIS FOR THE CHILD WHO "JUST WON'T EAT"

Rather than nag, force or coax a child into eating the food placed before him, treat your child as adults at the table are treated. Serve them as near as possible as the adults are served and make no comments or threats, no praise or discouraging words on the amount of food consumed.

Make no remarks when the child dawdles. Assume that the food will be eaten. The child soon discovers that he is not gaining attention by his actions and so will be eager to finish his meal, especially when the food is attractively served in a colorful setting.

141

Keep the table conversations cheerful and as gay as you can, letting the children enter into the conversation.

Older Children. Playing informative and guessing games at this period helps to make mealtime more interesting as well as educational.

Be an example to your child. How can you expect your child to eat the foods you do not care for yourself?

Variety should be stressed.

Coaxing, urging, forcing, punishing, rewarding does more harm than good in feeding your child.

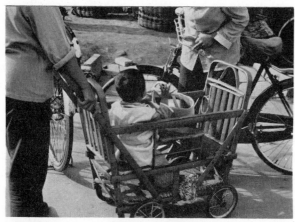

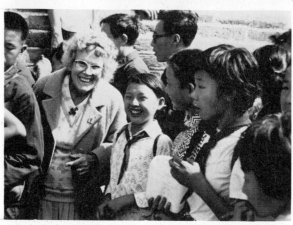

Mothers should know how to wean and raise their children. It is in the formative years that we begin to raise a good body for the future. Children are the same all over the world. These pictures were taken on our last trip to China.

─────10─────

A Great Discovery—
The Wheat Story

Over twenty years ago in London, England, I talked to doctors working on celiac disease, which is a serious intestinal disorder. It is caused by the gluten in wheat and other grains. Celiac disease is an extreme reaction to wheat in some individuals, but I feel wheat has some effect on all those who eat large amounts of it (29% in the average American diet).

Here is the picture story of what wheat can do to the small intestine, which is lined with millions of microscopic fingerlike projections called villi, as shown in our following illustrations. Food from the stomach passes into the small intestine, and as it comes in contact with the surface, tiny food particles are absorbed through the bowel wall, by way of the villi.

Illustration 1 is a section taken directly from *Taber's Cyclopedic Medical Dictionary* and shows the definition of celiac disease. Normally, the intestinal wall is made up of folds and changes in muscular structure. The normal bowel is not simply round as we often think of it. Each of the villi that coat the bowel wall has blood and lymph vessels that carry away food particles. Electron microscope photographs have shown that each villus is coated with thousands of microvilli, through which food must pass to get into the villus and into the blood and lymph vessels inside each villus. This is the only way food can be absorbed into the body. Wheat gluten, however, causes a toxic reaction in the villi, extreme in celiac cases, more moderate in other cases, down to a mild inflammation. A chemical in the gluten causes the villi to begin to shrink and shrivel up. This reduces the food absorption surface in the small intestine and is the beginning of nutritional deficiencies.

143

celery [Gr. *selinon*]. The edible stalks and leaves of the plant Apium graveolens. Food value of 100 gm. (raw): Cal. 17; protein 0.9 gm.; trace of fat; carbohydrate 3.9 gm.; calcium 39 mg.; ascorbic acid 9 mg.

celiac (sē'lǐ-ăk) [Gr. *koilia*, belly]. Rel. to the abdominal regions.

c. artery. The first branch of the abdominal aorta. Branches supply the stomach, liver, spleen, duodenum, and pancreas.

c. axis. C. artery, q.v.

c. disease. Intestinal malabsorption characterized by diarrhea, malnutrition, bleeding tendency, and hypocalcemia. TREATMENT: Gluten-free diet which may have to be continued for an indefinite period.

c. plexus. Sympathetic plexus lying near the origin of celiac artery. SEE: *plexuses* in *Appendix*.

celialgia (sē'lǐ-ăl'jǐ-ă) [Gr. *koila*, belly, + *algos*, pain]. Abdominal pain.

itis, inflammation]. Inflammation of muscles of the abdomen.

celioncus (sē'lǐ-ŏn'kŭs) [Gr. *koila*, belly, + *onkos*, tumor]. An abdominal tumor.

celioparacentesis (sē'lǐ-ō-păr''ă-sĕn-tē'sis) ["+ *para*, beside, + *kentēsis*, puncture]. Puncture of the abdomen for purposes of tapping or drainage.

celiopathy (sē'lǐ-ŏp'ă-thǐ) ["+ *pathos*, disease]. Any disease of the abdomen.

celiopyosis (sē'lǐ-ō-pī-ō'sis) [Gr. *koila*, belly, + *pyōsis*, suppuration]. Purulent peritonitis.

celiorrhaphy (sē'lǐ-ōr'ă-fǐ) ["+ *rhaphē*, suture]. Suture of wound in the abdominal wall. SYN: *laparrhaphy*.

celiosalpingectomy (sē'lǐ-ō-săl''pǐn-jĕk'tō-mǐ) ["+ *salpinx*, tube, + *ektomē*, excision]. Removal of the fallopian tubes through an abdominal incision.

celiosalpingotomy (sē'lǐ-ō-săl''pǐn-gŏt'ō-mǐ) ["+ "+ *tomē*, incision]. Opening of the

Figure 1.

Notice the definition of celiac disease above, as taken from Taber's Cyclopedic Medical Dictionary.

In the final stage of celiac disease, the villi have been destroyed down to the mucosal wall of the small intestine. Malnutrition is extreme and dangerous at this point. The only solution known to doctors is a gluten-free diet.

At lower levels of toxic reaction than that of celiac disease, inflammation due to wheat cause catarrh, and catarrhal problems encourage the use of suppressant drugs such as aspirin, antihistamines and antibiotics. The overuse of milk (25% of the average diet) and sugar (9%) also transgresses the law of excess and produces catarrh. Use of drugs to suppress catarrh destroys the normal bowel flora and leads to abnormal bowel conditions, causing a dilemma for gastrointestinal specialists.

No drugs used today can produce recovery of tissue, and the body is no better off than before. We believe there is a better way, an alternative way. By balancing the diet and providing the chemical elements needed for repair and rebuilding, we can provide a remedity with full tissue recovery. The illustrations used here are based on medical photographs in textbooks such as *Principles of Anatomy and Physiology* by Tortora and Anagnostakos, *Functional Human Anatomy* by James E. Crauch, and the *Cecil Textbook of Medicine* (see page 728), edited by James B. Wyngaarden, M.D., and Lloyd H. Smith, Jr., M.D.

Figure 2 (a)

Figure 2 (b)

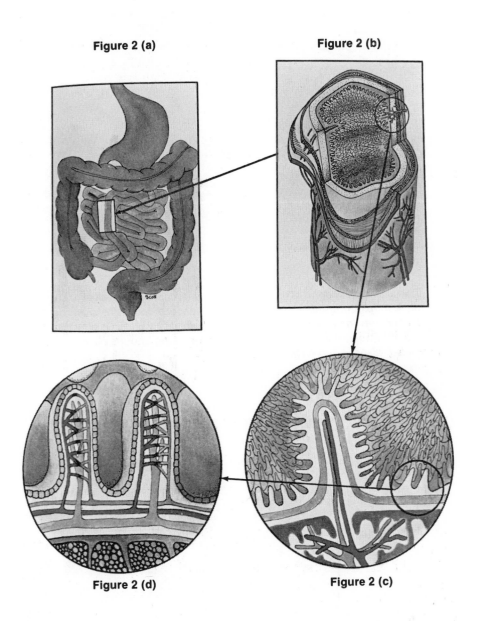

Figure 2 (d)

Figure 2 (c)

Figure 2.

These pictures present successive enlargements of cross-sections of the small intestine, showing; **(a)** the stomach, small intestine and colon, **(b)** cross-section of the small intestine, **(c)** cross-section of a villus, and **(d)** microvilli with arterioles, venules and lymph capillaries. The coating of the intestinal wall with villi increases the surface area for food absorption by thousands of times.

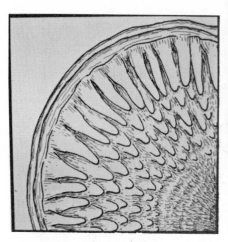 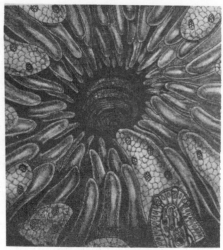

Figure 3.

    This is a cross section of the small bowel, magnified by the artist to show the villi, microscopic fingerlike projections that absorb food. This is the most important activity in the body (together with disposal of waste). Over twenty years ago, I visited England when doctors there were talking about a bowel condition called celiac disease, which interested me greatly.

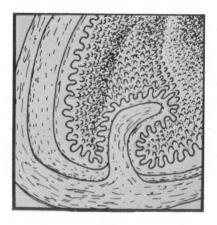

Figure 4.

    I had become convinced that bowel problems were at the root of many disease conditions. The normal bowel is not exactly round, as in the first illustration, but in folds, as above. Besides food, toxins filter through the bowel wall into the bloodstream, and I believe these same toxins damage the small intestine in the process of absorption.

146

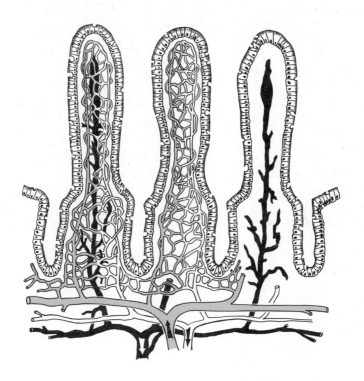

Figure 5.

Normally each villus (singular of villi) acts as a "little factory" in the final processing of food in the small intestine. As shown in the illustration, each villus has its own network of tiny blood capillaries and lymph vessels ready to receive and transport nutrients to the portal vein for the next step toward distribution. What is not shown here is the layer of microvilli, called the "brush border," that covers each villus (see 6), and it is the microvilli that draw food from the small intestine into each villus. Chemical reactions between digestive enzymes and food particles are going on even as the food is being drawn into the villus. Lymphatic tissue such as the tonsils, appendix, and breasts is especially subject to inflammation, infection, swelling and the development of lumps (breasts), and these conditions are nearly always related to digestion and assimilation, problems with the chemical process going on in and around the villi. Excess exposure to wheat over a long period of time seems to trigger a toxic reaction in the villi of the small intestine, in which the villi are gradually destroyed by some kind of interaction between the gliadin protein in the gluten of wheat, and the enzymes and chemical elements of the villi. Celiac disease comes on suddenly in many cases, but this can happen at any age, and researchers aren't sure what goes on in the body before symptoms appear. It seems that villi tolerance to wheat may break down suddenly, as in celiac disease, or more gradually over the years from using too much wheat, day after day.

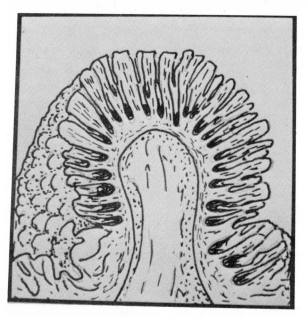

Figure 6.

    This is an enlargement of a single villus showing the microvilli (also called "brush border") coating its surface. As the chyme (pulverized food particles in semi-liquid form) washes against the microvilli, nutrients are removed and assimilated into the villus. Damage to microvilli precedes damage to the villi, reducing the amount of nutrients taken through the bowel wall. This is why we have to take such good care of our eliminative function.

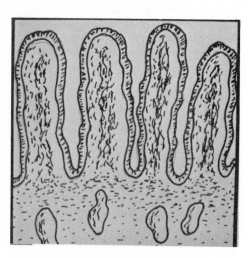

Figure 7.

    Gluten is in all wheat products, all white flour and in other grains such as rye and oats to a lesser extent. A chemical called gliadin in the gluten begins to damage the wall of the small bowel, causing villi to wilt and shrink.

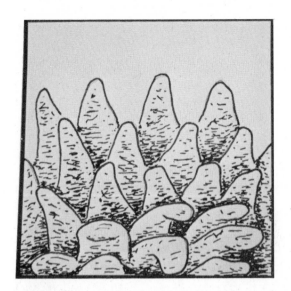

Figure 8.
  Villi damaged by gluten begin to collapse and disappear into the bowel wall, no longer able to absorb much food. This is the beginning of malnutrition and nutrient deficiencies.

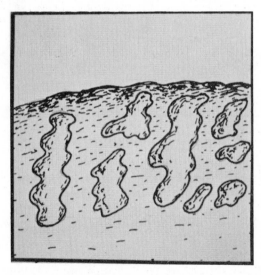

Figure 9.
  In the final stages of celiac disease, the villi are gone and only the mucous lining remains. I believe wheat may cause serious bowel problems in many people, even though they may not be as severe as celiac disease. The average American uses 29% wheat in the diet, and this amount can produce toxic reactions, trigger allergies, cause catarrh and encourage drug use to counteract unpleasant symptoms.

149

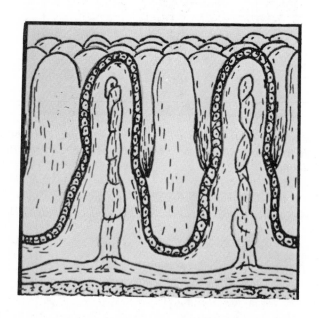

Figure 10.

Bowel underactivity and catarrh are often at the beginning of any disease. Drug use to counteract catarrh and other symptoms does not restore the bowel structure and function to a healthy condition. Drugs are remedies without tissue recovery. Only a properly balanced diet and the elimination of wheat from the diet can restore the bowel as it should be.

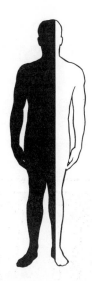

Figure 11.

63% of the average American diet is made up of wheat (29%), milk (25%) and sugar (9%). This proportion is detrimental to the chemical balance and well being of the body, violating the Law of Excess, the Law of Proportion, the Law of Variety and, indirectly, the Law of Deficiency (an excess of a few foods means we are creating deficiencies because we are neglecting other foods necessary to health).

Nature's garden provides a great variety of foods, and we need this variety to meet the nutrient needs of the many specialized cells, tissues and organs of the body. Without variety we can't be healthy, we can't meet the chemical needs of the body. This is where our allergies, catarrhal discharges, aches, pains, rheumatic conditions and some excess weight problems come in. They result from wrong proportions.

I believe wheat, milk and sugar should be no more than 6% of the total diet. I am not against wheat, milk or sugar, but we find that when they are used in such great amounts, they create problems in the body. Large proportions of wheat, milk and sugar weaken the immune system, lower our resistance to disease and compromise the integrity of the cells, making it almost impossible to stay healthy. A chemically imbalanced body cannot rebuild, repair or rejuvenate as well as it should.

Of all the thousands of people at my lectures that I have polled, 90% say they have been raised most on milk, wheat and sugar products. It is no coincidence that these foods that are eaten the most are sold most because they are among the most heavily advertised foods we have. With this predominance of 3 foods in the average diet, we are crowding out seeds, nuts, berries, fruits and vegetables that would normally help keep our bodies chemically balanced and well.

A chemically imbalanced body invites a future chronic disease, but this can be reversed by following my Food Laws in Chapter 2 and my Health and Harmony Food Program in Chapter 7. It may take years to rebalance the body chemically by correct diet, but improvement will be noticed within a month.

151

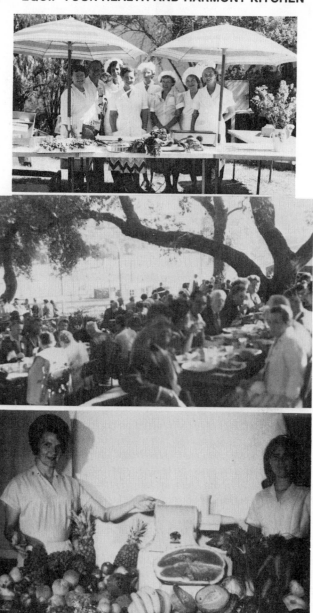

Top: Ranch kitchen staff. Middle: Outdoor dining area. Bottom: Lynne & Eleanor Johnston of Mesa, AZ, and their family practice natural food planning.

11

Equip Your
Health and Harmony Kitchen
Let's Get Ready
for Business

The most important kitchen gadgets, in my view, are a blender, a juicer, a shredder and stainless steel, low-heat cooking utensils. My book *Blending Magic* gives many wonderful recipes for healthy living, and we'll be presenting a variety of other lovely recipe ideas as we go along. Be innovative, create new ideas.

You will find that the following devices will be very helpful and time saving in your kitchen. Check different stores for price, quality and service before you buy.

Stainless Steel, Low-Heat Cookware. Look for a high-quality set of waterless, low-heat, stainless steel cookware. This is the best possible way that I know of to cook vegetables and retain the most nutritional value.

Juicers. The Champion juicer is possibly the most useful, since it not only makes as much juice as you want while ejecting the pulp, but it can make nut butters and natural "ice cream," too. The Acme is good for smaller quantities of juice. The most superior juicer is a hydraulic press type and is especially good for those on juice diets.

Blenders/Liquefiers. These come in many makes and models, from 3 speeds to 10 or more. A blender can mix liquids, puree, chop, liquefy and may be able to grind nuts and seeds into meal or powder, depending on the model.

Nut/Spice/Coffee Grinders. The small ones are handy for grinding almonds, sesame seeds, flaxseed, pumpkin seeds and other nuts and seeds into meal or powder to sprinkle on cereals, salads, vegetables—just about anything. You can also grind nutmeg, licorice root and carob pods in them.

Crockpots. The slow-cooking feature preserves the vitamin and mineral values in soups.

Electric Frying Pan. You can use it as a roaster.

Grain Mills. Freshly-ground grains are more nutritious than flour or meal that has been sitting around a while because the oils in these grains can become rancid. Small, home-sized grain mills are not cheap, however, and whole grain meal and flour are usually available in natural food stores, health food stores and even some supermarkets.

Graters/Grinders/Shredders. There are electric or hand-operated models to choose from. Crank-handled grinders have been around a long time, but some of the new stainless steel graters/shredders are much easier to operate. There are many to choose from, so shop around and pick a good one. These will shred vegetables, cheese, nuts, fruits and so on, in a variety of shredding sizes, and may have a slicer attachment, too.

Sprout Jars and Lids. You can make your own sprouts at home. Sprout jars are usually only one- or two-quart jars with screen lids to allow air to circulate. Most health food stores have them. If you are a heavy user of sprouts, you may want a good sprouter for your kitchen use.

Steamers. These vary from "spaghetti cookers" to the adaptable "flower petal" stainless steel steamer inserts that fit inside a variety of sizes of pans. The latter have short legs to keep the food above the water. Most people like to have both types of steamers.

Casserole Cookware. These are nice for the oven.

Double-Boiler. The best way to cook whole grain cereals is in a double boiler. The food is never cooked above 212 degrees F., as this is the temperature of boiling water.

Wide-Mouth Vacuum Thermos. Useful for cooking cereal overnight. Put cereal in preheated thermos jar, add boiling water, put on cap and in the morning, presto! Delicious whole grain cereal perfectly cooked in low heat to retain maximum nutritional value.

Parchment Paper. These special papers are wonderful and can be reused many times. Food put in them is wrapped to cook in its own juice. Different foods, packaged separately, can be added to boiling water at different times, so they will all be done at once.

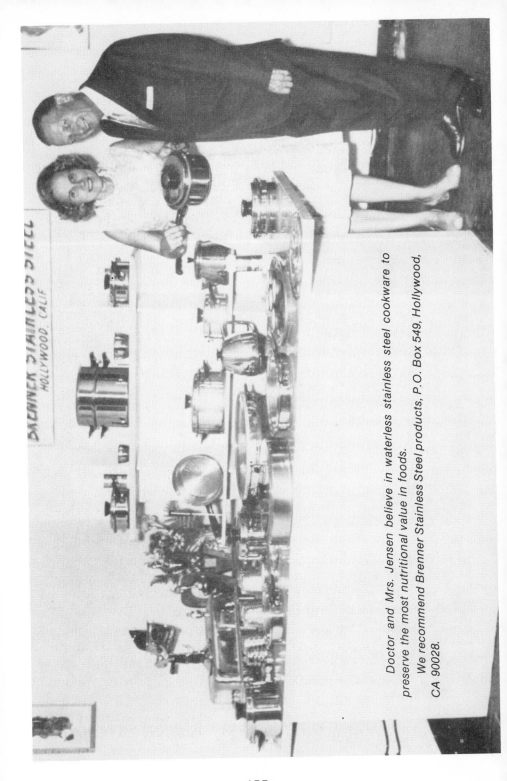

Doctor and Mrs. Jensen believe in waterless stainless steel cookware to preserve the most nutritional value in foods.

We recommend Brenner Stainless Steel products, P.O. Box 549, Hollywood, CA 90028.

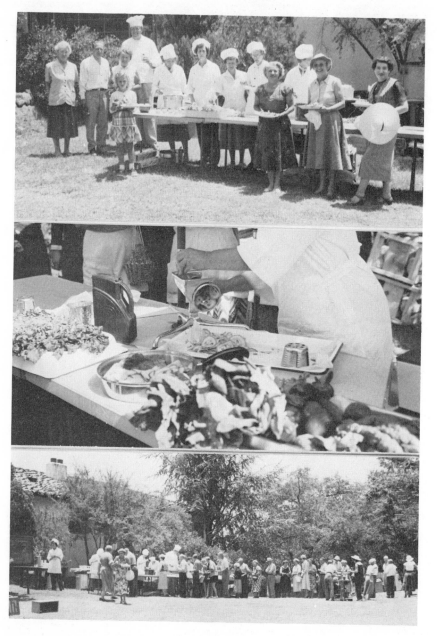

Top: Our staff of good cooks. Middle: Food demonstration. Bottom: It's time to eat all the good foods learned about in classes.

Miscellaneous Gadgets. Keep a variety of wooden spoons, knives, chopping and cutting boards, measuring cups and spoons, mashers, stirrers, strainers, plastic storage containers and a ceramic teapot.

Keep your eyes open in the stores. There are many wonderful things being developed for the kitchen these days.

Microwave Ovens. I am often asked what I think of microwave ovens. My first thought on this matter is that it is not a natural form of cooking. Secondly, I don't believe exposure of food to intense levels of radiation can be done without the possibility of unnatural changes in the chemical structure of some foods. Often it takes years or even decades to detect the dangerous side effects, cumulative effects and time-bomb effects of a new process or product on the body, especially radiation.

Wok. The wok is a good kitchen utensil for preparing Chinese food, but it is often used in cooking with hot oils which are not acceptable. It would be okay to use the wok to steam-cook foods, then add a good vegetable oil just before serving, if desired.

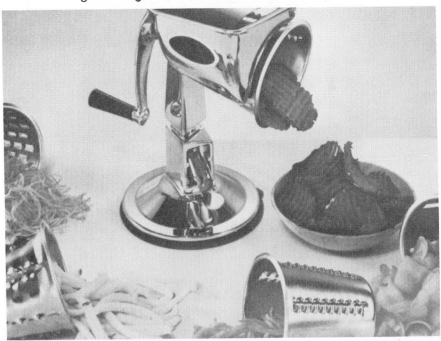

This handy shredder with interchangeable inserts should be in every health and harmony kitchen.

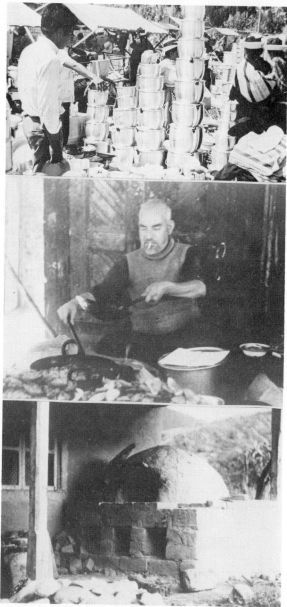

Top: Aluminum utensils in a South American market. Mid: This cooking oil had not been changed for months. Bottom: Baking bread over slow heat in an Indian oven in New Mexico.

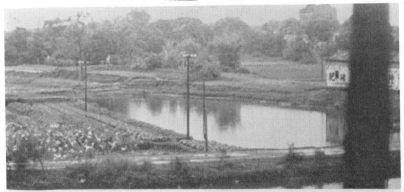

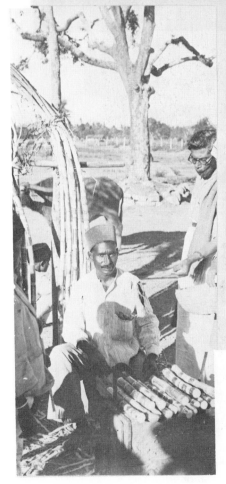

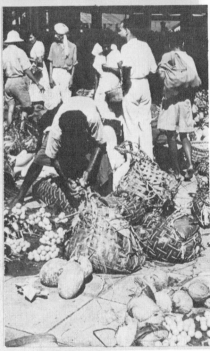

Top: Chinese rice paddy. Lower left:
Sugar cane loses the vitamins and
minerals when it's refined. Lower rt:
Marketplace in Papeete, Tahiti.

159

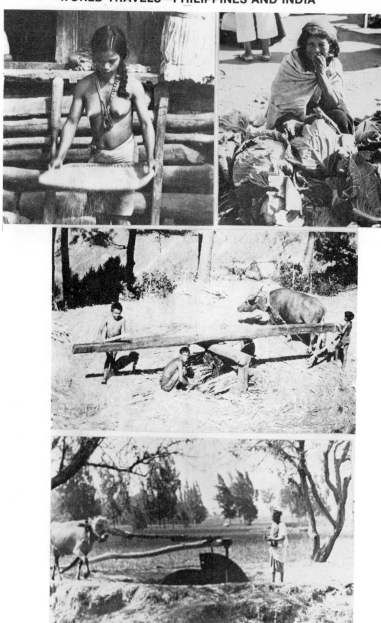

Preparing grain in the Philippines, upper left and middle. Top rt: Street market in India. Bottom: Water wheel for irrigation in India.

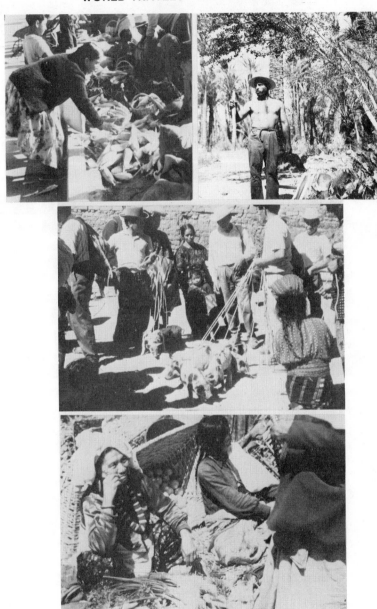

Top left: Street market in Mexico. Top rt: The heart of the palm tree is eaten in Mexico. Mid: Farmers trade pigs for other foods in Guatemala. Bottom: Tibetan markets abound with natural foods.

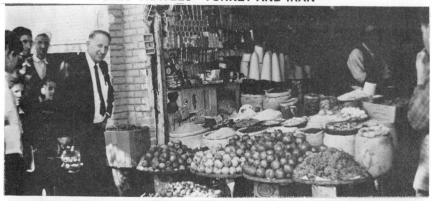

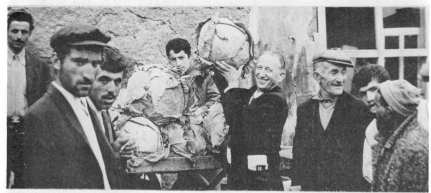

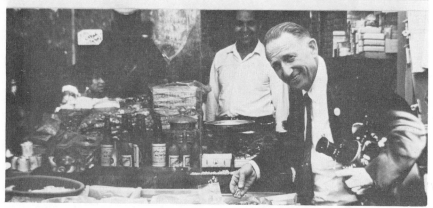

We've traveled through 55 countries, to learn and to understand the living habits and foods of other people.

─────12─────

Shopping for the Best Nutritional Values

My food philosophy can be summed up in one statement: ***Our health and well-being are best when we eat LIVE foods.***

WHAT ARE "LIVE" FOODS?

Live foods are foods with the enzymes still alive and intact, found best in raw foods. Fruits, vegetables and meats should be fresh. Nuts, grains, seeds and legumes should be in such condition that if you planted them, they would still grow. This can be accomplished even in slow, low-heat cooking. If we eat these kinds of foods, our bodies will be clean, healthy and full of vitality because they still contain nutrition as close as nature can provide it.

In contrast, dead foods are preserved foods, foods embalmed in sugary syrup, salt or chemicals; they are foods with the life "refined" out of them; they are foods fried, baked or heated at such high temperatures that the life has departed from them; they are the spoiled or rancid foods that have begun to decompose. We can't live well on dead foods. We can live wonderfully well on "live" foods.

Another important part of my philosophy is that foods must be *natural, whole* and *pure.*

LOOK FOR LIFE IN FOODS

The "live" foods in most stores are found around the outside perimeter. Here is where we find the bins of vegetables and fruits, the dried beans, lentils and split peas, the fresh eggs, the milk and other dairy products, and the meat counter.

First, let's turn our attention to leafy green vegetables. We need green vegetables for nature's sunshine energy, stored in the chlorophyll. Chlorophyll is a healing, cleansing substance.

We must have at least one green leafy vegetable every day, and it is important to have them as fresh as possible. Look for crispness and avoid wilted leafy vegetables. Buy a variety at different times. Don't stick to one or two favorites all the time. Consume them within two days. And always wash them thoroughly first. Watercress, beet greens, turnip greens, asparagus, bok choy, cauliflower, sprouts, red and green cabbage, Brussels sprouts, broccoli and parsley are lovely greens that we don't always think of using. All summer squashes, all leaf lettuce, spinach, Swiss chard, mustard greens, collard, curly cabbage, onions, leeks and celery root. *Have a variety.* Watercress and beet greens are never sprayed. Eat them often. I believe broccoli is our finest vegetable to use. It is made up of flower buds and is very easy on the digestion.

Underground vegetables such as carrots and beets last considerably longer in storage than leafy vegetables, but they have their limits, too. Softness and suppleness in underground root vegetables mean they are not too good. Most underground vegetables are not sprayed, so their leaves are good foods to use. Carrot tops, however, are usually too bitter. Outside leaves are to be desired. The outside leaves of cabbage have 40% more calcium than the inside leaves.

The potato skin is the most important part of the potato. The skin should be unblemished. Use the Idaho potato or the Idaho russet.

The most frequently sprayed vegetables seem to be cabbage and celery, so these have to be washed the most carefully. Parsley, actually an herb, is never sprayed. Most herbs are not sprayed. Nor are garlic, onions and leeks.

If you can get unsprayed vegetables and fruits, by all means, do it.

MOST FRUIT MUST BE RIPE

I can't think of a single fruit that isn't better to eat when it has been allowed to sun ripen on the tree, vine or bush. Bananas and tomatoes will ripen after being picked green, but the flavor is not

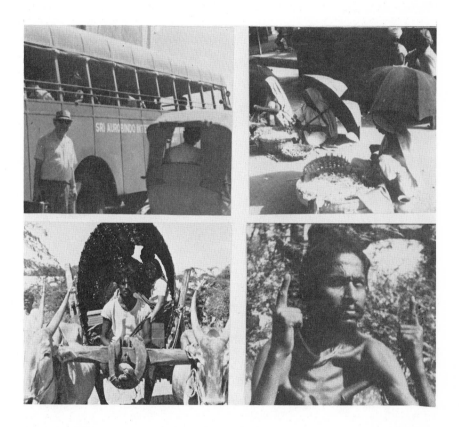

We visited various ashrams in India, using many means of travel, studying the customs. We visited with Sai Baba in Puttaparti and stayed at Sri Aurobindo's ashram.

THE NATURAL LIFE IS NOT THE EASIEST!

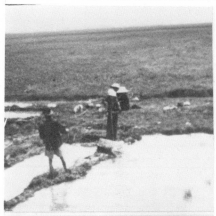

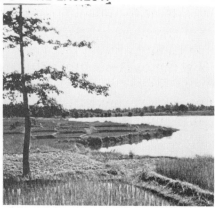

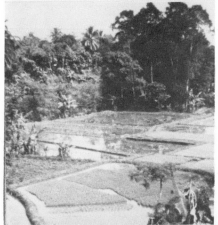

Rice is the main food throughout much of the Orient. Farm life is hard, but healthier than city life.

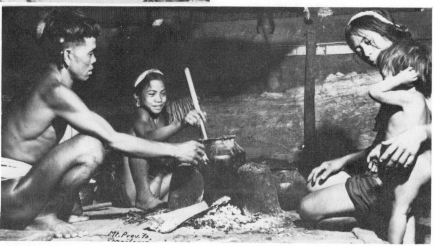

as nice as the fully sun-ripened fruit.

The sun is a sodium star, and its light is necessary to bring out the full nutritional value and sweetness in fruits. Sun-ripened fruit is at the peak of nutritional value. It also becomes a sodium food when ripened by the sun, otherwise we eat a green acid food unfit for human intake. It is more nutritious than fruit ripened in a shipping box.

Vegetables are different. You can pick lettuce early—or carrots, beets, chard and others. They're still nutritious. But immature fruit is green. The green fruit acids are not good for us.

Many fruits are picked 6 to 8 days early to allow time for grading, boxing, shipping, storing and, finally, selling. Grapefruit and oranges may be picked up to 2 months early. I do not recommend citrus, because green citric acid isn't a good thing. If you can get sun-ripened oranges, cut them in sections to eat. Be careful not to use too much citrus juice as it stirs up the acids in the body.

Cherries ferment soon after picking, so freshness is very important if you buy them at a market.

Pears should be yellow with no green tint on the skin and not much brown either. Soft or mushy spots indicate overripeness. They should be firm at peak ripeness but not so firm that they are hard.

Cabbage and cauliflower are best when the head is heavy, uniform in color and crisp. The outside green leaves of the cabbage are highest in enzymes. They should be washed thoroughly and eaten raw or cooked.

The best celery has deep green outer stalks, crisp and firm.

Bell peppers, both green or red, should be shiny, firm and deep in color. Avoid wrinkled or soft bell peppers.

Bulb onions should be whole (unsplit), dry, firm and without sprouts.

String beans picked right off the vine and for the next 5 days are alkaline forming. After the 6th day, they are acid forming.

Corn is sweet when first picked but its sugars immediately begin turning to starches and, by the 6th day, most of it is starch, unless it is refrigerated.

HOW TO TELL WHEN FRUIT IS RIPE

You can tell ripe pineapple because the top fronds can be pulled out by hand. If you get a pineapple that isn't fully ripe, turn it upside down and let it set on the fronds evenly. You'll be surprised how sweet it is throughout.

To tell when red apples are ripe, look them over. If the blossom end is green or if there is green elsewhere on the skin, it isn't fully ripe.

Watermelons are ripe when you thump them and they sound hollow. That's because the seeds are loosened as the melon ripens. Another way to tell is to run your thumbnail over the top of the watermelon rind. If a thin layer of green comes off, it is ripe. Cantaloupes and other similar melons are ripe when the outer skin is a uniform color and texture and when the blossom end smells sweet. It is harder to tell ripeness in the casaba and crenshaw melons.

We get most of our minerals from vegetables and our vitamins from fruit.

Hydroponic fruits and vegetables are very good, generally, in nutritional quality. These are plants such as tomatoes and cucumbers grown with the roots in a recirculating nutrient solution. In the ground, plants get nutrients from the earth, but they get them dissolved in water in the hydroponic method. Nutrients are simply added to the water alone.

Sprouts are one of our best buys. They are high in vitamins, minerals, enzymes and prostaglandins. The best are alfalfa sprouts and mung bean sprouts, but others are good also.

As for dairy products, eggs are our best protein and very economical. People often ask how many eggs they can eat. I realize eggs have been drawn into the cholesterol controversy, but if they are poached or soft boiled, the average person can have two a day without problems.

Milk and milk products make up 25% of the American diet, and this (as I have **repeatedly stated)** is too much. We use far too much milk in this country, which is why we see so many allergies to milk. If you must have milk, raw goat milk is best and raw cow milk is second. Goat milk is chemically balanced more like mother's milk than any other animal's milk and it is easily digestible.

As for cheese, I recommend only hard cheeses that crumble. Cheese that breaks is the best. In spite of the fact that cheese is pasteurized, the aging develops a bacteria that is friendly to the intestinal tract and helps to develop the friendly intestinal flora.

I do not advise eating wheat bread or any other wheat products because we've had too much wheat in the U.S., or in our growing up period. For the best health, use other whole cereal grains and products made from them—cornbread, rice crackers, Ry-Krisp and others. If you must have bread, use a variety of breads with no preservatives or additives and try to avoid using wheat as much as possible. There are good reasons for using whole grain flours and breads instead of white flour and bread, cakes and pastries made from it. It's been found that there are 30 micrograms of B-1 in 100 gm of white flour, 550 micrograms in the same amount of whole wheat flour and 2667 micrograms in an equal amount of wheat germ. This tells us why we should use the whole grain instead of denatured foods—those foods that have left us without the right materials to build a good body.

When we get to the meat counter, I work with very simple, sensible principles. Select only lean meat, poultry or fish with white meat, fins and scales. Recent studies published in the **New England Journal of Medicine** indicate that eating fish once or more a week lowers heart disease. I have visited so many of the old men in different countries to find out their secrets for health and long life. For most, living in moderation was the key—but one old black man, Charlie Smith (135 years old at the time), really blew my mind. Charlie was an American, and at 135 he took a walk with me and sang songs, but refused to believe the news when astronauts walked on the moon. When we finally came to diet questions, I still haven't recovered from his answers. "For the last 30 years," he said, "I've been living on sardines and crackers." No disease, no senility—on canned sardines! I found out two things about this that made sense. First, Dr. Benjamin Frank once said the highest food in RNA, the long-life factor, was yeast. Five years later, he discovered that sardines were 10 times richer in RNA than yeast! Secondly, Charlie was eating the whole fish—bones, skin, scales, fins—all of it. From the chemical standpoint in nutrition, **whole foods** are our best source of all the chemical elements we need. Use no pork, no fat meat, no shellfish, clams and so forth. This leaves poultry, lamb and fish. That is plenty. We only need meat 2 or 3 times a week at most. In fact in a recent Gallup Poll, 52% of those surveyed said, "No one really needs to eat meat more than once or twice a week." There are other good proteins we can use.

Honey is one of the natural sweeteners we should use instead of sugar. Buy the unheated kind for greater food value. Try to get the kind of honey made from flowers least likely to have been sprayed, such as Idaho clover, buckwheat, cactus flower or wildflower. Do not use the orange blossom or apple blossom honey. Residues of toxic insecticide sprays have been found in many kinds of honey. When spray-contaminated honey is used by people, it tends to trigger allergy problems. Usually, darker honey has greater mineral value. Tupelo honey is wonderful for those who can't handle sweets well. In using honey, remember that is is a concentrated sweetener and should be used sparingly.

HOW TO SHOP IN A "HEALTH FOOD" STORE

What will we find in a health food store?

1. Unprocessed cereal grains and their products: Whole grain breakfast cereals, breads and flours. They have no additives or preservatives.

2. Seeds and nuts in the raw natural state: Peanuts, sunflower seeds, squash seeds, chia seeds, almonds, sesame seeds, etc., and nut and seed butters. All are unprocessed and without additives.

3. Special diet foods such as low sodium foods and foods low in sugar, low in gluten, low in cholesterol. Such diet foods as are prescribed by physicians.

4. Naturally sweet foods: Honey, carob powder, syrup and flour; maple sugar and syrup; dried fruits, raw sugars, fruit concentrates.

5. Herbs, herb teas and other tea and coffee substitutes: The leaves, seeds and blossoms are unprocessed parts of trees, shrubs and plants. Coffee substitutes are often made from cereal grains.

6. Fruit and vegetable juices and fruit juice concentrates. These are unsugared and unprocessed. They should contain no additives or preservatives.

7. Vitamin and mineral supplements and herb remedies. Also miscellaneous supplements such as protomorphogens, chlorophyll, whey, algae, amino acids and so forth.

8. Organically grown fruits and vegetables produced without the use of chemical fertilizers and pesticides. (Found in some health food stores—not all.)

STANDARD PRODUCTS IN YOUR HEALTH FOOD STORE

Alfalfa seeds
Almonds
Apples
Baking powder (Royal or
  cream of tartar type)
Beans, dried
Bonemeal
Brewer's yeast
Butter
Carob chips
Carob powder, flour, syrup
Cashew nuts
Cheese
Chickpeas
Coconut
Dates
Dulse
Eggs
Swiss muesli
Filberts (hazelnuts)
Fruits, dried
Granola
Herbs and herb seeds
Honey
Kelp
Lecithin
Lentils
Maple syrup

Millet
Milk, cow, raw
Milk, goat, raw
Molasses
Mung beans
Nut butters
Oils
Peanuts, peanut butter
Peas
Pecans
Pumpkin seeds
Raisins
Rice, brown
Rice, wild
Rose hips, powder
Sea salt
Seed butters
Soybeans
Tofu
Soy margarine
Soy milk and products
Miso (soybean paste)
Sunflower seeds
Tahini
Vegetable broth powder
Vegetable and herb seasonings
Whole wheat berries
Yeast

There are usually many more products than these, varying with the type and size of the store and the food philosophy of the owner.

SEEDS, GRAINS AND LEGUMES

Alfalfa Seed. Use untreated seed for sprouting and teas. It is high in minerals. Very alkaline.

Arrowroot Starch. Use it in place of corn or tapioca starch. It is said to have an alkaline ash and contains calcium.

Hulled Barley. It is natural barley, not pearled or polished; only the very outer chaff is removed. Use in soups, cereals, casseroles and other dishes (Barley is a winter food).

Barley Grits. They are made of whole, hulled barley by cracking and removing flours. Add barley grits to soups, loaves, cereals, casseroles, burgers and patties as an extender for meats and other proteins.

Barley Flour. It is a finely ground hulled barley that blends well with other flours for baking breads, muffins, cakes, cookies, pancakes, and so on. It is a good substitute for restricted wheat diets.

Buckwheat Groats. They are made from whole, roasted buckwheat. Use them for cereals, stuffing, soup and puddings. Buckwheat groats are used in many Russian Jewish dishes (called Kasha).

Buckwheat Flour. It should be pure with no additives. It makes good pancakes and waffles and can be used in other recipes also.

Carob Powder. It may be referred to as "St. John's Bread", "Honey Locust," "Locust Bean" and many other names. It is delicious and ideal as a replacement for chocolate and cocoa for confections, cakes, frostings, milk drinks, syrup, cookies, candy, etc. It is alkaline, high in calcium, natural sugars, low in starch and fat.

Corn Meal. Yellow is preferable. Stone ground is best because excess heat is not applied. The grinds can be from fine to coarse. All the corn germ and flour is left intact, so other flour should be added to prevent crumbling in making cornbread. Use it for cornmeal cereal, cornbread, hotcakes, waffles, tamale pie, etc.

Corn Flour. Again, yellow is best. Whole corn is ground by the cool method. Use is as flour in breads, cakes, hot cakes, waffles and many other dishes; add to other flours.

Popcorn, Yellow. Popcorn can be made without the use of heated oil. Pop in hot container.

Flaxseed. It should be untreated. Add to cereals before cooking, grind for adding to cooked cereals, make into a tea for intestinal disturbances. Add small amounts to many recipes.

Flaxseed Meal. Whole flaxseed is ground to a medium meal consistency. Blend with cereals, flours, drinks and other recipes.

Garbanzos (Chick Peas). They should be untreated and large sized for cooking. Use in soups, casseroles and loaves or sprout them. They are alkaline usually.

Lentils. They should be untreated. Sprout or add to soups, loaves, casseroles. They tend to be alkaline. King of all beans.

Hulled Millet. Untreated, freshly hulled millet is best. It is alkaline forming, easy to digest and one of the four best starches or cereals. It absorbs three to four parts of water when cooking. Use in casseroles, puddings and as an excellent hot cereal alone.

Millet Meal. It is ground to medium consistency from hulled millet. Use with corn meal in equal parts for many dishes. Use as a cereal. It has an alkaline ash and is high in protein and lecithin. I consider it the No. 1 cereal.

Millet Flour. It should be made from pure, hulled, untreated millet. It is alkaline, easily digested and excellent for breads and wheatless diets. It is high in B-2, potassium, lecithin, silicon, iron, magnesium, calcium, phosphorus and some amino acids.

Mung Beans. They should be untreated, select quality. Use for sprouting or in cooking. They are excellent for sprouting because of their high content of vitamins C and B. Add sprouts to salads, omelets, soups, sandwiches and many oriental dishes.

Steel Cut Oats. They are natural, unrefined and make an excellent hot cereal. Blend with other cereal grains such as millet, wheat, rye for variety.

Rolled Oats. They cook into a flaky cereal and should be steamed slowly for best results. Use in cookies, bars and alone as cereal.

Oat Flour. Use in combination with other flours in baking breads, muffins, cakes, hotcakes or for thickening. Use in infant feeding. It is good for wheat restricted diets.

Green Split Peas. They should be untreated, natural green peas. Use in soups.

Potato Flour. It can be used in soups, bread, gravies, hotcakes, waffles, muffins, etc. To prevent lumping, blend with other flours before adding liquids.

Natural Brown Rice. It should be specially hulled to prevent loss of germ. All the bran and polishings should remain for maximum nutrition. It is one of the four best starches.

Brown Rice Flour. Natural brown rice is reduced to flour; use by blending with other flours in baking. It is good in hot cake and waffle batters.

Rice Bran. It is the outer layer removed from brown rice, a by-product of polishing and refining. Use as rice polishings or wheat germ.

Rice Polishings. They are the inner layers from brown rice, obtained from the refining and polishing process of white rice. Add to any foods as you would wheat germ. They are good in health "cocktails." High in silicon.

Rye, Whole. Use for home grinding and cereal. It is one of the best starches.

Rye Grits. Use as other grits or as a cereal alone.

Rye Meal. It is the consistency of coarse cornmeal. Blend with other meals or flours for baking. Use as cereal or alone.

Rye Flour. Use for bread, rolls, muffins, waffles. Mix with other flours. It is great for wheat restricted diets.

Hulled Sesame Seed. It should be untreated and ground cool to retain the oils. It is high in lecithin, protein, vitamins and minerals. Add to cookies, cakes, candies, other cereals, cooked vegetables and desserts; add to salad dressings. Blend with liquefied drinks. Keep refrigerated for best results. It is made into "tahini" or sesame butter. I consider these seeds the best.

Soy Beans. The soy bean is power packed with protein. It contains all the essential amino acids, lecithin, low carbohydrates, low fat, is rich in vitamins and has an alkaline reaction. Use it in place of meat as a protein. Serve them cooked, baked, sprouted, as soy milk, in soups, casseroles and loaves. Tofu, miso and soy sauce are made from soy bean.

Soy Meal. Use as an extender for all kinds of loaves and casseroles. Use as cereal.

Soy Flour. It is toasted or untoasted soy bean flour. Toasted, it has a nutty and sweet flavor that adds richness and smoothness to many dishes. It can be used to partly replace other flours, one part soy flour to five parts other flour.

Soy Powder. It is like soy flour, except more finely ground and higher in protein. Readily mixed with liquids. Use as milk substitute or powdered milk.

Hulled Sunflower Seeds. They can't be beat for energy-giving food additives or as a wholesome snack. Raw sunflower seeds contain rich oils and many vitamins and minerals. Add to cereals, cookies, cakes, salads, soups or almost any recipe. They can be ground into meal and added easily to many solid and liquid foods. They are excellent as a supplement in cereals.

Sunflower Seed Meal. It can be bought, or you can grind your own. It is rich in oils and nutrients. Blend with many dishes and drinks. Add to flours in baking, up to 50% replacement. It is quick baking. Add to soup after cooking or on salads.

Wheat Grits. Use them for cereals, loaves, burgers, patties, etc. Use as cereal alone.

Whole Wheat Flour. It should be stone or cool ground. Nothing should be removed—all bran and germ should be intact. Use wherever white flour is called for—baking breads, rolls, thickening, hotcakes, waffles, etc. Where pastry flour is called for, a whole wheat pastry or unbleached whole wheat flour is available. Be careful in using whole wheat in any manner to an excess. Use to a minimum.

Graham Flour. It is a whole wheat flour with the inner part of the kernel ground to fine flour and the bran layers are left flakey and coarse. Use for bread, cakes, rolls, etc.

Bran Flakes. Bran is from the outer layers of hard, red wheat. Use flakes in muffins, cereals, breads, health drinks and teas, etc.

Wheat Germ. It should be natural, untreated and vacuum packed for freshness. Refrigerate to keep freshness; to prevent rancidity always make sure it is carefully packaged. Use in omelets, breading fish and other meats, in drinks and cookies or candy. Add to nearly any food. It is a basic supplement for every diet.

Wheat Germ Flour. It is made from finely ground, pure and raw wheat germ. About 2% wheat germ flour adds the germ to flour that has been refined. Add to cakes, pies and health "cocktails".

"Unbleached" White Flour. It is a refined flour made without bleaching, additives or chemical preserving. It is still a "live" food, cream colored with much more flavor than regular white refined flour. Use in breads and other dishes except for cakes.

"Unbleached" White Pastry Flour. It is a refined flour made from soft wheat. Use for cakes, pies and general pastries.

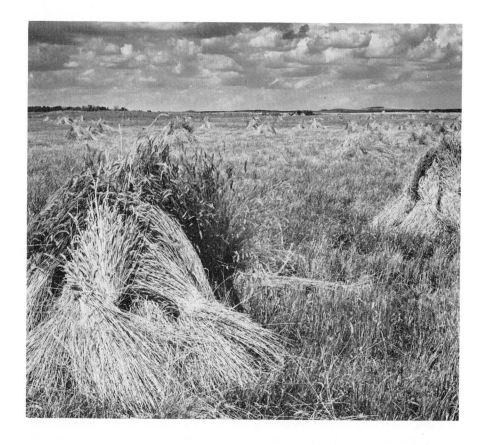

Grains can be the mainstay of our civilization, but its use can be overdone. Grains usually go through a processing program that can be detrimental to our health.

MAKING THE MOST OF YOUR HEALTH FOOD STORE

A number of foods have always been equated with health in general. They symbolize the "health food" philosophy. They include yogurt, blackstrap molasses, wheat germ, powdered skim milk and brewer's yeast. Add sprouts, whey and vegetable broth powder and seasoning to the family for their highly nourishing qualities and versatility, plus their natural goodness. Nutrition is a serious business, but it should also be enjoyable and enlivening.

To derive the utmost from nutrition, stress sense appeal of taste and sight in order to stimulate the flow of digestive juices and cause the "mouth to water."

Make these foods an indispensible part of any dietary regime. Remember the adage: "Variety is the spice of life." Listed are a few extra health ideas with which you may not be acquainted.

Acidophilus Culture. A wonderful aid for the bowel.

Arrowroot. A good thickening powder—high in calcium and alkaline in reaction.

Bran Water. An extract of minerals from simmering common wheat bran.

Carob. Chocolate-flavored powder with none of the disadvantages of cocoa and with higher nutritional value.

Dandelion Root Coffee. Has a "coffee taste"—made from roasted root of dandelion. Good for the liver.

Desiccated Liver. For building the blood.

Dulse. A powdered seaweed very high in iodine and manganese. A good supplement for underactive thyroid. Can be used as a salt seasoning.

Flaxseed Meal and Tea. Healing for intestinal tract; good natural laxative.

Fruit Juice Concentrate. Pure concentrates of whole fruits prepared by a special vacuum method, without high heat application. Cherry, apple and grape are usually available.

Gelatin. Use 100% pure gelatin. Gelatin is a valuable protein supplement, handy for reducing and normal diets.

Herb Teas. Healthful drinks made from steeping various herbs in boiling water.

Kefir. A wonderful "liquid yogurt" type drink, easily digested and good for the bowel.

Molasses. High in iron and sugar. Use unsulphured blackstrap variety.

Oils and Fats. Use only cold pressed, unrefined varieties. Avoid fats.

Raw Cheese. (Aged and unprocessed.)

Rice Polishings. High in silicon, good sources of B-complex vitamins.

Soy Milk. A milk substitute, noncatarrh forming.

Soy Sauce. Flavoring derived from the soybean. Use in broths, in cooking vegetables, in gravies and vegetarian loaves, in place of salt.

Seaweed. For seasoning and supplements, there are several varieties of edible seaweed, all high in iodine and mineral salts from the sea.

Sprouts. High in B-complex vitamins; add to soups just before serving; use in salads or eat them plain.

Unsulphured Dried Fruit.

Vegetable Broth Powder and Seasoning. Excellent seasoning to replace salt. High in organic minerals.

Vegetable Bouillon or Vegetable Stock or Vegetable Broth. Juices in which vegetables have been cooked, free from meat stock. Rich source of minerals.

Whey (Powdered). A high sodium food, good for arthritis and reducing diets, in handy powder form, made from fresh raw milk.

Yeast. Excellent source of B-complex, high in protein and RNA. Brewer's or primary grown yeast may be sprinkled on cereals, fruits, added to drinks.

Yogurt. Contains "friendly bacteria," good for the bowel. Good protein source.

BEST SUPPLEMENTS TO USE

Rice Bran Syrup. High in vitamin B-complex.

Lecithin. Balances cholesterol in the bloodstream; is a great heart support and a brain and nerve food.

Niacin. Vitamin B-3, flushes blood to the skin and extremities, especially the head, aiding circulation.

Chlorophyll. Best natural tissue cleanser and blood builder.

Chlorella. One of greatest foods for balancing the body

chemistry; high in chlorophyll.

Beet Tablets. Slightly laxative; good for sluggish liver and gallbladder; brings down the bile.

Acidophilus. Used to increase "friendly" bowel flora.

Bee Pollen. Blood builder; increases stamina, vigor and builds health.

Sesame Seeds: (King of the seeds), a whole food and a wonderful strength builder.

Megadophilus. High-potency acidophilus product.

Alfalfa Tablets. Brings fiber and chlorophyll to the bowel.

Digestive Aid Tablets. For digestive disturbances.

Pancreatin. For gas and poor starch tolerance.

Millet. King of all cereal grains.

Whey. Highest sodium food; needed in stomach and joints; neutralizes acids; helps some arthritis cases.

Sardines. One of the best "whole foods"; has 10 times as much RNA (the long-life factor) as yeast.

BioStrath. A liquid herbal extract, prepared to provide all elements needed for building a good body. (Made in Switzerland.)

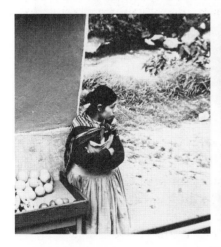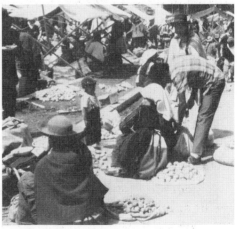

Left: A vegetable market on the way to Machu Picchu in Peru. Right: A market outside Lima, Peru.

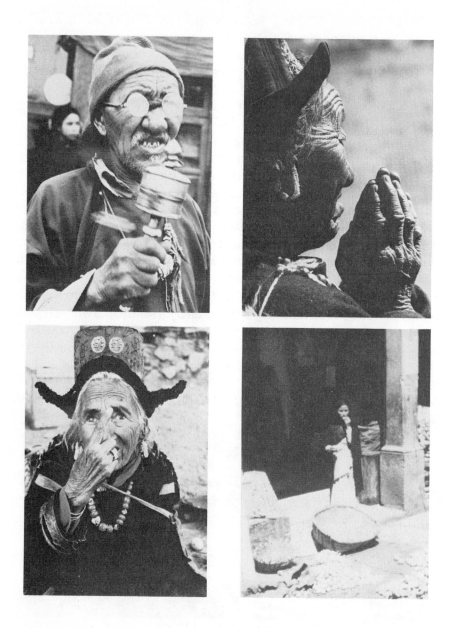

In Tibet, religion and natural food both were considered important. Top: Prayer wheel and direct prayer. Bottom: Street markets.

—13—

Raw Juices,
Tonics and Broths

There have been times when I have seen broths literally bring persons up out of their deathbeds. There have been other times when I have seen raw juices used to get rid of chronic diseases in people that doctors had given up on. And at still other times, I have seen natural tonics work wonders on people where drugs had not helped them. The power and effectiveness of foods in healing and in keeping people well is sometimes astonishing.

When you go over the following descriptions of juices, tonics and broths, remember the idea that what we need is variety in our foods. Each one is good for certain things and not for others. You should know when to use each of them. These are food remedies, but it is always best to be under a doctor's counsel if you are not well. You should also have a doctor's counsel to keep you well.

FRUIT JUICES

Fruit juices have more of the vitamin values. And some of them, like vegetable juices, are rich in particular minerals. I do not recommend citrus juices because they stir up too much of the acids in the body.

Blackberry. A good cleanser and blood builder (iron in iron) but can be constipating.

Cherry. Good for the bowel; high in potassium, sodium and iron salts. If you have an acid stomach, leave cherry juice alone.

Prune. Laxative to most, not all, people.

Mulberry. Nerve soothing, calming (especially to young people); brings down fevers; quiets the passions and emotions.

Strawberry. High in sodium and iron.

Elderberry. Vitalizes the female sex glands and organs if taken daily over a period of time. Seems to attract blood to the pelvic area.

Pineapple. Very good for throat ailments.

Currant (Black or Red). Builds bloodstream; detoxifies; acts as germicide.

Mango. Mild disinfectant; reduces body heat and perspiration; reduces body odors; somewhat binding to the bowel.

Peach. Laxative.

Nectarine. Same as peach.

Pomegranate. Tonic for kidneys; excellent cleanser; cooling on hot days.

Lemonade. Hot lemonade is good for colds, especially if mixed with clam juice. Stimulates perspiration and moves the blood; constipating to some persons.

Apple. Good hot or cold. Rich in potassium, sodium, magnesium, phosphorus. Can be mixed with other juices that are too sweet, sour or bitter to be taken alone.

Watermelon. An effective kidney cleanser, especially when put in juicer or blender with seeds, white rind and green skin, then strained through cheesecloth. Should be used within a half an hour of taking other foods.

Grape. For catarrh; laxative; should be juiced with skins and seeds, then strained.

VEGETABLE JUICES

Celery. Tones nervous system and sexual system. Good for stomach and bowel. Taken with whey, it helps some cases of rheumatism and arthritis.

Carrot. One of the best juices I know, the least allergenic, the easiest to tolerate. High in pro-vitamin A.

Spinach. Very high in mineral salts, especially potassium. High in iron and sodium; a good cleanser.

Tomato. Good for the blood; cooling; refreshing.

Cucumber. Cooling tonic; promotes healing, antiseptic; a blood purifier.

Beet. Very good liver cleanser but usually too strong to take alone. Dilute with water, celery juice or other mild juices.

Horseradish. Kidney stimulant and cleanser; mix or dilute with other juices.

Cabbage. Good for asthma.

Juice of any kind can be pressed or ground from any vegetable and mixed with other vegetable juices for flavoring. To add more flavor or to improve flavor, use grated orange rind, lemon peel, apple peelings, cloves, vanilla, banana, mint, sassaparilla, spearmint and/or honey.

Nuts and seeds can be blended with juices for a highly nutritious drink, but they should be soaked overnight in apple or pineapple juice before blending. Try almonds, sesame seeds, sunflower seeds and others.

RAW GOAT MILK

Many babies, intolerant of cow's milk or formula who couldn't breast feed for one reason or another, have taken raw goat milk very well. Older persons, invalids and those with stomach troubles or digestive problems do well on raw goat milk. For invalids, it is best taken foaming fresh from the goat. Cow milk has much larger fat globules so is harder to digest, and many have become allergic to it.

MILK SUBSTITUTES

The main nutrients in milk can be obtained from seed and nut milk drinks or soy milk, for those who want or need to eliminate regular milk from the diet.

Soymilk. Add 4 tablespoons soymilk powder to 1 pint water, sweeten to taste with honey, molasses or maple syrup. Refrigerate, as this milk sours easily.

Almond Nut Milk. Soak 1/3 cup of almonds overnight in enough apple or pineapple juice to cover plus an inch or so more allowed for absorption. Blend with 1 or 2 cups water or apple juice. This is an easily digestible protein drink.

Sesame Seed Milk. Add 1/4 cup hulled sesame seeds to 1 pint water or apple juice; let soak several hours or overnight. Blend until finely mixed. If you only have access to sesame seeds with hulls, strain the mixture through cheesecloth (several layers) or a fine wire-mesh strainer.

The same process can be used in about the same proportions

to make other nut and seed milk drinks.

To flavor these drinks, you may want to add a tablespoon of carob powder, dates, banana, reconstituted dried fruit, honey, fruit concentrates, strawberries or a combination of several of these.

MIXED DRINKS

Meal-in-a-Drink. To 1/2 cup each of mint tea, apple juice, unsweetened pineapple juice, orange juice, diced carrots, fresh fruit, add 1 pitted revived prune, 3/4 cup cashews, 1/2 celery stalk (diced), 2 sprigs parsley, 2 comfrey leaves, 1/2 ripe banana, 1 egg yolk, 1 tsp wheat germ and blend until smooth. Sip slowly.

See my book *Blending Magic* for many other delicious, healthful blender recipes.

A Travel Idea—When we travel and have to eat out, we order tomato, apple, unsweetened pineapple or V-8 juices. Another travel hint is to carry your own teabags and order hot water. You can also have Tea Kettle Tea, which is cream added to hot water. You can add honey or raw sugar.

BROTHS AND SOUPS

I do not believe in meat soups or meat broths—they are overloaded with uric acid from the meat. However, there is no uric acid in bone broths or vegetable broths.

There are two broths I have used with such wonderful results in patients that I recommend them highly.

You can drop a beaten egg yolk into any hot soup or broth which makes this a very good protein broth. You can also add a tablespoon of nut or seed butter to the broth before serving.

Vital Broth

To be used with any heavy catarrhal or acidic condition. Take peelings, 1/4-inch deep from 2 potatoes; simmer in 3 cups of water for 15 minutes. Strain and drink broth only, 1 cup twice a day for a month.

184

For a tastier, but equally potent, drink try the following recipe:
2 cups potato peelings
2 cups carrot tops
1/2 tsp vegetable broth powder
3 cups celery
2 cups celery tops
2 qt water
Onion, as desired, for flavor

Chop or grate vegetables and greens, add water, bring to a slow boil; simmer 20 minutes; strain off broth and drink 2 cups each day. I advise adding a teaspoon to a tablespoon of rice polishings either before cooking or after straining this broth to enrich it with B vitamins and silicon.

Veal Joint Broth

This broth is high in sodium, excellent for rheumatism, arthritis and catarrhal elimination. It is good for the stomach bowel, ligaments, joints and glands.

Buy a fresh, uncut veal joint and wash thoroughly in cold water. Put in large cooking pot, cover half with water and add the following:

1-1/2 cup apple peelings
2 cups potato peelings
1/2 cup okra or
1 tsp powdered okra
1 stalk celery, chopped
1 large parsnip
1 onion
2 beets, grated
1/2 cup chopped parsley

Simmer all ingredients 4-5 hours and strain off liquid, throwing solids away. You should have about 1-1/2 qt liquid when done. Drink a cup hot, store the rest in refrigerator.

Broths may be made of any meat, fish or bones, if they are fresh, with the addition of various vegetables and grains as desired.

Soups and salads seem to go together, and here I want to present a few of my nicest soups.

Barley and Green Kale Soup. This is a high calcium soup that

185

can easily be assimilated. Soak 1/2 cup of barley in 1 cup of water overnight. Add 1 quart water, 2 stalks of chopped celery, 1 chopped onion, bring to a boil, then simmer 1 hour. Add finely-chopped or ground fresh kale (frozen is all right) and simmer 20 minutes more. Just before serving, add chopped parsley and a little butter or sour cream.

Asparagus Soup. In blender, combine 1 bunch fresh, young asparagus spears, 1 cup each of tomato juice and celery juice, 1 slice onion, 1/4 cup rice polishings, 2 teaspoons vegetable seasoning and blend until smooth. Strain out coarse fibers. Reblend with 1 tablespoon chives and sprig of chopped parsley. Heat in top of double boiler. Before serving, add 2 tablespoons butter and sprinkle with paprika.

Raw Spinach Soup. Follow same directions as for asparagus soup, using a fresh bunch of raw spinach instead.

Mushroom Soup. To 1/2 cup water, add 1-1/2 cups sliced mushrooms, 1/2 small onion and 2 cloves garlic chopped finely, 2 teaspoons vegetable seasoning and 1/2 teaspoon paprika. Cook until mushrooms are tender, then add 1/2 cup raw cream and 1/2 cup raw milk; blend until smooth and heat in top of double boiler.

Fresh Corn Soup. Blend 1-1/2 cups raw cream (or half raw milk and raw cream), 1-1/2 teaspoons vegetable seasoning, 2-3 basil leaves and 1-1/2 cups corn off the cob. Blend until smooth. You may strain hulls off if desired. Heat in double boiler, sprinkle with chopped parsley and dash of paprika and serve.

Sleep Tonic. Soak barley bran in cold water and skim off the oily substance that floats to the top. Add to juices of celery, parsley, thyme, beet greens and spinach.

Keep in mind that most of your body weight is liquid. These liquid drinks, broths, etc., can bring a good deal of improvement to anyone's health.

Celery Broth

1 small bunch celery
1 Tbsp sweet butter
Chop celery fine, cover with water and cook slowly for 20 minutes. Season with broth powder, add butter and serve.

Soy Tomato Broth

1 C. cooked soybeans
1 small onion, cut fine

4 C. tomato juice
1 small green pepper, cut fine

Mash soybeans to pulp. Steam onion and green pepper 10 minutes and add to soybeans and tomato juice. Heat, but do not boil. Add butter and serve.

Onion Consomme

6 lge onions
4 C. water
1/4 C. vegetable broth powder
Sweet butter to taste
Put onions through a food chopper and simmer about 15 minutes. Strain the onions from the broth, add butter and broth powder and serve.

Tomato Consomme

10 fresh ripe tomatoes
Sweet butter to taste
1/4 C. vegetable broth powder
1/2 C. water
Wash and cut fresh ripe tomatoes in small pieces. Rub through a sieve. Heat but do not boil. Add broth powder, mixed to paste in water, sweet butter and serve.

Tomato Celery Broth

3 C. tomato juice
1 C. celery juice
Heat celery and tomato juice, but do not boil. Season with butter and vegetable broth powder and serve.

Vegetable Broth Delight

1 C. chopped okra
1/2 C. peas
1 C. string beans; string and cut fine
Tbsp broth powder
1 clove garlic, cut fine
1/2 C. chopped celery

Vegetable Broth

1 C. carrots
1 C. turnips
2 sprigs parsley

2 potatoes
4 sticks celery

Parsley and Potato Broth

2 C. diced potatoes
1 C. chopped parsley
Cover potatoes and parsley with cold water and simmer for 20 minutes. Strain, add a little milk and butter and serve.

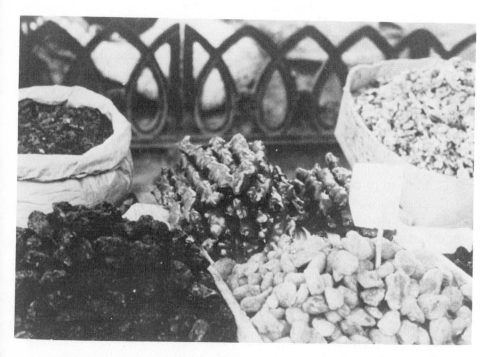

Using dried fruits and nuts in drinks can help you gain weight. Nut milk drinks should be used as substitutes for regular milk.

14

What Our Foods Are Made Of

My definition of good personal nutrition is *a food regimen which matches a person's needs in such a way as to build the body's natural defenses, to prevent disease, to repair and replace tissues and to produce maximum well-being.*

Definitions from **Webster's New World Dictionary:**

FOOD: Any substance taken into and assimilated by a plant or animal to keep up its life and growth; nourishment. Solid substances of this sort: distinguished from drink. A specified kind of food. Anything that nourishes or stimulates (food for thought).

Nutrition: A nourishing or being nourished; esp., the series of processes by which an organism takes in food and uses it living and growing and in repairing tissues. Nourishment; food. The science or study of proper diet.

To know what foods our bodies need, we should understand what it is about foods that makes them useful to the body.

There is much more to foods and diet than we realize, because there is much yet to be discovered. All natural foods get their life energy from the sun and get their physical structure from the dust of the earth, and each food has its own energy vibration, which man knows little about. These vibrational energies can be destroyed in handling, processing and cooking of foods. It is possible that we will find out in the future that we live more on the vibrational life energy of foods than on the physical substance they provide.

PROTEIN

We find that proteins are the building blocks of tissue, used to repair and replace tissue. Proteins are needed by virtually every tissue and system of the body, especially the brain, nerves and glands. Protein foods include meat, poultry, fish, eggs, cheese, milk, tofu and so forth. Nuts, seeds, grains, legumes and many vegetables have a little protein.

CARBOHYDRATES

Foods primarily made of carbohydrates are energy foods. People with jobs requiring physical labor need more carbohydrates than those with desk jobs or sitting jobs. Complex carbohydrates are found in fruits, vegetables, nuts, seeds, grains and sprouts. *These are whole foods.* When digested, they release energy in a steady, constant stream. Refined carbohydrates include sugar, white flour, white rice and products made of them. All these substances are lacking in vitamins, minerals, oils and natural food values because they have had much of the good "refined" out of them. They are not whole foods, and using them can create nutritional deficiencies in the body, contributing to conditions that invite disease.

FATS AND OILS

Fats and oils are either animal or vegetable in source. We need fats to make hormones, feed the brain and nerves, keep the skin supple and provide energy. We get sufficient fats and oils from our foods, such as meat, chicken, fish, milk, grains, nuts and seeds, and should avoid using the concentrated fats or oils in cooking or baking. Saturated fats, taken from animal sources, are hard to digest and are solid at room temperature. Unsaturated fats are from plant sources and are liquid at room temperature

CHOLESTEROL

We get cholesterol in meat and dairy products, but our bodies make enough for our needs. Cholesterol is needed to make steroid hormones, as a brain and nerve fat and for bile. If we balance our cholesterol intake with lecithin, we will not usually have a problem with it. *The problem comes in overcooking or cooking at too high a heat,* which destroys the lecithin needed to balance cholesterol in the body, allowing cholesterol to deposit in the arteries.

LECITHIN

Lecithin, found in eggs, meats, legumes and grains, is needed to keep cholesterol in solution and in the brain, nerves and the sexual fluids.

FIBER

Fiber is indigestible cellulose found in all vegetables, fruits, nuts, seeds and whole grains. Without enough fiber, bowel problems occur, especially constipation. Fiber keeps the bowel clean and regular. There is no fiber in meat, dairy products or refined carbohydrates. Good fiber supplements are alfalfa tablets, psyllium husks, wheat bran and oat bran. These are available at most health food stores.

CHLOROPHYLL

All plants and especially green leafy vegetables contain chlorophyll, the pigment that stores concentrated sunshine and gives leaves their green color. Chlorophyll is one of our greatest survival foods because of its cleansing effect on the blood and tissues, especially the bowel. The chemical structure of chlorophyll is almost exactly the same as the hemoglobin in red blood cells which carry vital oxygen to the tissues.

ENZYMES

Although our bodies make most of the enzymes we need, *live foods contain enzymes that can aid digestion* and other processes. Overcooking kills enzymes and so do many of the chemical additives in processed foods.

MINERALS

Chemical substances in the form of salts play a vital role in the body. We couldn't live without iron, iodine, calcium and many others. Some, like cobalt, are needed to form vitamins. Calcium and phosphorus are needed to build the bones. Many elements such as sodium, potassium and calcium neutralize acids in the body. We will go into this more in the next chapter.

VITAMINS

These powerful and essential elements of nutrition have only been discovered in the past century, mostly in the last 50 years. Vitamins protect tissues, enhance the immune system, speed up healing, aid in hormone production and do many other things. We'll have a closer look at them in the next chapter.

You cannot build a body with vitamins. Vitamins are like gasoline in an automobile. It runs the car, but it takes minerals to make the car. It also takes minerals to build a human body.

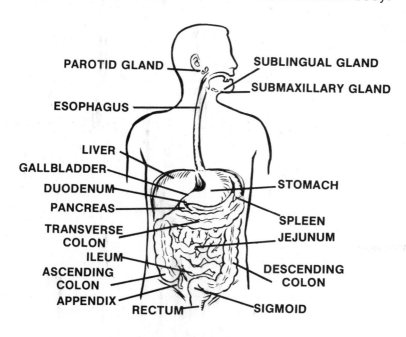

PAROTID GLAND
SUBLINGUAL GLAND
SUBMAXILLARY GLAND
ESOPHAGUS
LIVER
GALLBLADDER
DUODENUM
PANCREAS
TRANSVERSE COLON
ILEUM
ASCENDING COLON
APPENDIX
STOMACH
SPLEEN
JEJUNUM
DESCENDING COLON
RECTUM
SIGMOID

Digestive system.

HISTORY OF—

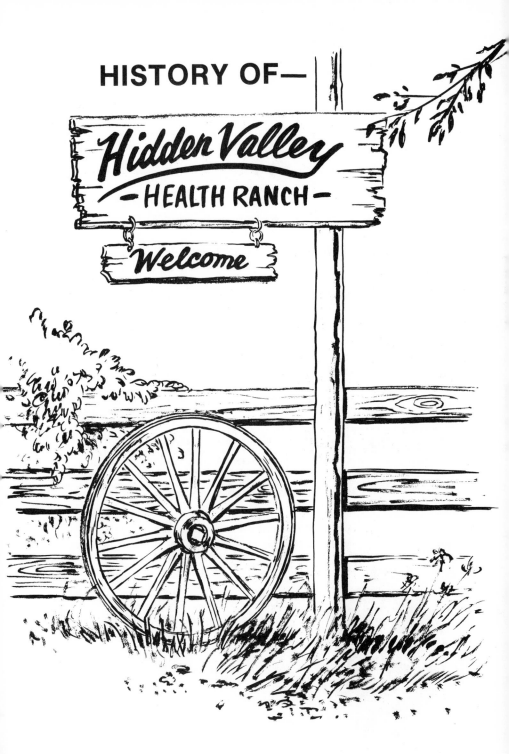

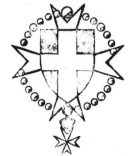

" Pro Fide, pro utilitate Hominum "

W E

MARQUIS DON K. VELLA HABER, HON.D.LITT.

Grand Bailiff, Hereditary Grand Cross

of the

SOVEREIGN ORDER OF SAINT JOHN OF JERUSALEM
- KNIGHTS OF MALTA -

BY THE GRACE OF GOD and in virtue of the Constitutions of the Order

GRAND PRIOR INTERNATIONAL
Head of the Executive of the Sovereign Council

HAVE DECREED as We do hereby Decree:-

IN RECOGNITION of his extensive works and endeavours in the humanitarian field
of the healing of man, the natural way; in view of his extensive studies a n d
research; his numerous publications; his lectures round the world and further-
more in the HIDDEN VALLEY HEALTH RANCH, at Escondido, California, U.S.A.,......
REMEMBERING also his visit to MALTA, along with a party of followers, purposely
for his ceremony of investiture at the historical Basilica of Our Lady of t h e
Victories, WE DO HEREBY GRANT, for his devotion to the Order and in view of his
willingness and vow to serve humanity under the auspices of the Order,...... We
GRANT our Beloved Confrere, KNIGHT COMMANDER Dr. BERNARD JENSEN, D.C., Ph.D.,-
the grace of operating, both his endeavours and his Hidden Valley Health Ranch,
under the auspices of the Order and therefore to use the ensign of the Order
for all same purposes thereof.

SO BE IT
One for all and all for one: non nobis

GIVEN UNDER OUR OWN HAND in MALTA, on the seventeenth day of the month of Feb-
ruary, in the year of Our Lord, one thousandninehundered and eightysix a n d
registered in Our archives with Doc. Symbol:G.P.D. I/86.

Grand Prior International S. O.S.J.

Countersigned:
Knight of Grace Jos. Camilleri, KGSJ.
SIGNATORY of t h e   O r d e r.

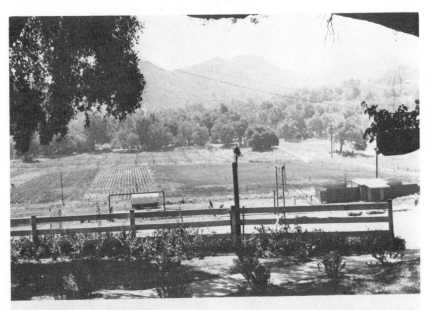

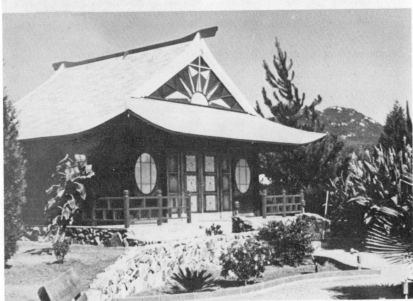

Proper foods, natural living, meditation, quietness, freedom from stress, a new lifestyle—these are the means for recovering our health. Bottom: Our Color and Meditation Center.

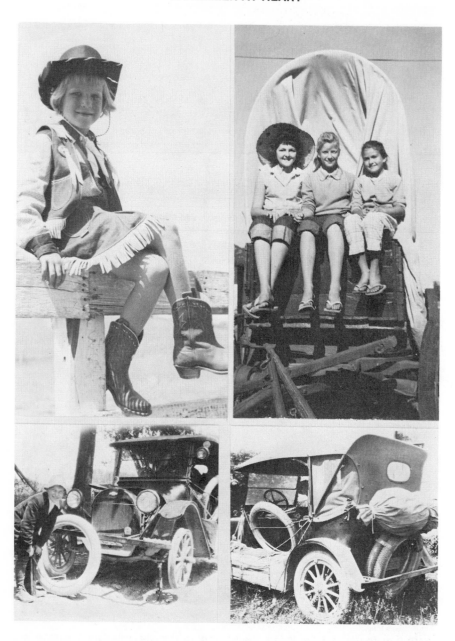

Top: My daughter in cowgirl outfit and with friends on the wagon. Bottom: "Go West, young man!" The car that brought us here from Detroit.

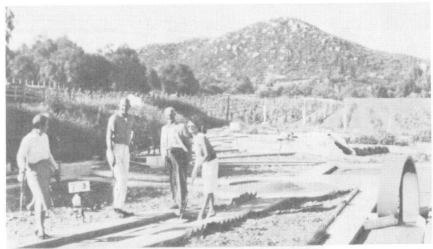

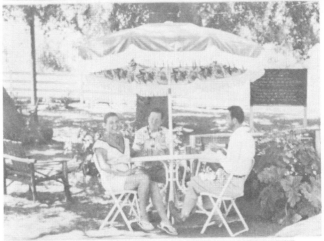

The climate at the Ranch was a great help to many who came to recuperate and recover their health. Diet, exercise and rest are the main factors, but climate and the beauty of the surroundings are also important healing factors.

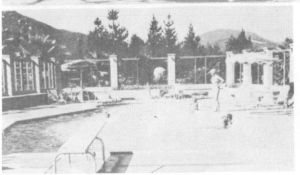

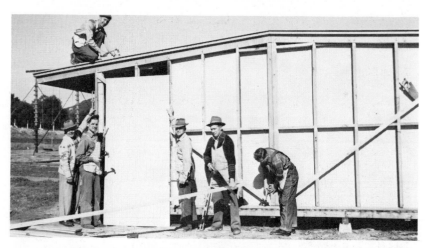

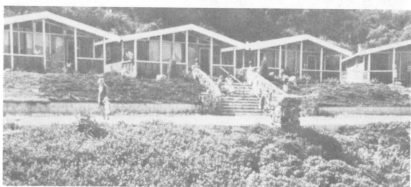

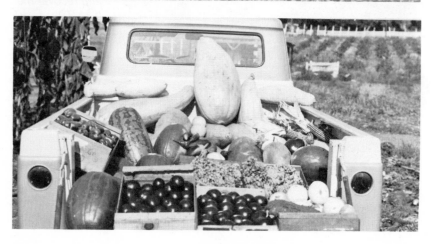

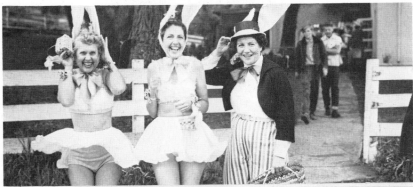

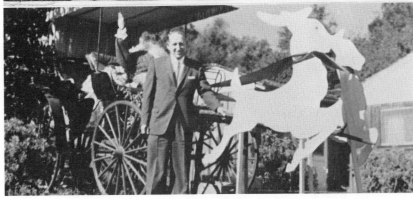

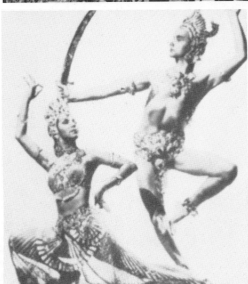

We had world famous entertainers such as Fujata and Asoka at the Ranch, and many guests provided entertainment on special occasions.

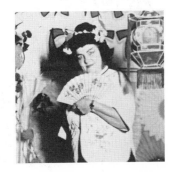

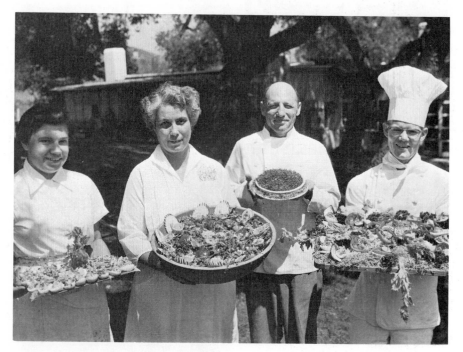

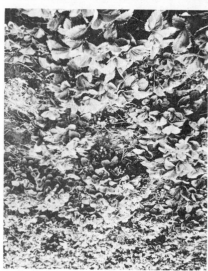

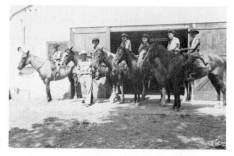

The art of living the wholistic life was practiced at the Ranch. My whole family (bottom right), 5 boys and 1 girl, enjoyed it. They ate most of my strawberries (bottom left).

WORK, PLAY, REST AND RECREATION

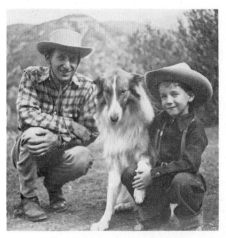

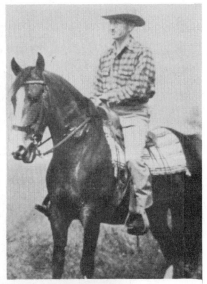

My home and family life and my
work life in the early years.

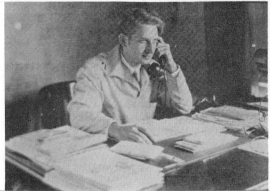

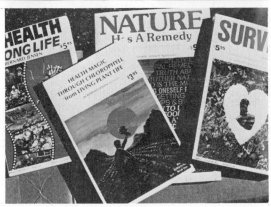

THE RANCH WAS ALWAYS BUZZING WITH ACTIVITY

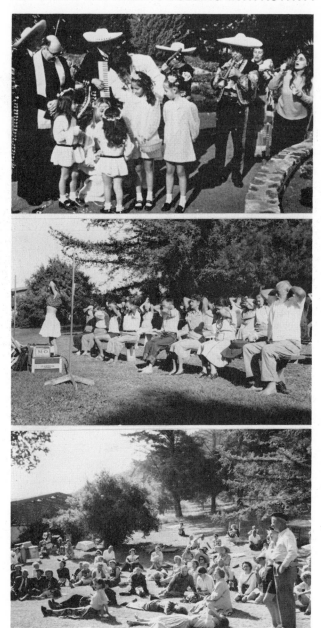

Weddings were performed, posture and breathing exercises and inspirational lectures were given.

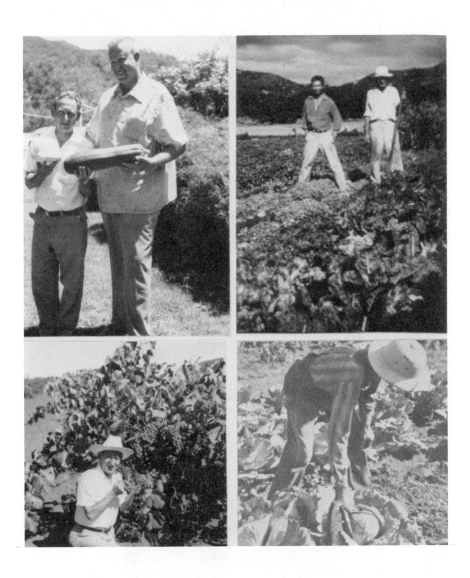

Food grown on organic, well-mineralized soil, eaten with a positive attitude and healthy appetite, builds the best bodies.

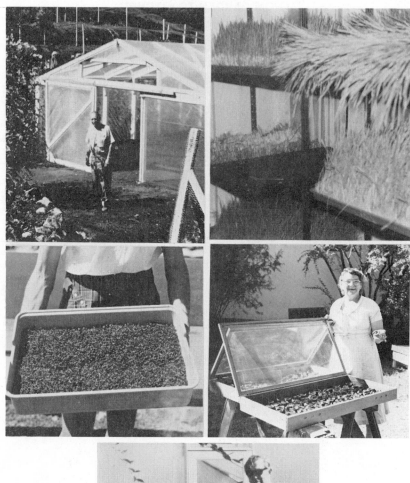

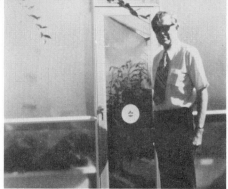

In our greenhouse on the Ranch, we grew special grasses and sprouts. Mid rt: Drying fruit. Bottom: A visitor looks over our work.

204

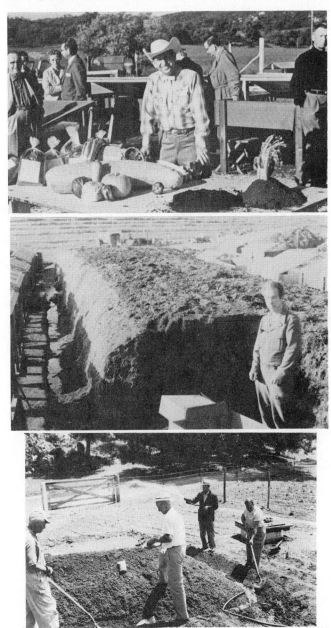

Minerals first come from the earth before becoming part of our foods and our bodies. We replenish the earth.

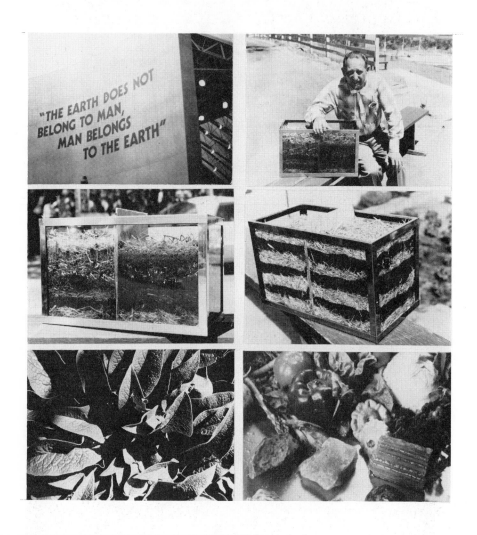

We did experiments with worms at the Ranch. Worms produce nutrient-rich castings, aerate the soil and help break down organic matter. Bottom Left: Comfrey. Bottom Right: Minerals build the foods we eat.

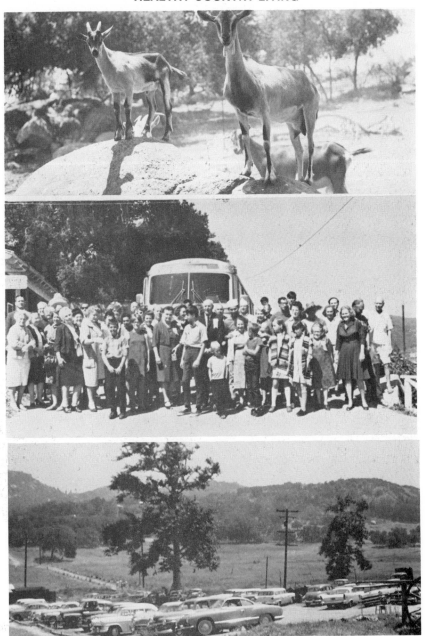

People came from all over the world to Hidden Valley Health Ranch to improve their style of living to a more natural way.

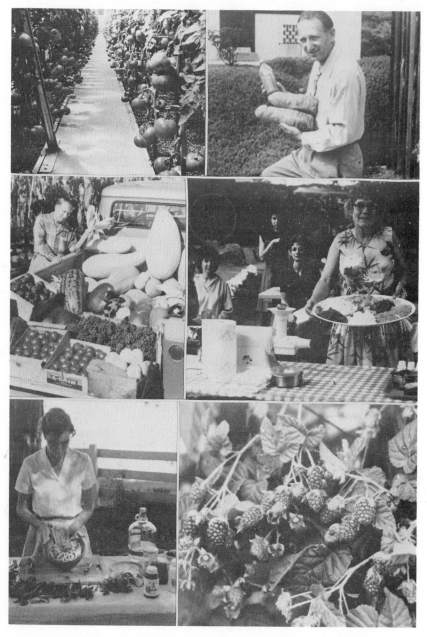

*Foods grown from hydroponics and our organic gardens—and food
demonstrations were going on all the time for patients' knowledge.*

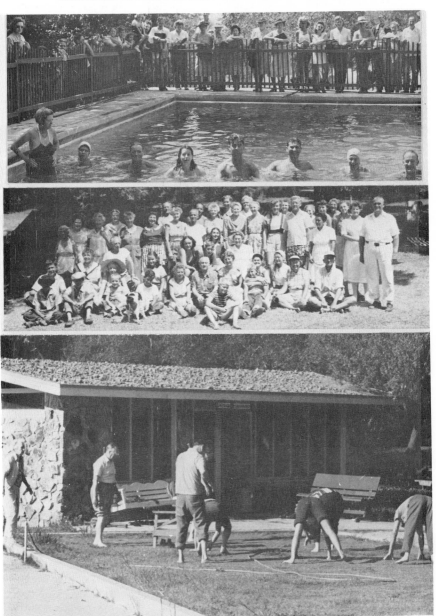

Top: Swimming lessons at Ranch with Paul Bragg and Clark Irvine, founder of Let's Live magazine. Middle: A morning hiking group. Bottom: Our Kneipp water cure house with grass and sand walks.

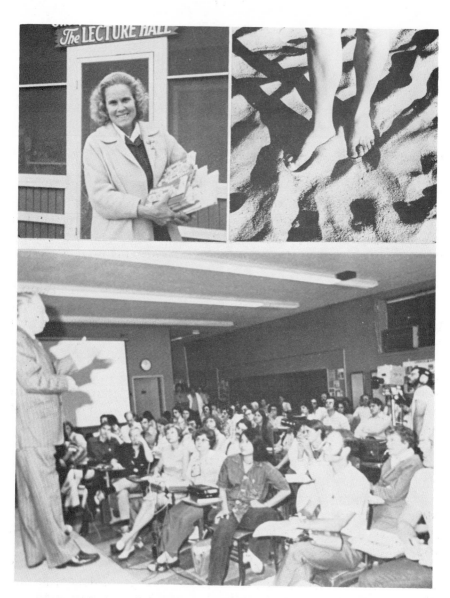

We learn by doing. Sand walks for the leg muscles and circulation.

—15—

Vitamins and Minerals

I don't believe the discovery of all vitamins is over yet, and it is very likely that not everything is known about the vitamins discovered so far. The purpose of this chapter is to mention briefly the main functions of the known vitamins and minerals and their best food sources.

As we traveled throughout the world, we found those people who lived the longest lives and had the healthiest bodies didn't know anything about vitamins and minerals. These people lived on natural foods. All the vitamins and minerals are found in our natural foods, but in this book we have to learn to select. We have to learn to use the right proportions in our foods. We have to learn how much raw food to have each day. All of these ideas were taken originally from the long-lived people of the world who had the best health.

VITAMINS

Vitamins affect our emotions, attitudes, energy level, physical strength and resistance to disease. Some help control levels of mineral elements in the body and some work more powerfully in the presence of other vitamins or minerals.

The important thing to know about vitamins is that if we follow the natural regimen, in most cases, we are going to get all the vitamins we need. All the vitamins synthesized and made in laboratories were originally found in nature. Vitamin K was originally found in alfalfa, but now they make it. Vitamin A was originally found in butter and carrots. You cannot get the same results from a synthesized laboratory-made vitamin as you can from the natural one. Vitamin C is found in both vegetables and fruits and also in our nuts, berries and other natural foods. The B vitamins were found in wheat germ and rice germ. Vitamin E, in nature, was found in wheat germ and wheat germ oil. All vitamins in their natural state are an integral part of foods. None exists in nature as a separate substance. I don't think man was made to take vitamins or minerals individually, apart from foods. We should be taking them from natural foods, and this is what my whole book is based on. Supplements really should be a prescription given by a nutritionist who knows what shortages you have in the body and how to take care of them properly.

No matter what is available to you in the store in the way of vitamin and mineral supplements, always try to have the natural, because the body is meant to have vitamins and minerals in foods.

The following presentation is for your information and perusal, not to encourage you to buy and use vitamin and mineral supplements along with your foods. Before using vitamin and mineral supplements, you should be well eduated about them and about the right amounts to use. There is a good deal of controversy about vitamins these days. Large dosages of some of them are dangerous. It is said that some of the synthetic vitamins are treated by the body like drugs, with possible side effects and time-bomb effects.

Vitamin A. Protects from infection, needed for growth, helps keep skin smooth, keeps up normal vision. Best sources are fish liver oil, milk products, carrots, apricots and green leafy vegetables.

Vitamin B-Complex. The B vitamins support the nerves, help produce energy from foods and protect the liver. Foods highest in B-complex are brewer's yeast, molasses, liver (and other organ meats), eggs, milk, beef, green vegetables, alfalfa sprouts, whole grains, legumes.

Vitamin C. Builds resistance, healing and increases iron absorption. Best sources are citrus and other fruits. Vegetables have little vitamin C, excepting bell peppers and parsley.

Vitamin D. Helps control calcium and phosphorus in the body. Best source is sunlight on the skin or fish liver oil. Most foods, unless fortified, have very little vitamin D.

Vitamin E. Protects nutrients from oxidation, strengthens the heart, increases oxygen and supports the sexual system. Best

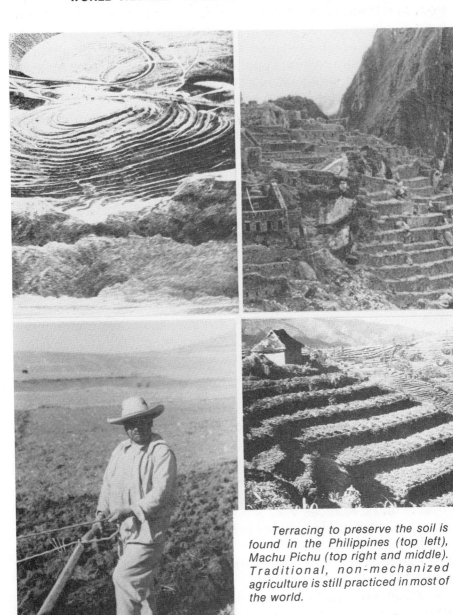

Terracing to preserve the soil is found in the Philippines (top left), Machu Pichu (top right and middle). Traditional, non-mechanized agriculture is still practiced in most of the world.

sources are wheat germ, whole cereal grains, milk products, eggs, seeds, nuts, legumes and green vegetables. The oil in these foods contains lecithin, the great brain and nerve food for the body.

Vitamin F. This vitamin is made of nutrients essential to growth, a healthy blood supply and strong nerves. Best sources are nuts, seeds, vegetable oils and fish liver oils. Vitamin F is found highest in flaxseed and flaxseed tea.

Vitamin K. Necessary for liver function and normal blood clotting. Best sources are soybeans, egg yolk, all green vegetables and molasses.

MINERALS IN THE BODY

Sodium, *The Youth Element.* Needed for the stomach, bowel, joints and ligaments. Contributes to good digestion, assimilation and limber joints. Neutralizes acids in the body. Best sources are whey, okra, celery and green leafy vegetables. (Table salt has the wrong kind of sodium.)

Potassium, *The Great Alkalizer.* Needed by the heart, muscles and nerves. Neutralizes muscle acids. Helps nerve conduction, needed to form secretions. Best sources: potato skins, olives, parsley, blueberries, peaches, prunes, figs, meat, green peppers, watercress.

Calcium, *The Knitter.* Needed for bones, teeth, acid neutralization, blood clotting, muscle function, vigor, endurance, strength, pain relief, healing of bone fractures. Best sources: cheese, fish, green vegetables (especially kale), milk products, prunes, figs, dates, soybeans, lentils, barley.

Magnesium, *The Relaxer.* Needed by bones, teeth and nerves. Aids in building protein, acts as natural laxative, helps prevent heart attacks, reduces mental disturbances. Best sources: Yellow cornmeal, figs, barley, wheat bran, egg yolk, goat milk, nuts and seeds.

Phosphorus, *The Light Bearer.* Needed by all cells but especially brain and nerve cells. Must be in balance with calcium. Best sources: Seafood, milk products, eggs, parsnips, whole cereal grains, legumes, meat, seeds and nuts.

Iron, *The Frisky Horse Element.* Needed by the blood cells to attract oxygen. Best sources are meat (especially liver), eggs, brewer's yeast, wheat germ, dried fruits, black raspberries, milk products, green vegetables, rice bran, whole grains.

Iodine, *The Metabolizer.* Needed by the thyroid to form hormones that affect general energy level of the whole body and the energy level of each organ. I believe iodine is one of the most necessary elements in dealing with the fast-paced life of our day. Poor circulation, symptoms of aging, change of life problems and loss of mental acuity can all come from a lack of iodine. We should have one or more iodine foods every day. Excess iodine intake is rare, especially in Western nations, but a type of goiter is found in about 10% of the people along the coast of the Northern Island of Japan believed to be caused by excessive use of a local seaweed for food, which is very high in iodine. Best sources: Nova Scotia dulse, kelp, seafood, legumes, mushrooms, green leafy vegetables, onions, garlic, leeks, cod liver oil.

Fluorine, *The Decay Resistance Element.* Needed to strengthen resistance to disease, cleanse the body, strengthen bones and teeth. Sources: Raw goat milk, cheese, dulse, seaweed, rose hips, raw vegetables such as cabbage, spinach, watercress, tomatoes. Easily destroyed by heat.

Chlorine, *The Cleanser.* Needed to form hydrochloric acid for protein digestion; keeps the body clean; forms secretions; purifies; disinfects. Sources: Raw milk, fish, sea salt, cheese, green vegetables. Destroyed by high temperatures.

Sulphur, *The Heating Element.* Needed by brain and nervous system. Sources: Eggs, meat, cabbage, cauliflower, onions, leeks, garlic, horseradish, asparagus, melons, tops of mustard, turnips and beets.

Silicon, *The Magnetic Element.* Needed by skin, hair, nerves, ligaments, membranes. Sources: Sprouts, whole grains, rice bran, legumes, figs, seeds, oat straw tea.

Manganese, *The Love Element.* Needed by glands and nervous system. Aids memory and production of hormones. Sources: Whole grains, green vegetables, nuts, seeds.

Cobalt, *Trace Element.* Needed to assist in glucose tolerance and to build vitamin B-12. Sources: Organ meats, meat, milk products, green vegetables, sea salt, seafood, seaweed.

Zinc, *Trace Element.* Needed for sexual system and skin. Deficiency in men may contribute to prostate trouble. Sources: Nuts, seeds, liver, wheat germ. Fatigue and loss of taste may indicate zinc deficiency.

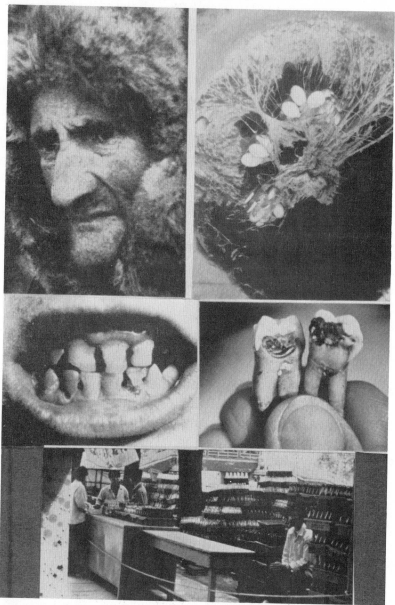

Upper left: This 27-year-old man was taken from a prison camp with great mineral deficiencies. Top rt: The minerals are rich in seeds, and every seed is connected by fibers to the outside of the food. Our teeth are made of minerals, and poor food habits can cause serious tooth decay. Bottom: Chinese cola stand.

STORAGE SITES FOR MINERALS

Every chemical element needed by the body usually has one main storage site in the body where most of it is kept. For example, iodine is mainly stored in the thyroid, where it is used to make thyroid hormone. When iodine is lacking, the thyroid enlarges to form a goiter. We find that the Chinese carried fish and other seafoods as much as 500 miles inland to those who had goiter. Natives in the Peruvian Andes brought kelp all the way from the coast and considered it a valuable food. They put it in ice cream, candy, bread and use it to flavor many other foods. It is a known fact that there isn't a single case of iodine-deficiency goiter in all of Japan. Iodine is seldom found in land vegetation over 50 miles from the sea, but can be obtained from pineapple, papayas, mangoes and other fruit grown near the sea.

When specific organs, glands or other tissues that serve as storage sites become depleted, we know the whole body is short. For example, when the blood is low in iron, the whole body is low. If the skin and hair are short of silicon, so is the rest of the body. If the joints and stomach are deficient in sodium, the whole body has been robbed of sodium. My book, **Nature Has A Remedy**, tells more about these shortages for the average person, while my book, **Chemistry of Man**, with over 500 pages, is for the student who seeks deeper understanding of the chemical elements.

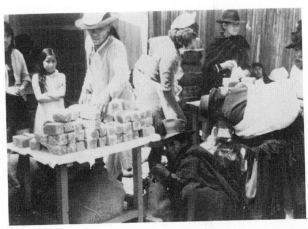

Natural cane sugar of South America. In white sugar, most vitamins and minerals are taken out.

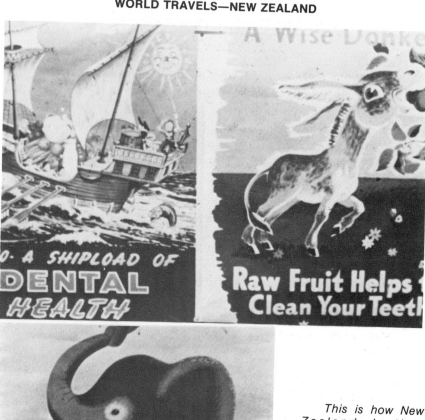

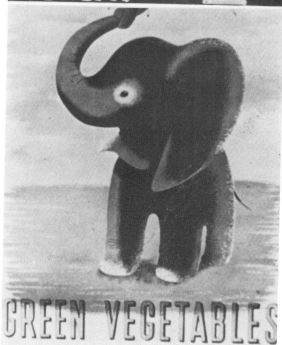

This is how New Zealand dentists advertise, to help people have better teeth. After going through a time of very poor dental hygiene, New Zealand had nurses in every school checking the childrens' teeth regularly and sending those who needed dental work to the dentist.

BODY SYSTEMS—THEIR FUNCTIONS
AND BIOCHEMICAL THERAPIES

A Reference Chart Designed to Provide
Greater Insight into the Human Body

- Biochemical therapies do not cover all aspects of wholistic treatment. For mechanical, mental or spiritual disorders, the appropriate disciplines should be utilized.

- Any so-called disease can involve several systems simultaneously.

- Vegetable juices are an all-around body system builder.

- Any program, consistently followed, requires three months to bring about change.

- Consider elimination channels on first visit, then specific problems on following visits.

- Single herbs are most efficient in healing crises, fevers and acute elimination processes.

- Universal medicine in the future will use all the constructive principles from the Wholistic Healing Arts.

- Remember that when you help one organ—every other organ benefits.

SKELETAL SYSTEM

STRUCTURE: All bones, cartilage, and joints.

FUNCTION: Support and protection of body, leverage, mineral storage, production of red blood cells.

FOODS: Sesame seed, kale, millet, celery, barley, okra, almonds, collards, turnip greens, raw goat's milk.

DRINKS: Black mission figs/raw goat's milk; black cherry juice; green kale juice; celery/parsley juice; veal joint broth.

VITAMINS: C, D, A, B-complex, B-2, B-6, B-12, E, F, folic acid, niacin, pantothenic acid, bioflavonoids.

MINERALS: Calcium, fluorine, copper, magnesium, iron, iodine, sulphur, zinc, silicon, phosphorus, potassium, sodium.

HERBS: Comfrey, kale, boneset, poke root, chicory, juniper berries, arnica flowers, elderflowers, oatstraw, alfalfa, irish moss.

MUSCULAR SYSTEM

STRUCTURE: All muscular tissue in the body.

FUNCTION: Facilitation of body movement, production of heat, maintenance of body posture.

FOODS: Olives, rye, lima beans, rice bran, bananas, sprouts, watercress, complementary proteins (grains, legumes, etc.), apples.

DRINKS: Potato peeling broth; dried olive tea; nut milk drink with liquid chlorophyll.

VITAMINS: B-6, D, E, A, B-complex, B-12, C, biotin, choline, pantothenic acid.

MINERALS: Calcium, potassium, magnesium, nitrogen, chlorine, iron, silicon.

HERBS: Juniper berries, rosemary, tansy, black willow, horseradish, wild cabbage, kelp, dulse, watercress, horsetail, black walnut.

INTEGUMENTARY

STRUCTURE: Skin, hair, nails, oil and sweat glands.

FUNCTION: Regulation of body temperature; elimination of waste; temperature, pressure and pain reception.

FOODS: Raw goat milk, black bass, rye, avocados, sea vegetables, whey, apples, cucumbers, millet, rice polishings, rice bran and concentrate, sprouts.

DRINKS: Carrot/celery/lemon juice; cucumber/endive/pineapple juice.

VITAMINS: Pantothenic acid, PABA, D, A, B-complex, B-2, B-6, B-12, B-1, C, E, F, K, biotin, choline, folic acid, niacin, bioflavonoids.

MINERALS: Silicon, calcium, fluorine, iron, phosphorus, potassium, sodium, sulphur, iodine, copper, manganese, zinc, magnesium.

HERBS: Oatstraw, shavegrass, horsetail, comfrey, aloe vera, burdock.

LYMPHATIC SYSTEM

STRUCTURE: Spleen, thymus, appendix, tonsils, lymph nodes, lymph vessels and fluid.

FUNCTION: Filtration of blood, production of white blood cells, protection against disease, return of protein to cardiovascular system.

FOODS: Green leafy vegetables, watercress, celery, okra, apples.

DRINKS: Potato peeling broth; celery juice; blue violet tea; parsley juice; carrot juice; apple juice.

VITAMINS: A, C, choline, B-complex, B-1, B-2, B-6, biotin, pantothenic acid, folic acid.

MINERALS: Potassium, chlorine, sodium.

HERBS: Blue violet tea (leaves), chaparral, burdock, echinacea, blue flag, poke root, golden seal, cayenne, mullein, black walnut.

REPRODUCTIVE SYSTEM

STRUCTURE: Testes, ovaries, sperm, ova, mammaries.

FUNCTION: Reproduction of the organism.

FOODS: Sesame seeds, pumpkin seeds, seed and nut butters, cod roe, lecithin, egg yolk, raw goat milk.

DRINKS: Black cherry concentrate/chlorophyll/one egg yolk drink; pineapple juice/egg yolk/wheat germ/dulse drink; 3/4 cup carrot juice/1/4 cup coconut milk/one tablespoon wheat germ oil/one teaspoon rice polishings drink.

VITAMINS: B-complex, E, A, B-2, B-6, C, D, F.

MINERALS: Zinc, calcium, iodine, phosphorus, iron, sodium, chlorine, potassium, fluorine, silicon.

HERBS: Black cohosh, licorice, dong quai, ginseng, blessed thistle, blue cohosh, uva ursi, raspberry, squaw vine, chickweed, saw palmetto, false unicorn, raspberry.

RESPIRATORY SYSTEM

STRUCTURE: The lungs, trachea, bronchi, bronchial tubes, and alveoli.

FUNCTION: Oxygenation; elimination of carbon dioxide; regulation of acid-base balance of the body.

FOODS: Garlic, onions, leeks, turnips, grapes, pineapple, honey (eucalyptus), green leafy vegetables.

DRINKS: Celery/papaya juice; carrot juice; watercress/apple juice with one quarter teaspoon cream of tartar; rose hips tea; goat milk whey.

VITAMINS: A, C, D, B-complex, B-1, B-2, B-6, B-12, E, F, inositol, choline, bioflavonoids, folic acid, niacin, pangamic acid, pantothenic acid.

MINERALS: Calcium, iron, silicon, manganese, potassium, copper, fluorine.

HERBS: Mullein, elderflowers, peppermint, yarrow, lobelia, comfrey, cayenne, marshmallow, sage, coltsfoot.

220

GLANDULAR SYSTEM

STRUCTURE: Pineal, pituitary, thyroid and parathyroids, thymus, adrenals, pancreas, ovaries, testes.

FUNCTION: Regulation of body activities through transportation of hormones by the circulatory system.

FOODS: Sea vegetables, kelp, dulse, swiss chard, turnip greens, egg yolks, wheat germ, cod roe, lecithin, sesame seed butter, seeds and nuts, raw goat milk, RNA/DNA.

DRINKS: Pineapple juice/egg yolk/wheat germ/dulse drink; black cherry concentrate/chlorophyll/egg yolk drink.

VITAMINS: B-complex, E, C, choline, inositol, folic acid, pantothenic acid.

MINERALS: Iodine, silicon, phosphorus, calcium, chlorine, magnesium, sodium, potassium, sulphur, iron manganese.

HERBS: Kelp, dulse, ginseng, dong quai, licorice, echinacea, golden seal, dandelion.

DIGESTIVE SYSTEM

STRUCTURE: Gastro-intestinal tract with exception of large colon (eliminative). Salivary glands, liver, gall bladder, and pancreas.

FUNCTION: Mechanical and chemical (enzymatic) breakdown of foods for cellular use.

FOODS: Papaya, liquid chlorophyll, spinach, sun-dried olives, chard, celery, kale, beet greens, whey, shredded beet, watercress, yogurt and kefir.

DRINKS: Parsley juice; papaya juice; chlorophyll; carrot juice; potato peeling broth; whey drinks.

VITAMINS: A, C, B-complex, B-1, B-2, B-6, B-12, D, E, F, K, folic acid, inositol, niacin, pantothenic acid.

MINERALS: Sodium, chlorine, magnesium, potassium, iron, sulphur, copper, silicon, zinc, iodine.

HERBS: Papaya, alfalfa, aloe vera, peppermint, slippery elm, cayenne, burdock, comfrey, ginger, fennel, anise.

CIRCULATORY SYSTEM

STRUCTURE: Heart, blood vessels, blood.

FUNCTION: Distribution of oxygen and nutrients to cells, transportation of CO^2 and wastes from cells, acid-base balance, regulation of body temperature, formation of blood clots.

FOODS: Brewer's yeast, garlic, wheat germ, liquid chlorophyll, alfalfa sprouts, buckwheat, sun-dried olives, watercress, rice polishings.

DRINKS: Blackberry/parsley juice; black fig juice; watercress; parsley/grape juice; hawthorne berry tea.

VITAMINS: B-complex, B-6, niacin, B-12, C, E, bioflavonoids, choline, folic acid, inositol, pangamic acid.

MINERALS: Calcium, iron, silicon, cobalt, copper, magnesium, iodine, phosphorus, potassium, zinc, manganese, nitrogen, fluorine, sulphur.

HERBS: Hawthorne berries, cayenne, ginger, garlic, poke root, sassafras, burdock, chaparral, echinacea, red clover, oatstraw.

NERVOUS SYSTEM

STRUCTURE: Brain; spinal cord; nerves, and sensory organs such as the eye and ear.

FUNCTION: Regulation of body function through nerve impulses. Sensory perception and motor response.

FOODS: Egg yolks, kale, celery, fish, raw goat milk, veal joint broth, cod roe, rice polishings, brewer's and nutritional yeast, tryptophan.

DRINKS: Celery/carrot/prune juice; prune juice/rice polishings; raw goat milk/one teaspoon sesame, sunflower, or almond butter/one teaspoon honey/sliver of avocado; black cherry juice/egg yolk.

VITAMINS: B-complex, A, B-1, B-2, B-6, B-12, B-13, C, D, E, F, choline, folic acid, inositol, niacin, pantothenic acid, pangamic acid.

MINERALS: Calcium, phosphorus, manganese, sulplur, iodine, iron, magnesium, potassium, zinc, fluorine, silicon.

HERBS: Valerian, hops, scullcap, lobelia, lady's slipper.

ELIMINATIVE SYSTEM

STRUCTURE: Large colon.

FUNCTION: Completion of nutrient absorption, manufacture of certain vitamins, formation and elimination of feces.

FOODS: All squash, flaxseed, green and yellow vegetables, yogurt & kefir, alfalfa tablets, acidophilus, bran, clabbered milk, grapes, whey, psyllium seed, berries, sprouts, yellow cornmeal.

DRINKS: Chlorophyll, coconut milk and carrot juice; celery, parsley, spinach, carrot juice; flaxseed tea; black cherry juice.

VITAMINS: A, F, choline, B-complex, B-1, B-2, B-6, B-12, C, E, inositol, niacin, folic acid, pantothenic acid.

MINERALS: Magnesium, potassium, sodium, sulphur, calcium, chlorine, iron, phosphorus.

HERBS: Psyllium seed, aloe vera, cayenne, black walnut, flaxseed, comfrey, slippery elm, cascara sagrada, senna, barberry, golden seal.

URINARY SYSTEM

STRUCTURE: Kidneys, bladder, ureters, urethra.

FUNCTION: Elimination of liquid waste, regulation of chemical composition of blood, fluid and electrolyte balance and volume, maintenance of acid-base balance.

FOODS: Watermelon (including seeds), pomegranate, apples, asparagus, liquid chlorophyll, parsley, green leafy vegetables.

DRINKS: Celery/pomegranate juice; black currant juice/juniper berry tea; pomegranate juice/goat whey; celery/parsley/asparagus juice; beet juice, grapes.

VITAMINS: A, B-complex, B-2, B-6, C, D, E, choline, pantothenic acid.

MINERALS: Calcium, potassium, manganese, silicon, iron, chlorine, magnesium.

HERBS: Juniper berries, uva ursi, parsley, golden seal, slippery elm, elderflowers, ginger, dandelion, marshmallow.

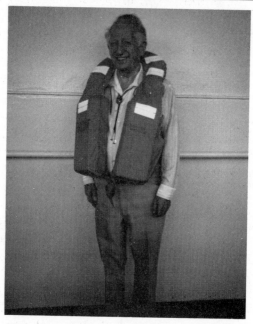

Nutrition—a lifesaving business, as my wife, Marie, and I can tell you.

—16—

What Our Bodies
Do With What We Eat

Breaking down food by chewing and digestion of starches begins in the mouth. Secretion of saliva, an alkaline solution, moistens our food and begins to break down starches. Food must be well chewed to be properly digested, and it is chewing that brings out the saliva. I believe a lot of salivary gland problems have come to people who did not chew their foods well in the past. It isn't until our food reaches the stomach that protein digestion starts. The stomach churns and mixes our food with pepsin and hydrochloric acid in the first step of protein digestion. Food is processed in the stomach for 2-3 hours, while small amounts of mixed finely broken-down food particles enter the duodenum of the small intestine through the pylorus valve at the bottom of the stomach every few seconds.

Thorough chewing of foods helps us get more of the good out of them. We must have good teeth. If you have missing teeth or a poorly-fitting bridge, you are not chewing well. This can lead to digestive disturbances. Bolting down food like a starving animal means that some foods will be incompletely broken down and incompletely assimilated. When we chew our foods well, we aid digestion and assimilation, building a better, healthier body.

When our food reaches the duodenum of the small intestine, it is called chyme. Pancreas and liver secretions are released into the bowel, and other digestive enzymes come from glands in the bowel wall. These substances complete the process of breaking down proteins, carbohydrates and fats as they can be taken into the bloodstream through the bowel wall. Millions of villi, tiny fingerlike projections, line the wall of the small intestine. Digested food particles are absorbed by these villi, from which they enter the bloodstream. What remains after this is indigestible fiber, cellular wastes and food residues. The wastes pass through the ileocecal valve into the colon or large intestine.

The main job of the large intestine is to extract water from the waste before it is eliminated and absorb the water back into the body. But we find that toxic materials can also be absorbed through the bowel wall if proper eating and lifestyle habits are not followed.

Food is moved along the length of the bowel by rhythmic wave-like motions. The importance of fiber in the diet is that it gives the bowel some bulk to push against. Bulk helps develop muscle tone and keeps the bowel clean and regular. Without enough fiber in our foods, bowel contents move too slowly, allowing toxic materials, fats and cholesterol to be reabsorbed into the body. A healthy bowel contains millions of friendly bacteria, fungi, yeast and viral organisms, from 400 to 500 varieties. Some varieties of bacteria produce some of the B vitamins. Other organisms assist in keeping the bowel wall clean. Gas-producing, putrefactive bacteria begin to take over in an underactive, constipated bowel as a direct result of poor food habits, too little exercise and an unwise lifestyle. The toxic waste products of these undesirable bacteria pollute the bowel, invade the bloodstream and create conditions favorable for disease.,

Everything taken into the bloodstream is brought to the liver where it is detoxified and prepared for assimilation before being sent to the cells. *The liver is the great detoxifier of the body.*

THE IMPORTANCE OF A PLEASANT MEALTIME

Because the nerves to the digestive system are associated with nerves that deal with the emotions, it is very important that mealtime be a calm, relaxing and pleasant time.

The table is no place to argue or discipline the children. This interferes with the digestion of everyone present and creates nerve acids. It can also cause a nervous condition called spastic colon and may cause constipation.

Normally, we will have a bowel movement after every meal, triggered by the peristalsis which accompanies digestion, unless we have been trained differently or unless we have allowed sluggish bowel habits to develop.

17

Analytical Food Guide

The following chart has taken many long hours to put together, but it might be interesting to see how each food is earmarked for the various parts of the body.

We have drugs that are earmarked for the kidneys, the heart, for pain of various types, for tranquilizing effects and for stimulation, for reducing, for hormonal balance, for internal fevers and so forth.

We also have foods and herbs that are earmarked for various organs that can actually accomplish the same thing. While they may take more time, it might be well to realize that as we live with these things, all things will be taken care of. In other words, the kidneys will be fed; the heart will be nourished; the bowel will eliminate on time; our brain will be fed with the nerve foods and so forth. So, we find we have to know that all foods have their effect on the nourishment, on the replenishment of tissue broken down and for the regeneration of new tissue to take the place of the old.

Food & Type	Predominant Chemical Elements	Best Way Prepared and Served for Digestion	Remedial Measures
Almond Nuts Protein Fat	Manganese Phosphorus	Serve with vegetables or fruits. Almonds, celery, and apple: a complete meal.	Muscle, brain and nerve food. Best of nuts to use.
Apples Mineral Carbohydrate	Potassium Sodium Magnesium	Wash, eat alone, in salads or with proteins. Give to children in between meals.	Apple skins used for tea. Fine for kidney and urinary tract.
Apricots Mineral Carbohydrate	Potassium Phosphorus Iron Silicon Copper	Use only fresh or dried (unsulphured), alone, with whipped cream, or in salads. Make into apricot whip, add flaked nuts.	Good for anemia, constipation and catarrh.
Artichokes Mineral Carbohydrate	Iodine Potassium Iron Silicon	Wash and steam. Use as cooked vegetable.	Good for soft bulk and minerals and general body builder.
Asparagus Mineral Carbohydrate	Calcium Iron Silicon	Cut tender portion from woody base. Remove scales if sandy. Cut up fine and steam.	Good for kidney and bladder disorders.

226

Avocado
Mineral
Fat

Chlorine
Phosphorus
Sulphur

Wash and peel. Eat alone, have in salads and soups. Good in sandwich filling. Goes well in any combination.

Body builder. Because of its non-irritating consistency it is good for colitis, ulcers. Patients can use as natural oil and bulk in intestines. Slightly laxative and good mineralizer for the body.

Banana
Carbohydrate

Potassium
Calcium
Chlorine

Buy when spotted and no green tops. Wash. Eat alone or in salads, serve as a starch. Eat dead-ripe or baked.

Good for gaining weight. Used as natural bulk for irritated bowels, such as colitis, ulcers or diarrhea.

Barley
Carbohydrate
Protein

Potassium
Silicon

Use unpearled. Wash, steam and serve as a starch, alone or in soups.

For gaining weight. Excellent for children up to ten years for silicon content.

Bass
Protein

Phosphorus
Chlorine
Iodine

Broil, bake or steam. Serve with natural sauces, or lemon.

Brain and nerve food. Use head, fins, and tail in broth for nerves and glands. Refer to Broths.

Beans, Lima
Carbohydrate
Protein

Potassium
Phosphorus
Calcium
Iron

Shell and wash fresh limas, steam or use in vegetable and protein loaves.

Pureed for stomach ulcers. Good muscle-building food.

227

Food & Type	Predominant Chemical Elements	Best Way Prepared and Served for Digestion	Remedial Measures
Beans, String Mineral Carbohydrate	Manganese Nitrogen	Wash, remove ends and strings. Cut once lengthwise and cut crosswise in one-inch strips. Steam.	Good body mineralizer.
Beef Protein	Phosphorus Potassium Chlorine	Should be broiled or roasted. Serve with green vegetables and tomatoes or grapefruit.	Brain and nerve food. Good in anemia, especially for those over twenty, and for those who use up surplus energies.
Beets Mineral Carbohydrate	Potassium Fluorine Chlorine	Cut off leaves, leaving one-inch stems. Steam. Also shred and steam for variation.	Beet juice when combined with blackberry juice is a good blood builder. Use leaves like spinach.
Beet Greens Mineral Carbohydrate	Potassium Magnesium Iodine Iron	Clean and wash thoroughly. Use stems if tender. Cut up fine and steam like spinach.	Body mineralizer.
Blackberries Mineral Carbohydrate	Potassium Magnesium Iodine Iron	Wash and serve alone, with other fruit, or with protein.	Blood builder. Used for dysentery or diarrhea. Good for anemia.
Blueberries Mineral Carbohydrate	Potassium Calcium Magnesium	Wash and serve alone, with other fruit, or with protein.	Blood purifier and body mineralizer.
Bread, Whole Wheat Protein Carbohydrate	Phosphorus Chlorine Calcium Silicon	To be eaten once a day with raw vegetable juices and salads. Sandwiches allowed but vegetable filling should be used.	When used discriminately, good for teeth, muscles, bones and anemia.

228

Broccoli Mineral Carbohydrate	Potassium	Remove tough leaves, tough part of stalk. Wash thoroughly and steam.	Body mineralizer.
Butter, Cow Fat Mineral	Sodium Calcium Chlorine	Eaten on toast and served with cooked vegetables in moderation. Use sweet butter.	Good for eyes and supplying vitamin A, if not used in excess. Easiest fat to digest.
Buttermilk Mineral Protein	Sodium Calcium Chlorine	Best with citrus fruit or protein.	Good for diarrhea, gas, intestinal gas normalizer, and for acidity.
Brussels Sprouts Carbohydrate	Potassium Calcium Sulphur	Remove wilted leaves. Leave whole. Wash and soak in salt water 30 minutes. Steam.	Good mineralizer.
Cabbage Mineral Carbohydrate	Potassium Sodium	Remove wilted outside leaves. Cut in fourths. Wash, soak in salt water. Boil seven minutes in uncovered pot. Also use raw in salad.	Good mineralizer.
Carrots Mineral Carbohydrate	Potassium Calcium Sulphur Silicon	Clean with vegetable brush. Shred fine, use in salads, raw or steamed. A raw whole carrot daily develops children's teeth and and jaws.	Eye food. Good for hair, nails. Easy to digest. One of the best foods to break a fast. Shred finely.

Food & Type	Predominant Chemical Elements	Best Way Prepared and Served for Digestion	Remedial Measures
Casaba Mineral Carbohydrate	Potassium Sodium Chlorine Iron Silicon	Eat like other melons. Fill center with berries or sour cream. Good on hot afternoons.	Blood cleanser and cooler.
Cauliflower Mineral Carbohydrate	Potassium Calcium Sulphur Silicon	Remove leaves and woody base. Break flowers apart. Soak in salt water thirty minutes. Steam.	Good intestinal cleanser.
Celery Mineral Carbohydrate	Chlorine Sodium Potassium Magnesium	Best eaten raw or in vegetable juice. May also be used steamed or in vegetable broth.	For arthritis, neuritis, rheumatism, acidity, high blood pressure, and for nerves. Use in juice form in good health and for every disease. Good blood cleanser.
Chayote Mineral Carbohydrate	Potassium Magnesium Silicon	Wash, peel, cube, or slice and steam.	Non-fattening and a good mineralizer.
Cheese, Cow *Cottage* Protein	Calcium Phosphorus Chlorine	Eaten as protein. Always serve with fruit and vegetables.	Hard to digest, but good source of complete protein. Dry or Farmer Style best.
Cheese, Goat *Cottage* Protein	Calcium Phosphorus Fluorine Chlorine	Always serve with fruit or vegetables.	Has fluorine in abundance. Good for bones, teeth, beauty, especially for children.

Cheese
Roquefort
Protein

Calcium
Phosphorus
Fluorine
Chlorine

Always serve with fruit or vegetables.

Has fluorine in abundance. Good for bones and teeth.

Cheese,
Swiss
Protein

Calcium
Phosphorus
Chlorine
Sodium

Always serve with fruit or vegetables.

Good body builder.

Cherries,
Wild Black
Mineral
Carbohydrate

Potassium
Iron
Magnesium

Eat alone or serve with protein.

For anemia, catarrh. Use one glass for three days in succession twice a month for chronic gall bladder trouble.

Chervil
Mineral
Carbohydrate

Potassium
Iron
Phosphorus
Sulphur

An herb eaten with salads, vegetables, protein, or carbohydrates

Body mineralizer.

Chicken
Protein

Phosphorus
Potassium
Chlorine

Serve with non-starch vegetables and tomatoes or grapefruit.

231

Food & Type	Predominant Chemical Elements	Best Way Prepared and Served for Digestion	Remedial Measures
Chicory Mineral Carbohydrate	Iron Sulphur Chlorine Potassium	A green to be served in salad.	Body mineralizer.
Chinese Cabbage Mineral Carbohydrate	Sodium Calcium Magnesium Iron	Serve raw or in salad, or prepared like cabbage.	Body mineralizer.
Chives Mineral Carbohydrate	Potassium Calcium Sulphur	Served in salads, with vegetables, or in cottage cheese.	Body mineralizer, good for catarrh.
Coconuts Protein Fat Mineral	Potassium Magnesium Phosphorus Chlorine	Milk and coconut meat eaten with fresh or diced fruit or vegetables.	Body builder and for weight building. Good for bones and teeth.
Corn Carbohydrate Protein	Potassium Phosphorus Silicon	Remove husk and silks with a stiff brush. Steam. Eat with green vegetables. Yellow corn better than white corn.	A great brain, bone, and muscle building food.
Cranberries Minerals Carbohydrate	Calcium Sulphur Chlorine	Eat with proteins.	Use as pack in rectum for hemorrhoids.
Cream, Cow Fat	Calcium Phosphorus Fluorine	Eat with fruit or vegetables.	Weight builder. Put on chapped or sunburned skin.

Food	Elements	Preparation	Benefits
Cucumbers Mineral Carbohydrate	Potassium Calcium Phosphorus Silicon Iron	Eaten in salad. Serve with a starch or protein.	Good for skin troubles, and for blood cooling.
Currants, *Black* Mineral Carbohydrate	Phosphorus Magnesium Potassium	Used as a sweet dried fruit; juice of fresh currants makes a refreshing drink.	Blood builder.
Dandelion *Greens* Mineral Carbohydrate	Potassium Calcium Manganese Chlorine	Discard greens with bud or blossoms as they are bitter. Cut off roots. Clean and wash thoroughly. Mix with sweet vegetables. Eat raw in salad or steam.	Cleanse liver and gall bladder. Body mineralizer.
Dates, Dry Carbohydrate	Chlorine	Wash, eat alone, or with sub-acid fruits or vegetables. Candy substitute.	Good for undernourishment.
Duck Protein	Potassium Phosphorus Chlorine	Broil or roast. Serve with green vegetables and grapefruit or tomatoes.	An easy protein to digest.
Eggplant Mineral Carbohydrate	Potassium Phosphorus Chlorine	With protein or starch as a vegetable. Wash, steam or bake whole, sliced or cubed. May be stuffed or used in roasts and loaves.	Good form of bulk. Good mineralizer.

233

Food & Type	Predominant Chemical Elements	Best Way Prepared and Served for Digestion	Remedial Measures
Egg Yolk, Raw Mineral Fat Protein	Sulphur Chlorine Iodine Iron	Slowly cook, never fry, and serve with green vegetables, grapefruit, tomatoes, or fruit.	Excellent food for children. Brain, nerve, and gland food.
Endive Mineral Carbohydrate	Potassium Calcium Sulphur	Wash and serve in salads.	Body mineralizer.
Figs, Black Carbohydrate	Potassium Magnesium	Wash and eat alone, or with fruits. Good candy substitute.	A natural laxative. Good for constipation. Fig juice is a drink when acid fruit juice cannot be taken.
Grapefruit, *Fresh* Mineral Carbohydrate	Sodium Potassium Calcium	Eaten alone, or with fruit or protein. Buy grapefruit when it has a brownish-yellow cast.	For fevers and reducing. Blood cooling, and catarrh eliminator.
Grapes Mineral Carbohydrate	Potassium Magnesium	Wash and serve alone or with other fruit or protein. Concord grapes are best.	Blood purifier. Grape diet once or twice every year should be taken. Good for intestinal cleansing. Especially good in all catarrhal conditions.
Halibut, *Smoked* Protein	Phosphorus Potassium Chlorine	Serve with green vegetables and grapefruit or tomatoes. Steam, bake or broil.	Good source of complete protein. Good source of brain and nerve fat.

Honey
Carbohydrate

Potassium
Calcium
Phosphorus

Because it is a concentrated sweet, use starches and green vegetables.

Honey in conjunction with onions makes good cough syrup when allowed to stand overnight. Eucalyptus honey is good for throat ailments.

Horseradish
Mineral
Carbohydrate

Sulphur
Fluorine
Potassium

Used in seasoning salads, salad dressings, sandwich filling and sauces.

Gall bladder and liver cleanser. Body mineralizer.

Kale
Mineral
Carbohydrate

Calcium
Potassium

With green vegetables in salad. Wash, cut fine, and use raw, or in soups.

Green kale broth for supplying body calcium. Best source of calcium. Makes teeth and bones hard. Body mineralizer.

Kohlrabi
Mineral
Carbohydrate

Calcium
Magnesium
Potassium

Wash, peel, then cube, slice, or shred, and steam.

Body mineralizer.

Lamb
Protein

Potassium
Phosphorus
Chlorine

Bake or broil. Serve with green vegetables and tomatoes or grapefruit.

Good source of protein. Brain, gland, nerve food.

Food & Type	Predominant Chemical Elements	Best Way Prepared and Served for Digestion	Remedial Measures
Leeks Mineral Carbohydrate	Sodium Calcium	With green vegetables. Wash and use in salads.	Good for catarrhal conditions. Body mineralizer.
Lemons Mineral Carbohydrate	Calcium Magnesium Potassium	To be used alone as a drink or in salads served with a protein meal. Use instead of vinegar. Cuts sweetness of grape juice when added.	Catarrh elimination. Best used in fevers and liver disorders. Used in douches, enemas. High in lime salts. Blood cooler and weight reducer. Good germicidal agent. Use as a skin bleach.
Lentils Protein Carbohydrate	Phosphorus Potassium	To be served with a green salad. Soak and cook until soft.	Muscle builder. Good when pureed for stomach ulcers and colitis.
Lettuce, Head Mineral Carbohydrate	Sodium Calcium Chlorine Potassium Iron	Wash well and use in salads. Green outside leaves are always best.	Slows up digestion. Good for sleeplessness. In severe gas conditions stop using in diet.
Lettuce, Romaine Mineral Carbohydrate	Calcium Sodium Potassium Chlorine	With green vegetables, in raw salads, with starches or proteins.	Mineralizer of the body.,
Lettuce, Sea Mineral Carbohydrate	Iodine Potassium Phosphorus Iron	Use powdered over salads, in drinks, or sprinkled on steamed vegetables.	Good source of iodine.

236

Limes Mineral Carbohydrate	Calcium Magnesium Potassium	To be used in a drink or on salads served with a protein meal.	Limes in whey, good as a blood cooler. Marvelous in congestion of the brain.
Mangoes Mineral Carbohydrate	Potassium Calcium Chlorine	Eaten like melons or served in salads.	Good for irritated intestinal disorders.
Milk, Cow Protein	Calcium Sodium Phosphorus	To be served with fruits. Served as a protein.	Complete protein. Use on eyes as a pack for inflammation.
Milk, Goat Protein	Sodium Fluorine Calcium Phosphorus	Use in place of cow milk. Always have raw.	Better source of fluorine than cow milk. Easier digested than cow milk. Use raw.
Mushrooms Mineral Protein Carbohydrate	Potassium Phosphorus Iodine	Used as flavoring in meat substitutes, roasts, and in sauces.	Body mineralizer.
Muskmelon Mineral Carbohydrate	Sodium Potassium Silicon	Eat alone or with protein, or cut up in salads with other fruit.	Good mineralizer, blood cooler. Use instead of artificial soft drink.

237

Food & Type	Predominant Chemical Elements	Best Way Prepared and Served for Digestion	Remedial Measures
Mustard Greens Mineral Carbohydrate	Sulphur Potassium Calcium Magnesium	Wash thoroughly, cut fine, and use in salads, or steam as a green vegetable. May be mixed with other greens.	Good body mineralizer, or source of calcium. Good liver and gall bladder cleanser.
Oats, *Steel Cut* Mineral Carbohydrate	Silicon Iodine Magnesium	Use with green vegetables, or raw salad. Must be well cooked. Soak before cooking.	Excellent children's food, especially when they lack silicon. Good source of silicon.
Okra Mineral Carbohydrate	Sodium Chlorine	Wash pods. Cut off stems. Use in broth and soups or steam. Serve separately with butter.	Good for stomach ulcers, irritated intestinal tract. Use in all broths for stomach disorders.
Olives Mineral Fat	Potassium Phosphorus	Serve with green vegetables, raw salad, or fruit.	Best source of potassium. Good brain and nerve food found in oil.
Onions, White Mineral Carbohydrate	Sulphur Potassium	Peel onions under water to keep eyes from watering. Serve cooked or raw in salads.	Good for all catarrhal, bronchial, and lung disorders.
Oranges Mineral Carbohydrate	Potassium Calcium Sodium Magnesium	To be used alone, with nuts, raw egg yolk, or with a protein meal.	Good to stir up acids, catarrhal settlements and hard mucous.

238

Papaya Mineral Carbohydrate	Sodium Magnesium Sulphur Chlorine	Eat as a melon or serve in salads.	Good for stomach and intestinal disorders, especially the seeds made into a tea.
Parsnips Mineral Carbohydrate	Calcium Potassium Silicon	Wash, clean with stiff brush, cube, slice, or grate and steam.	Body mineralizer.
Parsley Mineral Carbohydrate	Calcium Potassium Sulphur Iron	Eaten raw with salads, meats, soups, and vegetables. Used as tea, and in raw vegetable juice.	Good for diabetes, for cleansing the kidneys, for controlling calcium in the body. Body mineralizer.
Peaches Mineral Carbohydrate	Calcium Phosphorus Potassium	Eaten alone, or in fruit salads with protein meal.	Good bowel regulator. Body mineralizer and blood builder.
Peanuts Protein Fat Carbohydrate	Phosphorus Silicon Potassium	Eaten with green leafy salad. Raw peanuts are best.	Hard to digest.
Pears Mineral Carbohydrate	Sodium Phosphorus	Eaten alone or in fruit salads with protein meals.	Good body mineralizer. Good intestinal regulator.

239

Food & Type	Predominant Chemical Elements	Best Way Prepared and Served for Digestion	Remedial Measures
Peas, Garbanzo Protein Carbohydrate	Magnesium Phosphorus	Eaten as protein. Cook as dried beans, such as lentils and navy beans. Soak before cooking.	Good source of vegetable protein.
Peas, Fresh Carbohydrate Mineral	Magnesium Calcium Chlorine	Shell and wash. Steam or use in broth. The pods also are good to use in broth with peas.	Body mineralizer.
Pecans Protein Fat	Phosphorus Calcium Potassium	Best eaten with green vegetables or fruit, or flaked on breakfast fruits.	Good nut protein. Used in weight building with celery and apples.
Persimmons Mineral Carbohydrate	Phosphorus Calcium	Eaten with other fresh fruit, protein, or alone.	Good body mineralizer. Good for irritable intestinal tract.
Pineapple Mineral Carbohydrate	Sodium Calcium Magnesium Iodine	Eaten alone, with other fresh fruit, as in salad, or with protein.	Good for sore throat, catarrhal conditions, good blood builder, aids digestion.
Plums Mineral Carbohydrate	Magnesium	Eaten with other fresh fruit, alone, or with protein.	Good laxative and bowel regulator.
Pomegranate Mineral Carbohydrate	Sodium Magnesium	Squeeze out juice and drink very fresh.	Pomegranate juice with whey is good in brain and nerve congestion, and is a blood cleanser. Pomegranate juice is beneficial in bladder complaints.

Popcorn Carbohydrate	Phosphorus	May be eaten with green leafy vegetable salad and a cream dressing.	Good for intestinal roughage.
Potato, Baked Mineral Carbohydrate	Potassium Phosphorus Magnesium Silicon	Clean with a stiff brush. Parboil two minutes. Butter skins and bake in slow oven.	Best source of starch. Use potato peeling in broths. Use for poultices.
Prunes Mineral Carbohydrate	Potassium Phosphorus Magnesium	Wash, place in clean water, bring to boil, and let stand overnight. Use as dried fruit for breakfast, whipped for a dessert, or in salads.	Good bowel regulator. Good source of nerve salts.
Pumpkin Carbohydrate	Sodium Iron Phosphorus	Eat with vegetable meal. Can be made into custards.	Body builder.
Radishes, Black Mineral Carbohydrate	Potassium Phosphorus Magnesium	Use as seasoning.	Has Raphanon which is extremely good in gall bladder and liver disorders.
Radishes, Red Mineral Carbohydrate	Potassium Phosphorus Magnesium	Use raw in salads, with green vegetables and starches.	Good source of sulphur. Good for catarrh.

241

Food & Type	Predominant Chemical Elements	Best Way Prepared and Served for Digestion	Remedial Measures
Raisins Mineral Carbohydrate	Potassium Phosphorus Chlorine	With vegetables, starch, or protein. Wash well. Soak. Use in cereals for sweetening or in salads.	Concentrated sweet. Good body builder and good energy food.
Raspberries Mineral Carbohydrate	Sodium Iron	Wash well. Serve alone or with fruit or protein.	Blood mineralizer. Neutralizes acidity. Good for anemia.
Rice, Natural Brown Carbohydrate	Phosphorus Sodium	Steam and serve with green vegetables.	Good body building food. Good for bones, teeth, etc.
Rye, Whole Carbohydrate	Phosphorus Magnesium Silicon	Use with raw green vegetables.	Good source of silicon.
Spinach Mineral Carbohydrate	Potassium Silicon	Cut off roots and dead leaves. Wash, cut fine, and use raw or steamed.	Body mineralizer.
Squash Carbohydrate Mineral	Sodium Magnesium	Cut into pieces, or leave whole, and bake or steam.	Body builder, and bowel regulator.
Strawberries Mineral Carbohydrate	Calcium Sodium	Wash, and use fresh with or without fruit or protein.	Acid neutralizer when eaten ripe.

Swiss Chard
Mineral — Sodium, Calcium, Magnesium, Iron
Carbohydrate

Wash thoroughly. Cut up in one inch pieces. Steam. Tender sections may be used raw in salads.

Body mineralizer.

Tomatoes
Mineral — Potassium, Sodium, Chlorine
Carbohydrate

Use only ripest tomatoes. Use in salads, broths, or steamed. Use with proteins.

Consider canned tomatoes best. Always use with a protein. Use also in packs and poultices.

Turnips
Mineral — Potassium, Calcium
Carbohydrate

Wash and shred. Use raw in salads or serve steamed.

Body builder. White turnip juice good for asthma, sore throat and bronchial disorders.

Turnip Leaves
Mineral — Calcium, Magnesium
Carbohydrate

Serve raw, in salads in vegetable juices, or steam with greens.

Good for controlling calcium in the body.

Walnuts
Protein — Manganese, Phosphorus, Magnesium
Fat

To be used with fruit or vegetables in salads.

Black walnuts are best source of brain and nerve manganese food.

Watercress
Mineral — Sulphur, Chlorine, Calcium
Carbohydrate

Wash well and use as salad green or garnish.

Body mineralizer.

Food & Type	Predominant Chemical Elements	Best Way Prepared and Served for Digestion	Remedial Measures
Watermelon Mineral Carbohydrate	Silicon Calcium Sodium	Use in fruit salads and protein meals, or serve alone.	Good for kidneys. Blood cooler, and good source of silicon.
Wheat, Whole Carbohydrate	Phosphorus Silicon	Used in breads and cereals. Chew well, because starches must be mixed well with saliva in mouth to be digested properly.	Body builder of bone and teeth, especially for children. Best used in dry forms to promote vigorous chewing.
Whey Mineral Protein	Sodium Calcium Chlorine	Add fruit juices to whey and drink two or three times daily between meals, drink alone, or with meals.	Good source of mineral salts. Easy to digest, good blood builder. Important culture for the friendly bacteria in the intestinal tract.
Zucchini Mineral Carbohydrate	Potassium	Wash, cut into pieces. Steam as vegetable or cut up raw in salads.	Body mineralizer.

18

You Deserve the Best

In the many categories of foods and types of foods, there are a few that stand out as the very best. Here are some of them.

Best Proteins. Eggs, milk (raw), fish (white meat with fins and scales), cheese (hard cheese that crumbles), poultry, lamb, lean beef, nuts, seeds, lentils.

Best Carbohydrates. Brown rice, yellow cornmeal, millet, rye, sweet potatoes, yams, bananas, oatmeal (steel cut), baked potato, barley, wheat, buckwheat.

Best Sweets. Honey, maple syrup, maple sugar, fruit concentrates, dried fruits, fresh sweet fruits, carob powder.

Best Oils. Avocado, safflower, soybean, sesame, sunflower, apricot seed, olive oil, corn, almond, linseed, pumpkin and wheat germ oil. Try to have raw and uncooked.

Best Drinks. Whey, vegetable juices, green drinks, herb teas, soymilk, almond milk, sesame milk, fruit juices (except citrus), buttermilk (occasionally), raw goat milk, blender drinks.

Best Salad Vegetables. Leaf lettuce (no head lettuce), carrots (grated), beets (grated), celery, cucumbers, parsley, watercress, green onions, green bell peppers, zucchini, tomatoes, sliced radishes, raw spinach, cauliflower, young peas, parsnips (grated), turnips (grated), sprouts. The outside leaves of our green leafy vegetables such as lettuce and cabbage are highest in calcium, chlorophyll and other nutrients. They are the best part.

Best Salads. Cole slaw, mixed greens topped with grated carrot, beet, etc., fruit salad, shredded carrot and raisin, potato salad, gelatin salad, Waldorf salad.

Best Salad Dressings. Bleu cheese, Roquefort, vinegar and oil, avocado, nut butter, oil and lemon with honey, mayonnaise with

245

seasoning, yogurt, vinegar and caraway seeds, vinegar and oil with raw egg yolk, fruit concentrates (for children).

Best Legumes and Beans. Lentils, lima beans, soybeans, peas, garbanzos, black beans, split peas, pinto beans, fava beans, aduki beans, kidney beans, blackeyed peas, horse beans.

Best Herbs (and foods they are best used with). Mint (fruit, lamb, vegetables), thyme (meat, sauces, stocks, fish, most vegetables), rosemary (lamb, duck, veal and vegetables), basil (tomatoes, fish, eggs), dill (salads, vegetables, potatoes), sage (sparingly with meats and cheeses), bay leaves (soups and sauces), parsley, caraway, savory and marjoram.

Best Seasonings. Vegetable broth powder, cayenne pepper, paprika, nutmeg, carob, cinnamon, ginger, poppy seed, allspice, vanilla and almond extracts, kelp, dulse.

Best Soups. Vegetable soup, borsch, onion soup, split pea, potato, miso, barley and mushroom, lentil.

Best Nuts. Almond, Missouri black walnut, cashews, pignolias, pecans, coconut, hazelnuts.

Best Seeds. (Butters or finely ground) Sesame, sunflower, squash, pumpkin, melon (put in blender with water, strain out hulls), chia, alfalfa.

Best Fruits. Peaches, bananas, apples, pears, berries, pineapples, apricots, nectarines, avocados, papayas, mangoes, cherries, persimmons, grapes, plums, melons.

Best Dried Fruits (unsulphured). Black Monnuka raisins, prunes, figs, dates, apricots, peaches, pears, apples, pineapples, bananas.

Best Herb Teas. Alfalfa and mint, comfrey, lemon grass, oat straw, chamomile, papaya, cornsilk, hawthorne berry, parsley, blueberry, KB-11 (diuretic tea), shavegrass.

This is a shortened version of a section of my book *Creating A Magic Kitchen.*

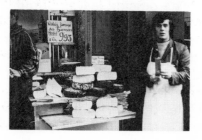

Markets of France. Cheese is considered a protein, high in calcium, but an excess can lead to cholestrol deposits in the body.

─────19─────
Summer
and
Winter Foods

One of the great ideas I have followed in my work is how to make foods act as our medicine. We should be well and happy, but most of us are not because we don't have the right food knowledge. In this chapter, I want to share some fascinating food facts with you, so you can see a little farther along the path to better health.

We find that the world of foods always has somethig nice to teach us if we are open to a new and better way.

When we stop and think about it, our bodies were designed to eat seasonal foods. It is only in the past century that man has had transportation, distribution and preservation technologies capable of making many foods available all year round. For several thousand years before that, man had to eat what was locally available by season or what could be kept by primitive preservation ways such as sun drying, keeping in root cellars or smoking.

SUMMER FOODS AND HEALTH IDEAS

Summer is preparation time for winter. The abundance of available fruits and vegetables allows us to cleanse the body and build up our stores of minerals, especially calcium. Calcium is the chemical element for healing, strength, stamina and long life. Outdoor activity and summer sports expose us to the sunlight that makes vitamin D in our bodies, the vitamin that controls calcium. We need plenty of calcium to carry us through the Fall, Winter and Spring.

The warm summer weather brings on perspiration, and the fruit acids and vitamins clean out last year's toxins. We build and rejuvenate our tissues for the coming winter. We should have as many of our summer fruits and vegetables as possible in their natural raw state so we can get the most good out of them. Fruits thin the blood and bring on elimination, but vegetables are more cooling.

Have plenty of salads in the summer in unlimited combinations. Those who have digestive difficulties should take raw vegetable juices before a meal of cooked vegetables, preferably cut finely or shredded to shorten cooking times. If you need fiber, try liquefying raw vegetables or steaming until slightly done and still a little crisp.

Use plenty of tops of root vegetables—beet greens, turnip greens and so forth. Plant a little herb garden to season them.

Make protein salad dressings such as yogurt, roquefort and bleu cheese to keep the summer fruit you are eating from becoming too much of an elimination program.

Avoid heavy starches such as barley and rye, and don't eat much of the dried fruits in summer.

Sodium (organic) is the "cooler" in the body. Whey and celery drinks are nicely cooling and should be taken by all who perspire freely. Lime juice and whey make a refreshing drink that cools the blood and brings down the blood pressure.

Use vegetable broth powder instead of table salt to help the body keep from "holding" too much water. Salt tends to attract water. Surprisingly, hot drinks cool the body better than cold ones. All iced drinks are hard on the stomach.

There are several common mistakes people make in the summer. At the top of the list is eating ice cream, which heats the blood. Ice cream is primarily a winter food. Artificial ice cream robs the body of calcium, which we need to be storing up for winter. Drinking iced drinks of any kind is the second mistake. Iced drinks interfere with digestion.

Another common error is letting the body dry off in a cool or cold wind after a swim.

Avoid extreme glare from the sun reflecting off water, as it is hard on the eyes.

WINTER FOOD WISDOM

Our wintertime objectives will be completely different from those of summer, and traditional seasonal foods give us something

248

to think about. In centuries past, dried fruits, seeds, nuts, grains, legumes, potatoes, meat, poultry and fish were the winter staples of the diet. These are foods that heat the blood and help the body keep warm. In cold winters, we spend more energy keeping warm and doing work than in summers. We wear heavy clothing, which prevents the skin from eliminating as it should. We get less sunshine, so we may have to take a little cod liver oil.

Cod liver oil has both vitamins A and D. To build the blood, we also need vitamin C, bone marrow capsules, liquid chlorophyll, bone meal and lecithin. We could use an all-around vitamin and mineral supplement at this time of year.

Winter is a time for hearty soups, heated blender drinks, hot cereals in the morning, baked potatoes, yams and sweet potatoes. Winter squash is good, and a hot baked apple with cinnamon and raisins is a special treat for dessert. We should still keep up our salads and green vegetables, not so much because they are heating, but because of the fiber and mineral values. Eggs are a good winter protein because of the fat content along with it, but we must have them boiled or poached to keep the food value.

Nuts are a good winter food, and they can be used in casseroles as well as eaten plain or ground into meal and sprinkled on other foods. Don't eat too many, since they are high in oils (but not cholesterol).

Rye and barley are good heating cereals for winter.

Barley and green kale soup is one of the best winter soups, high in calcium. (See recipe in other chapter.) Kale is available frozen.

Another good winter soup is Borsch. Vegetable soups to which a little cream is added after cooking are also good. You may add nut butters or seed butters to any soup to make it a good winter, health-building protein soup. Seed and nut butters should be added at the table. Do not cook them.

In winter, it is well to avoid rushing from a warm house to a low temperature outdoors. Move slowly; dress warmly. Avoid heavy outdoor perspiration from hard work and sudden chill from ceasing work while still standing in the cold. Keep the feet, hands and head warm and dry.

Most doctors will tell you that March is the worst month for pneumonia, with many deaths each year. Toxins in the body, lack of sunshine and fresh air, breathing stale indoor air and lack of fresh vegetables all take their toll on the body.

Muesli, first popular in Switzerland, is an excellent winter breakfast combination. (Soak raisins for 10 minutes in boiling water before using.)

Muesli

1/2 cup flaked whole (steel-cut) oats
1 tbsp ground almonds
1 tbsp (heaping) dried apricots or apples (cut small)
1 tbsp (heaping) reconstituted raisins
1 tsp date sugar

Add 2/3 cup warm or cold water, raw milk or raw cream. You can add fresh fruit such as bananas, berries, peach, etc.

In the summer time, we can drink more juices, because we need higher sodium foods to take care of perspiration. "Cool as a cucumber," the saying goes. The sodium foods are your cucumbers. They help keep us cool. This is one of the old myths that probably is more true than we give it credit for being. Cucumbers, being high in sodium, will help keep anyone "cool as a cucumber." Strawberries, strawberry juice and all of the fruit juices are high in sodium.

Summer is really a time when we can cleanse more. In winter time, we build and usually put on weight. We are usually more active in the summer. We have longer sunshine days. We wear less clothing and our skin is more active. We're in the sunshine more. We're in the active air. We find that these are all conducive to elimination through the skin in the summer time. If we have not been well, we should plan to get well in the spring and summer months. Those who still have problems at the end of summer should go South like the birds to complete their healing. They can do this best in warm weather.

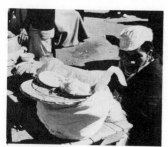

Peru—rice is a food for all seasons, and for all people.

20

The Cook's Department—
Food Tips and Recipes

It is in the hands of the cook that we have the birth of a new nation. It is the hands of the cook that we have the destruction of our bodies. The demineralization, the breakdown of our digestion, the upbuilding of our health. The new body of tomorrow comes from the kitchen. The opportunity we can give our bodies to be regenerated and rejuvenated is in the hands of the cook and Mother. The well and healthy family starts at the kitchen table.

There are many cook books written today, but if we could only realize that possibly someone in these cook books is trying to make a gourmet dinner. Or, if possible, we are trying to see what new mixtures we can put together. We try to see what new brands of foods we can possibly put together. We try to make exotic looking foods with abnormal and synthetic flavors. We use excessive sweets that are detrimental to our bodies; acid producing for instance. We go to the extreme to make things taste good, so that they have that extra flavor, so that you would rather have certain foods than others because of the looks and the taste.

We would like to say that it is the simple meal. It is how close we can have it when it comes out of the garden that means the most. It is right here that the health will be our salvation. But, our salvation is in the hands of the cook. We are going to make things simple, and give simple ideas to follow in your cooking to make the art of cooking more natural, more pure and more whole. You can take any cook book or recipe and substitute the natural things to be used instead of all the processed de-mineralized foods we are using today.

We found that these natural foods abound in every country. That is the reason we have shown the markets that every country has. Is there any reason why we should take these natural foods from the farm, from the garden, from the vine, from the bush, and then take it home and, in the kitchen, destroy it? We demolish all of the natural enzymes, the natural food properties, the mineral elements, the vitamin values - right in our kitchen. Much of our life today is built around the kitchen. The fast food departments have come in and we have tried to see how we can cut down in our work in the kitchen and if we could keep it more simple. I believe we could get out of the kitchen in less time. Some people spend too much time in the kitchen. As we scramble everything together, it is almost impossible for our digestion and our elimination to unscramble it. Our fast foods have given us an inspiration to go out and get a career, to do extra work, to do some of the other things in life that other people are doing. There is a competition that we are trying to keep up with. The Joneses are able to do this, why can't I? So, we find that the kitchen has been neglected in our thinking.

We are going through this suggestive chapter to help us realize that if we are going to have only half of the nutritive values in our kitchen, we are only going to have half a body. We are going to have half the mineral material in our body. So, we are going to have half-body health as the result. We will give some suggestions that you should think about. You could go to any food market and recipe book and see how it should be prepared and eaten in your own home. Make it simple, not too many heavy flavors, no frying and without unnatural processing methods. We must get as natural a food as possible to the table, and then to the body. Good food - natural, pure and whole - is going to be our salvation.

SALADS

Most meals start out with a salad. Salads are usually pretty good in every country in the world. There are many salads and vegetables served throughout the world that could be used in any country. Just remember that the basis of all salads should be raw and as natural as possible. Let us not destroy the value by adding sauces, dressings and so forth that will interfere with that first natural thought we have. While we list salad dressings, we make them simple. As far as salads are concerned, you make up your own combinations. Always consider the seasons. Seasons bring in colors. A salad should always be a rainbow salad. A rainbow has all the chemicals, all the minerals. I will feed the whole body better than any of the other foods that you serve on your table. The salad should be the main part of any meal.

Here are a few suggestions for salad combinations:

FRUIT AND VEGETABLE SALADS

Cabbage and Pecan Nut Salad

1 Cup shredded Raw Cabbage
1/4 Cup freshly grated Coconut
1/4 Cup chopped Pecan Meats
Mayonnaise
Lettuce

Mix the above thoroughly with mayonnaise and serve on the lettuce. Grated turnips may be substituted for the cabbage for variation.

Lettuce and Tomato Salad

2 Cups shredded Lettuce
4 Tablespoons Cream Cheese
1 Hardboiled Egg Yolk
4 ripe Tomatoes
4 Walnut meats

Place the lettuce lightly on salad plate. Cut the tomatoes in eighths and arrange on the lettuce to resemble petals of a flower.

Stuffed Tomato with Cottage Cheese

1 Tomato for each serving
Chopped Celery
Broth Powder
Unpasteurized Cottage Cheese
Spinach leaves, to garnish
Celery curls, to garnish

Stuff one tomato per serving with a mixture of chopped celery and cottage cheese, seasoned with broth powder. Garnish with spinach leaves and celery curls. Add chopped nuts, if desired.

253

Carrot and Raisin Salad

Shred 3 carrots fine and add 1/2 cup raisins. Mix with 1/4 cup mayonnaise and serve on crisp lettuce. Garnish with slices of unpeeled red apple.

Waldorf Salad

3 Delicious Apples
1/4 Cup Mayonnaise
4 sticks Celery
3/4 Cup chopped Walnuts
Lettuce leaves to garnish
Whipped Cream dressing

Dice the apples in 1/4 to 1/2 inch pieces. As they are diced, mix with mayonnaise to keep them from turning brown. Add the celery chopped medium fine. Add nuts last and serve on crisp lettuce leaves with whipped cream dressing.

The Herb-Lover's Salad

Equal parts of: Endive, Escarole, Romaine, Spinach
1 clove Garlic
Chives, minced
Parsley, minced
Firm Tomatoes, sliced
Few sprigs of: Thyme, Tarragon, Marjoram, Mint

Toss together the green leaves of crisp endive, romaine, escarole and the fine tender inner leaves of spinach in your favorite salad bowl, first rubbing bowl with clove of garlic. Mince parsley and chives and add to greens. The choice of herbs may be the small sprigs of marjoram, thyme, mint and tarragon. Choose those whose particular odors tempt you. Slice firm tomatoes and add to the salad. Make a lemon and oil dressing and pour over salad. Toss all together lightly and serve in 20 minutes.

Chinese Salad

1 Cup Beansprouts
1/2 Cup cooked Brown Rice
1 or 2 Apples in small slices
   or equal amount of Chinese Water Chestnuts
1 Cup chopped Celery
1/2 Cup shredded Lettuce

(continued next page)

1/2 Cup Mayonnaise
Radish roses, to garnish

Mix all together with mayonnaise and serve. Garnish with radish roses.

Maroon Salad

6 small Beets, cooked, peeled after cooking
1/2 bunch Watercress
3 hardboiled Eggs
1 head shredded Lettuce
Russian dressing

Grate the beets over shredded lettuce and place slices of hard-boiled eggs on beets. Garnish with watercress. Serve with Russian dressing.

FRUIT SALADS

Avocado in Half Shell

Cut avocado lengthwise and remove the seed. Place on salad plate garnished with watercress and red pepper rings. Serve with lemon juice.

Date Cheese Nut Salad

1-1/2 Cup Dates
1 small head Watercress
1 Cup Pecans, Walnuts, Brazil Nuts, chopped
1/4 Cup Cream Cheese or Cottage Cheese
Juice of one Lemon
2 Teaspoons Olive Oil

Remove the pits from the dates and fill with cream cheese. Place on watercress leaves that have been dipped in lemon juice and olive oil. Place nuts that have stood a short time in lemon juice, between the dates.

Date or Raisin, Apple Celery Salad

2/3 Cup Dates or Raisins, chopped
4 Apples, unpeeled and diced
4 sticks Celery
Romaine leaves

(continued next page)

Green Pepper rings
1/2 Cup Banana dressing

Chop the celery fine. Mix with the apples and dates. Raisins may be substituted for dates. Mix with banana dressing, serve on romaine leaves, garnished with pepper rings.

Carrot Pineapple Liquid Salad

1/2 Cup cubed Celery
1/2 Cup cubed Carrots
1-1/2 glasses Pineapple Juice

Put all through liquefier and serve.

RECIPES FOR SALAD DRESSING

Sour Cream Dressing

1 Cup Sour Cream
1/2 Cup Lemon Juice

Mix together. This dressing is best with fruit salads, but may be used with vegetable salads, too.

Honey Lemon and Cream Dressing

2 Teasponns Lemon Juice
1/2 Cup Sour Cream
1 Teaspoon Honey

Mix lemon and honey until smooth. Add cream and mix well. Proportions may vary according to tart taste and thickness desired. Coconut milk may be used.

French Dressing

1/2 Cup Olive Oil
1/4 Cup Lemon Juice
Juice of one Tomato or 1/4 Cup Tomato Juice

Mix ingredients thoroughly and serve.

Coconut Dressing

1/4 Cup Coconut Milk
2 Teaspoons Honey
1/4 Cup Salad Oil

(continued next page)

Mix ingredients to a paste and serve on salads. Coconut milk may also be used alone as an excellent dressing for lettuce and cucumber salads.

Fruit Dressing

3 Teaspoon Lemon Juice
3 Teaspoon Orange Juice
4 Teaspoon Oil
1 Teaspoon Honey

Mix all ingredients well, pour into a jar and shake well.

Avocado Dressing

1 Avocado
Juice of 1 Orange, Lemon or Papaya

Beat the pulp of the avocado to consistency of whipped cream. Add juice very gradually to season. The juice should be added slowly. Whip with a rotary beater until the consistency of whipped cream.

COOKING FOODS

The cook has the idea that foods have to be cooked. We do not always have to have cooked foods. In our laws that we follow, 60% of our foods should be raw. It is here that we have the natural mineral materials intact. The vitamins are there waiting to be taken into the body. It cannot be destroyed with heat, overheating or with frying. These are destructive methods. I am sometimes afraid of that old saying, that they are a "good cook." Sometimes we can cook too good and destroy the value that we should be getting from our foods.

SOUPS

Soups are found in practically every nation in the world. They all start out as broths. These broths are flavored and additions made, so that we do not get all the natural uncooked material we should. I think the worst thing we can put in soups is the oil, butter and the cream. We destroy the lecithin, fragile elements and vitamins when doing so. Any fat or oil that is cooked should never be in the kitchen. Wonderful is the Russian Borsch, but they use a lot of butter and cream. This should be added to the soup after it is cooked. We do not believe in meat soups as they are high in uric acid. If we want to make a protein soup, we follow the idea of the Chinese. We drop an egg yolk in the soup at the table, or we can take any nut or seed butter and put it in the broth at the table. We have to be careful of seasonings as we cook them. We can destroy all the good. For instance, if we are using honey in cooking, you must put it in the food, if possible, after it is cooked. Cooked honey is not of real value. If we want to sweeten our foods at the table, use dried fruits, finely cut, or date sugar. There are many substitute sugars, and always use them at the table. Finely cut up dried fruit, raisins, etc., can be used. We would use a lot less, and produce less acids in our body by doing so. We go around the world and see many cultures in every country. But I think we have to consider that the stomach needs the same mineral elements, the same care, the same natural minerals in Japan as the stomachs do in Germany or any other country. We have to find out what is right and not who is right. So many of our cultures today have their own individual ideas and it is very difficult for people to get away from French cooking, from Italian pasta, or the tea drinking ceremonies in Britain, or the flavoring of Mexican dishes. The idea is to make it simple, and as pure and natural as we possibly can. Fried foods, for example, are doing the greatest amount of harm throughout the world today. We find that cooking with oils is bringing more sickness and chloresterol problems in this world today than anything else. In many countries, the main dish is meat and potatoes or some heavy solid food. It does not always have to be a heavy solid food. There are many substitutes for meat. We do not always have to have a meat meal to have a complete meal. There are many substitutes for meat.

Barley Soup

2 Cups whole unpearled Barley
1/2 Cup chopped Parsley
1 large Onion
1 Cup chopped Celery

(continued next page)

Cook soaked whole barley about 2 hours. Add vegetables, more water if necessary, and a little vegetable broth powder. Cook until just tender, and serve.

Avocado Cream Soup

Avocado
Warm sweet Milk
Parsley
Celery
Little Brown Rice or Barley, cooked

Soup stock can be used for the base of this soup or you can put in a double boiler to heat, or just use warm milk and enjoy a soup that is not hot, but warm.

You can make a corn soup, carrot, asparagus, spinach and mushroom soup. You can add a little rice flour for thickening. You can make other combinations by using a little butter, beet greens, endive and occasionally some tomato.

Fruit Soup

2 Cups Prune Juice
2 Cups Pineapple Juice, unsweetened
1/2 Cup grated Pineapple
1/2 Cup Lemon Juice
3/4 Cup Honey
1/2 Cup diced Peaches

Serve hot or cold.

Vegetable Soup

1 bunch Celery
1 Pkg. Carrots
4 Potatoes with skins
Cabbage
Onions
Tomatoes

Dice all vegetables to about the same size, using celery green leaves as well as stalks. All or any of the above vegetables may be used. Steam all together for 25 minutes or until fairly tender. Add water to make soup. Stir well and season to taste.

LOAVES

Many people use soy bean loafs and so forth. As a suggestion, we have to be careful about using eggs in these loaves, which have a good deal of fat in them. To keep that fat at a high heat is one of the greatest cholesterol forming foods. We cannot heat oil too much. We cannot use a lot of nuts roasted or heated. Many loaves are really not the best as far as favoring good health. It is better to eat lentils plain that we use in loaves, it is best to keep it by itself and add flavorings such as tomatoes, celery, onions and herbs. Carrot and celery are wonderful additions to be used in loaves, to keep it as simple as possible. We have to remember that our diet must be at a minimum as far as cooked foods are concerned. Fried meats are going to be found to be causing a lot of trouble, even to the place of being cancer-forming from the charring. A good vegetarian has the least amount of cooked foods. Heating foods to no more than a boiling temperature will keep the heat down below 212 degrees. Most loaves are heated to 350 to 400 degrees and for a longer time than they should be. If it is possible in making loaves, use beans you have cooked ahead of time, so that whatever we add in smaller amounts are not cooked as much. It is going to take a lot of natural raw foods to offset all the cooked foods we have today. That is why we should follow the laws as given in our NATURAL FOOD HARMONY REGIME.

You know we should have eggs soft boiled. Never more heat that 212 degrees or boiling water. Always have 2 or 3 vegetables and salad when having most entrees. When we have potatoes, they must be baked, not fried. Fried potatoes and chips are an abomination to our bodies.

PROTEIN AND VEGETABLE DISHES

Baked Vegetable Loaf

1 Onion, chopped
1/2 Cup finely chopped Walnuts, Almonds or Pecans
1 Egg, well beaten
1 Cup Whole Wheat Crumbs, or cooked Rice
1 Tablespoon Tomato Juice or Water
1 Tablespoon Butter

(continued next page)

Mix all ingredients well and pack in greased baking dish. Bake 1/2 hour in moderate oven. Turn over on platter and serve with tomato sauce (homemade and without condiments).

Delicious Vegetable Roast

2 lbs. Spinach
1-1/2 Cups Carrots, grated
1 Onion, chopped
1 Cup Celery, diced
1 Green Pepper, chopped
1 Cup cooked Brown Rice

Mix and steam together, then add 1/2 cup nuts (walnuts, almonds or raw peanuts), chopped well. Mix 2 well-beaten eggs and 1/2 cup oil. Bake the whole mixture in a moderate oven approximately 1/2 hour. Serve with tomato juice or a sauce.

Soybean Loaf

1 Cup cooked Brown Rice
2 Tablespoons Soy Butter or 1 Cup of cooked Soybeans
2 hard-boiled Eggs, mashed
1/2 Cup Tomato Juice
1 Tablespoon Oil
1 heaping Tablesppon Soy Flour
1 Cup toasted, crushed Rye Krisp
1 Tablespoon minced Onions
Vegetized Salt to taste

Mix together well. Put in casserole dish and bake until well set.

Pine Nut Roast

1 Cup Pine Nuts	1 Teaspoon Vegetized Salt
1 Cup cooked Wild Rice	1/2 Cup Milk
1/2 Cup chopped Celery	1 Egg
1 Onion, finely chopped	

Combine ground pine nuts, rice, celery, onion, salt. Over these pour beaten egg and milk. Mix well and bake in oiled casserole 1/2 hour.

EGG RECIPES

Soft-Boiled Eggs

Drop eggs in boiling water with a spoon and cook for 4 minutes for very soft, or 5 minutes for medium soft eggs. Serve with sweet butter. Hard-boiled eggs should be cooked for 20 minutes. If a softer texture is desired, eggs may be coddled; or placed in boiling water, taken off the stove and let stand in the water for 7 minutes. Take out, break into a dish and serve with a little butter and vegetable salt.

Poached Egg

Break the egg into a sauce dish and gently lower into a pan of boiling water. Turn the heat low and let cook with water below the boiling point until done. Lift out and serve with sweet butter. As soon as the egg is put in the water, the pan may be taken off the fire and the egg left for about 7 minutes, then served with butter. This makes a very soft-textured egg.

Poached Eggs A La Jensen

1/2 Teaspoon Vegetable Broth Powder
2 large Eggs
2 Cups Water

Mix broth powder with water and bring to a boil. Break eggs in broth and poach lightly. Remove to dish and serve, garnished with parsley. Eggs may be dotted with butter if desired. Drink broth eggs were cooked in.

Mushroom Omelet

4 Eggs
1 Cup cooked Mushrooms, finely cut
4 Tablespoons raw Sweet Cream
1/2 Teaspoon Vegetized Salt
Parsley to garnish

Beat yolks and whites of eggs separately. Add mushrooms, cream, and salt to yolks. Fold in stiffly beaten egg whites. Pour into oiled pan. Bake in oven on low heat for 15 minutes. Serve garnished with parsley.

Walnut Lentil Loaf

1 Cup Lentils
1 Cup chopped Walnuts
1/2 Cup chopped Celery
1 small Onion, cut fine
1 Teaspoon Vegetized Salt
1 Egg
1/2 Cup Milk

Combine lentils, walnuts, celery, onion, salt. Over these pour milk to which beaten egg has been added. Mix lightly. Bake in oiled casserole in moderate oven 3/4 hour.

Beet Greens

Select young green leaves of 2 bunches of beets. Rinse in water several times. Cut in one-inch pieces. Place in a heavy utensil, add a small amount of boiling water, cover and cook for 5 minutes. Before serving, season with lemon juice and butter.

Italian Goulash

Steam together onions, red or white cabbage, sweet peppers, and chopped mustard green leaves. Add sliced tomatoes. Cook all until tender. Add a little celery salt and serve.

Riced Buttered Carrots

2 Cups riced, raw Carrots
1/2 Teaspoon Vegetized Salt
2 Tablespoons Brown Sugar
1/4 Cup soaked Raisins
2 Teaspoons Butter

Steam carrots in 1/2 cup water for 15 minutes. Place in casserole. Add brown sugar and salt. Brown top, remove from oven and cover with butter and raisins. Serve hot.

Eggplant-Okra-Tomatoes En Casserole

2 Cup cooked Eggplant, diced
1 Cup Okra, cooked
1 (2 lb.) can Tomatoes *(continued next page)*

1 Tablespoon sweet Butter
Mushroom Sauce
Vegetable Broth Powder
1 Cup cooked Rice

Alternate eggplant, okra and tomatoes in layers in oiled casserole. Sprinkle vegetable broth powder over each layer. Cover with rice and dot with sweet butter. Bake in moderate oven 1/2 hour. Serve with mushroom sauce.

Corn and Green Peppers

7 ears yellow Bantam Corn
2 large sweet Green Peppers
1/4 Cup boiling Water
3 Tablespoons Butter
1/2 Teaspoon Vegetized Salt

Boil corn on the cob 5 minutes, according to the variety. When cold, cut the kernels from the ears of corn. Remove seeds from green peppers, cut in small pieces, and combine with the corn. Add butter and salt or vegetable broth powder. Add 1/4 cup boiling water. Place in an iron skillet and simmer for 10 minutes.

Squash Surprise

2 lbs. summer Squash
1/2 Cup Cottage Cheese
1/3 Cup chopped Celery
1 Teaspoon Vegetable Broth Powder
1/3 Cup Walnut and Pecan Nutmeats
1/2 Cup shredded Cheese

Steam squash, scoop out center and mix with finely chopped celery, cheese and vegetable browth powder. Place a walnut and pecan nutmeat in the center of squash and fill over with the mixed filling. Sprinkle cheese over all. Place squash in pan and heat in oven.

Spinach and Mushroom Patties

2 bunches cooked Spinach
1 Cup Mushrooms, cooked
1 small Onion, chopped fine
1 Teaspoon Vegetized Salt

(continued next page)

1 Egg
1 Cup Coconut Milk

Chop spinach very fine or put through grinder. Combine with finely chopped mushrooms, onion and salt. To this mixture add beaten egg and milk. Mix well. Make into small patties and bake on an oiled baking sheet in moderate oven 30 minutes.

CHEESE RECIPES

Ways with Cheese

1. Cheese lends zest and variety to any healthful dinner.
2. If mold forms on cheese, do not throw away. Merely cut off moldy portion.
3. Grind or grate a quantity of cheese and store in refrigerator in a tightly covered glass jar. This will save time and labor in the preparation of a meal.
4. Place cheese souffles in a pan. Place this pan into another larger pan containing water to avoid too much heat. Be sure to bake long enough to be firm after taking from oven.
5. When melting cheese, use top of double boiler. Keep heat below boiling point.
6. Too much heat applied to cheese makes it leathery and hard to digest.
7. A hard cheese is preferable for grating. Use as a garnish on salads or vegetable dishes browned in oven; in omelettes, soups or sauces for additional flavor.

How to Make Cottage Cheese
(New Improved Recipe)

1/4 "Junket" Rennet tablet
4 Tablespoons cold Water
1 gallon Skim Milk
3/4 Cup Buttermilk or Sour Milk
1/2 Teaspoon Salt
1/2 Cup Cream *(continued next page)*

1. Dissolve 1/4 "Junket" Rennet tablet in 4 tablespoons cold water.
2. Combine skim milk and buttermilk and heat to remove chill only (75° F.).
3. Add 2 tablespoons of the rennet tablet solution and stir well (discard remaining part as solution will not keep).
4. Cover with a towel and let stand at room temperature until the curd shows the characteristic "clean break" and there is a slight whey on top (16-20 hours).
5. Heat curd slightly over hot water (in a double boiler) until the curd pulls away from the sides of the container and tiny bubbles start to rise around the edge of the curd. Cut the curd in 1-1/2 inch squares using a long knife. Continue heating until lukewarm (110-120° F.). Meantime, stir the curd gently with a wooden spoon (once in 3-4 minutes) so the curd will be heated evenly but still remain in large lumps. Hold the curd at this temperature for about 25 minutes, or until a handful of curds, when squeezed lightly, will be somewhat springy and tumble apart when released.
6. Drain in cheesecloth bag until the curd is free from whey.
7. Season with salt and cream according to taste.

NOTE: If a dry, crumbly type of cottage cheese is desired, use the higher temperature (120° *F.); if a soft cottage cheese is desired, use the lower temperature (110°* F.). Do not throw away whey -flavor into juice and drink.

VEGETABLE DISHES

Vegetable Chop Suey

1 Cup dried Mushrooms
1 Cup chopped Celery
2 Cups Bean Sprouts
2 large Onions, chopped
2 Tablespoons Broth Powder
1/2 lb. Tofu
1/2 Cup Walnuts or Water Chestnuts

Soak mushrooms 3 or 4 hours. Add water to cover. Add all ingredients and simmer until vegetables are tender. Do not use too much liquid. Use soy sauce, if desired, at the table.

Baked New England Dinner

4 medium sized new Potatoes
3 medium sized Carrots
6 small white Onions
3 small Beets
1 small Rutabaga
Sweet Butter
Vegetable Broth Powder

Cut potatoes and carrots lengthwise once. Slice beets and rutabaga. Leave onions whole. Place all in casserole with enough water to cover bottom of vessel. Bake in moderate oven until vegetables are thoroughly cooked. Add sweet butter and vegetable broth powder to taste and serve.

Vegetarian Croquettes

3 Tablespoons Olive Oil
3 Tablespoons Soya Flour
1/2 Cup Milk
1/2 Cup cooked Carrots
1/2 Cup cooked Peas
1/2 Cup cooked Beans
1/2 Cup cooked Spinach
1/2 Cup ground Nuts
1 Teaspoon Onion Juice
Parsley to garnish

Make a sauce in the double boiler of oil, soya flour, and milk. Put through grinder: cooked carrots, peas, beans, spinach. Add ground nuts. Blend with sauce and season with vegetable broth powder. If desired, add 1 teaspoon of onion juice. Shape into balls and flatten. Dip first into crumbs, then into egg, and back into crumbs again. Arrange on oiled pan. Place in medium oven until brown. Garnish with parsley and serve.

Stuffed Peppers with Rice

6 Green Peppers
3 Cups cooked Brown Rice
1/2 Cups cooked Pea Puree
2 Tablespoons sweet Butter
2 Teaspoons Vegetable Broth Powder

(continued next page)

1 Teaspoon Onion Juice

1/4 Cup grated Cheese

Cut peppers in halves lengthwise, remove the seeds. Soak in boiling water for ten minutes. Fill peppers with cooked rice and pea puree to which broth powder and onion juice have been added. Sprinkle grated cheese over each pepper half. Place in small pan and then place into large pan with small amount of water. Bake in oven for 20 minutes. Add sweet butter to each pepper.

SAUCES AND FLAVORINGS

Avoid all artificial seasonings, flavorings and stimulants such as table salt, black and white pepper, vinegar, mustard, hot sauces, alcoholic flavorings, artificial extracts, ketchup and mayonnaise. It is impossible to find a mayonnaise or salad dressing, except in health food stores, that does not contain some of the above-listed ingredients which are detrimental to good health.

Green peppers, red peppers, onions, garlic, celery salt, nuts, tomatoes, mushrooms, lemon, lemon peel, and all the herbs such as dill, thyme, mint, and bay leaf are delightfully delicious and healthful for flavoring sauces. Learn to enjoy natural foods meant for us to eat.

Herb Sauce

1 large bunch of Parsley, minced

1/2 as much minced Chives as the amount of Parsley used

Juice of 4 Lemons

1/4 teaspoon dried Thyme or Basil

4 Tablespoons Sweet Butter

1-1/2 Teaspoon Vegetable Broth Power

Allow the parsley, chives and lemon juice to infuse for 1 hour. Then add the thyme or basil, sweet butter and boiling water. Simmer for 5 minutes on low heat. Pour into a tureen, add vegetable broth powder and serve immediately.

Spanish Sauce

1 clove Garlic, finely chopped

1/2 Cup Rice Pepper, finely chopped

1 large Onion, finely chopped   *(continued next page)*

268

1/2 cup Celery, chopped
1-1/2 Cup Tomatoes
1 Teaspoon Vegetable Broth Powder
2 Tablespoons sweet Butter

Steam garlic, onion and pepper 7 minutes in double boiler. Add tomatoes, broth powder, celery. Steam over a low heat for 30 minuts. Add butter and serve.

Tartar Sauce

1 Cup Mayonnaise
5 Black Olives, ripe
1 small Cucumber, ground
2 Tablespoons Watercress
1 small clove Garlic, chopped very fine

Stir all ingredients into the mayonnaise.

SPREADS

Quick Tofu Spread

1 Cup Tofu
1 Cup canned Tomatoes, drained well
1/2 Cup raw Almonds
1 Teaspoon Salt

Blenderize all ingredients together until satiny. Add chopped celery and onions if desired. Chill and serve on crackers or sandwiches.

THE WORKING MAN'S LUNCH

Sandwiches

1. Cucumbers, sliced very thin, marinated with French dressing with lettuce on sprouted bread.
2. Watercress, cut into small pieces and marinated with dressing.
3. Watercress, chopped fine, creamed with butter, and spread on bread.
4. Cottage cheese, Spanish or green onion, mayonnaise if desired.
5. Cottage cheese or cream cheese with jelly or jam, health-made.
6. Cream cheese with shredded pineapple.

7. Cream cheese or cottage cheese and nuts.
8. Cream cheese, nuts, and raisins. Mayonnaise if desired.
9. Carrot, nut and celery with mayonnaise.
10. Nuts and chopped olives.
11. Nut spreads and raisins.
12. Olives, nuts, salad dressing, and lettuce.
13. Avocado or avocado with olive.
14. Chopped raisins.
15. Chopped raisins with nuts and cottage cheese.
16. Chopped raisins, dates and figs, with or without nuts or mayonnaise.

Salad, drink and dessert suggestions should be followed as in school lunches.

Add dry or fresh fruits to the lunch box to be eaten at ten or three o'clock to keep your man from starving while he waits to get at those fresh surprises in his lunch box or on the dinner table when he gets home. The evening meal should be especially planned with enough protein to offset the starch consumed at the noon meal, and to give sufficient energy.

Thermos Bottle variations:
1. Vital Broth, varied according to taste and desire.
2. Buttermilk or goat milk.
3. Oat Straw tea.
4. Thin cream soups and clear vegetable broths.

The ideal lunch for everybody where sandwiches are included also includes a raw vegetable salad and a health drink.

Instead of bread, try using lettuce or slices of zucchini to hold spreads.

Our children's lunches always had sticks of carrots, stuffed celery, slices of green peppers along with their sandwiches. The sandwiches had more filling and the bread was cut thin.

DRINKS

When you have drinks, it can be broths, vegetable juices, buttermilk and above all, I think that everyone should be using healthful herb teas. Everyone should have 2 cups of herb tea daily. Instead of coffee, use a coffee substitute.

TEA

Alfalfa Tea

This is the most alkalinizing of all foods. Use 1 teaspoon tea to 1 cup boiling water. Steep 5 minutes. Add honey to taste.

Mint Tea

This is an excellent cleanser of the alimentary tract, especially if taken before going to bed. Use 1 teaspoon mint tea to 1 cup boiling water. Steep 3 minutes and serve with a lemon ring.

Oat Straw Tea

Oat Straw is one of the highest silicon containing foods. Use 1 teaspoon oat straw to 1 cup boiling water. If the oat straw is coarse, boil 10 minutes. Serve with honey and lemon.

Silicon Tea with Mint

Boil water and add oat straw to the strength desired. Simmer slowly for 5 to 10 minutes, depending upon cut of oat straw. Strain into scalded pot to which 4 or 5 mint leaves have been added. Serve at once with added flavoring if desired. It is suggested that tea be made double strength and freshly boiled water added at table according to the strength desired by each individual.

Parsley Tea

This is an excellent skin and kidney cleanser. Chop parsley very fine, the finer the better. Cover the parsley with distilled water and simmer about 30 minutes. Strain, cool and serve with lemon.

Strawberry Tea

This tea is excellent for all intestinal difficulties. Use 1 teaspoon of tea to 1 cup of boiling water. Steep 3 minutes. Serve with lemon.

Senna Leaf Tea

Senna tea is a laxative, but must not be relied upon for this purpose. A teaspoon of senna leaves to 1-1/2 cups of Sparkletts spring water is suggested. Bring to a boil and steep about 5 minutes.

Flaxseed Tea

Flaxseed tea is very healing to stomach ulcers if used alone for about 3 days. Also very healing for any gastro-intestinal irriration. Wash 1/4 cup of flaxseed thoroughly. Drain, and add 3 cups boiling water. Let boil gently until well done, which will require from 1 to 2 hours. Drain and season the liquid with lemon juice.

FRUIT AND NUT MILK DRINKS

The addition of delicious and nutritious powdered coconut milk to any of the following is invaluable as a food for the body; goat milk, soybean milk, nut milks and coconut milk, fruit juices of all kinds, and prune, fig, and apricot juices.

Coconut and Pineapple Drink

2 Teaspoons of Coconut Milk Powder
1 or 2 Tablespoons Pineapple juice, or more according to taste
1/3 Teaspoon Honey
1 Cup boiling Water

Stir ingredients as you add water.

Nut Milk Drink

5 Tablespoons Nut Butter
5 Cups warm Water
2 Teaspoons Honey

Mix nut butter with warm water. Add honey. Beat together until foamy.

Almond Nut Milk

1 Tablespoon raw Almond Butter
1 Cup warm Water

Beat until well blended.

Orange Almond Milk

1 Teaspoon Almond Butter
1 Cup fresh Orange Juice

Beat 1 teaspoon almond butter into apple, grape, or pineapple juice, until frothy. This is a delicious building food.

272

Coconut and Carrot Milk

Use equal parts of fresh coconut milk and fresh carrot juice, or proportion according to taste. Serve this drink immediately upon extraction of juices.

Pecan Apple Fruit Drink

6 Pecans
1 Apple, diced, with skin
3 Teaspoons Raisins
1 Banana, cut
1 glass Pineapple Juice

Put all in liquefier when ready to serve.

Date Milk Drink

5 Dates, pitted and cut in half
1 glass of Milk and Cream
1 Teaspoon powdered coconut
1 Teaspoon Mal-ba Nuts

Put all in liquefier when ready to serve.

FRUIT AND VEGETABLE COCKTAILS

Body Building Cocktail

1/2 Coconut Milk
1/2 Fig Juice

Pickup Cocktail

1/2 Orange Juice
1/2 Pomegranate Juice
1 Egg Yolk to each cup
1/2 Teaspoon Honey
    to each cup

Brain Cocktail

1/2 Cabbage Juice
1/2 Pineapple Juice
1 Teaspoon Almond Butter
    to each cup

Pep Tonic Cocktail

1/3 Celery Juice
2/3 Orange Juice
1 Egg Yolk to each cup

Youth Cocktail

1/3 Cucumber Juice
1/3 Radish Juice
1/3 Pepper Juice

Carrot and Coconut Cocktail

1/2 Carrot Juice
1/2 Coconut Juice

273

Hair Beautifying Cocktail

2/3 Oat Straw Tea
1/3 Celery, Prune, or
   Fig Juice
1/4 Teaspoon powdered
   Nova Scotia Dulce
   to each cup

Building Cocktail

1/3 Beet Leaf Juice
1/3 Beet Juice
1/3 Pineapple Juice

Alkalinizing Cocktail

1/2 Grapefruit Juice
1/4 Spinach Juice
1/4 Pineapple Juice

Appetizer Cocktail

1/2 Dandelion Juice
1/2 Pineapple Juice

Skin Cocktail

1/3 Cucumber Juice
1/3 Parsley Juice
1/3 Pineapple Juice

JUICE FOR SPECIFIC AILMENTS

Vegetable juices are a great aid for the sick in regaining their health and for the well in maintaining their health. The vegetable juice idea is nothing new, but in late years it has become quite a commercial venture. Fast living today requires more concentrated and more easily assimilated foods. Consequently, vegetable juice therapy has come into its own, and is served right on our street corners for our health's sake.

Vegetable juices can be assimilated quickly and easily. In fact, the green, or chlorophyll, is taken up by the blood with little effort. We have seen a million red blood cells added to a blood count in a month and a half by adding vegetable juices to the diet.

But don't get the idea you should live on them entirely. Have them with meals and between meals. For best results, have at least one pint a day. There is no better organic water for your system than raw vegetable juice.

Many times diarrhea is experienced while taking vegetable juices. In most cases it is necessary, as nature is doing a little housecleaning. To bathe the tissues in your body with these juices will, in time, cleanse them and then rebuilt, rejuvenate, and feed a starved body.

Most people lose weight when taking juices. However in making a new body you must sometimes lose weight in order to rebuild.

Make these vegetable cocktail in proportions pleasing to the taste. Usually any juice mixed with an equal proportion of another juice will be about right. We find carrot, celery, and parsley good in nearly every condition and good in combination. They mix with any fruit or vegetable juice and can be had between meals, with most any meal, and any time during the day. However, when you mix fruit juices with vegetable juices, as pineapple and tomato, it is best not to mix with starches. Acid fruits and starches do not combine. Vegetable juices go best with them. When having carrot juice, drink with a straw and mix well with saliva.

There are many combinations of health cocktails that you can make. A bitter green taste can be made palatable by adding sweet vegetables, honey, pineapple juice, coconut milk, or a little sweet cream.

The following listed diseases can best be aided by using a vegetable cocktail or combination of juices for each ailment.

Nearly every disease responds much quicker by adding vegetable juices. Celery, parsley, and carrot juices are good for any condition. They can be mixed any way or can be had alone.

Disorders in the Body	Health Cocktail Suggestions
1. Anemia	Parsley and Grape Juice
2. Asthma	Celery and Papaya Juice
3. Bed Wetting	Celery and Parsley Juice
4. Bladder Ailments	Celery and Pomegranate Juice
5. Cancer	Carrot Juice
6. Catarrh, Colds, Sore Throat	Watercress and Apple Juice (add 1/4 teaspoon of Pure Cream of Tartar)
7. Constipation, Stomach Ulcers	Celery with a little Sweet Cream, Spinach and Grapefruit Juice

8. Colds, Sinus Troubles

Celery and Grapefruit Juices
(Add 1/4 teaspoon of Pure
Cream of Tartar

9. Colitis, Gastritis, Gas   Coconut Milk and Carrot Juice
10. Diarrhea, Infection   Carrot and Blackberry Juice
11. Fever, Gout, Arthritis   Celery and Parsley Juice
12. Gall Bladder Disorders   Radish, Prune, Black Cherry,
and Celery Juice
13. General House Cleaning   Celery, Parsley, Spinach, and
Carrot Juice

14. Glands, Goitre,
Impotence   Celery Juice, 1 teaspoon Wheat
Germ, and 1 teaspoon Nova
Scotia Dulce
15. Heart Disturbances   Carrot and Pineapple Juice
and Honey
16. High Blood Pressure   Carrot and Parsley Juice
and Celery
17. Indigestion, Underweight   Coconut Milk, Fig Juice, Parsley
and Carrot Juice
18. Insomnia, Sleeplessness   Lettuce nd Celery Juice
19. Kidney Disorders   Celery, Parsley and
Asparagus Juice
20. Liver Disorders   Radish and Pineapple Juice
21. Nervous Disorders   Radish and Prune Juice and
Rice Polishings
22. Nerve Tension   Celery, Carrot and Prune Juice
23. Neuralgia   Cucumber, Endive and
Pineapple Juice
24. Nerve Quieter   Lettuce and Tomato Juice
25. Overweight, Obesity   Beet Green, Parsley and
Celery Juice
26. Poor Circulation   Beet and Blackberry Juice
27. Poor Complexion   Cucumber, Endive and
Pineapple Juice
28. Poor Memory   Celery, Carrot and Prune Juice
and Rice Polishings

Disorders in the Body	Health Cocktail Suggestions
29. Poor Teeth	Beet Green, Parsley and Celery Juice and Green Kale
30. Reducing	Parsley, Grape Juice and Pineapple Juice
31. Rheumatism, Neuritis, Neuralgia	Cucumber, Endive and Goat's Whey
32. Rickets	Dandelion and Orange Juice
33. Scurvy Eczema	Carrot, Celery and Lemon Juice

(The juices suggested for a specific body disorder may be used separately or in combination with each other.)

DESSERTS

This is one department everyone seems to like and look forward to having at the finish of their meal.

There are 2 or 3 things we should be careful of concerning desserts. First, we are putting that extra amount of food in our body that we don't need and can't possibly use because we have had a good meal already. Most desserts are made with sugars, flavorings and synthetic colorings to make them look good. They look appetizing and teasing. We do not believe in desserts, unless a little fresh fruit occasionally. A person that gets used to desserts adds too much of the sugars, the acid forming food, to the body. Someday he will be treated for it in a doctors office.

Here are a few desserts that are natural. One or two a week is plenty.

Dessert Suggestions

A half teaspoon of cinnamon added to stewed peaches give zest to the fruit.

The juice of a lemon, the grated rind and a whole clove or two will enhance the flavor of stewed prunes.

Add a few shreds of lemon peel (not juice) to a rice pudding. You will find the flavor immeasurably improved.

277

BAKED FRUITS

Baked Apples

Rome Beauty apples are best for baking. Wash desired number of apples. Core, taking care not to cut through to the bottom. Remove black flower at end of apple and peel 1 inch of skin off the top away from center. Place in baking dish. Simmer the removed cores and skin about ten minutes. Fill the apple centers with this juice and a tiny piece of butter. You can then stuff cores with dates or raisins. Pour any remaining juice into bottom of baking dish. Bake apples in a slow oven for 1 hour. Cool and serve.

Stuffed Apples

Prepare the apples as above, filling the center with raisins, dates or figs. Serve with honey, almond chips, yogurt, coconut milk or soy milk.

FRUIT WHIPS

Prune Whip

Wash and soak 1/2 pound prunes in water 36 hours. Remove pits and put through fine sieve or a vegetable grinder. Combine prunes with equal parts whipped cream flavored with honey and almond extract. Top with a red grape or cherry. This recipe will serve 4.

Apricot Whip

Follow recipe for prune whip using fresh mashed, or dried and soaked and mashed apricots.

Banana Whip

3 mashed Bananas
1 Tablespoon Honey
1 Cup Whipped Cream

Mix mashed bananas with honey. Fold whipped cream into bananas, chill and serve.

Raw Apple Sauce

Grate washed, unpeeled Roman Beauty apples. Remove any big pieces of skin. Serve wth coconut milk powder.

SHERBETS

Many people are allergic to milk products and then we use the milk substitute such as yogurt, coconut milk or tasty soy milk.

Strawberry Sherbet

1 Package frozen or frosted Strawberries
1 Cup Orange Juice
1/2 Cup Water

Mash strawberries, add orange juice and water. Pour into refrigerator tray and freeze. Serve with heavy whipped cream.

Dr. Jensen's Cherry Concentrate
Cherry Fruit Delight

(A gelatin dessert)

1/4 Cup Cherry Concentrate
1/2 Cup Cold Water
1 Tablespoon Honey
1 Tablespoon Unflavored Gelatin
8 Ounces Diced Pineapple or 8 ounces Fresh Pitted Cherries
1/2 Cup Chopped Walnuts
1 Cup Boiling Water

Mix gelatin with cold water to dissolve. Add honey and boiling water. Stir well, add nuts and cherries. Place in refrigerator to thicken. Serve on organically grown leaf lettuce or romaine.

Dr. Jensen's Apple Concentrate
The Youth and Eye Delicacy

(A gelatin dessert)

1/8 Cup of Apple Concentrate
1/2 Cup Cold Water
1 Tablespoon Unflavored Gelatin
1 Tablespoon Honey
Juice of 1 medium Lemon
1 Medium-sized Apple, chopped
1 sliced Banana

Mix gelatin with cold water to dissolve, add honey with 1-1/2 cups boiling water. Stir well and add lemon juice to the chopped apples, which also aids in keeping the apples from getting dark in color.

You can also add grated carrots, then mix and pour into a dish and chill. If desired, add 1/4 cup of raisins. Serve on chilled leaf lettuce with a topping of 1/2 cup of yogurt, and 1 teaspoon of Dr. Jensen's Broth Powder Seasoning, if desired.

DELIGHTFUL SUGGESTIONS

1. **Shredded Apple Salad:** 1 large shredded apple; 6 apricots, cut up small; 1 tablespoon apple concentrate. Mix together and chill.

2. **Teas:** Pour 1 tablespoon apple concentrate into a cup of tea for a sweetener.

3. **Pick up:** 1 tablespoon apple concentrate in a glass of water. Serve to friends who drop in and to children after school.

4. **Pep up the nerves:** 1 tablespoon apple concentrate in a cup of celery juice.

5. **Regulator:** 1 tablespoon apple concentrate in a dish of yogurt.

6. **Cottage Cheese Salad:** 1/2 cup crushed pineapple; 1/4 cup chopped pecans; 1 tablespoon apple concentrate; 1 pint cottage cheese. Mix together and chill.

7. **Use as a base in the blender:** Use 1 tablespoon apple concentrate to 1/2 cup of water.

8. **Topping for Ice Cream:** Pour apple concentrate over a dish of ice cream.

SEASONINGS

Try to get your seasoning from herbs. They are healthy, body building and body correcting. They are for a regeneration purpose when used properly. We can have carob instead of chocolate. We use the natural sweets instead of white sugar products. Don't use too much salt. The minerals that you get from salt are very minor and produce side effects in arteries and various parts of the body. The best salt to use is sun evaporated sea salt if using any salt. We should be getting all of our mineral salts from our vegetables, fruit and berries we get from the garden foods. They have no side effects.

HEALTH BREADS

Grace's Yellow Corn Bread

3/4 Cup Whole Wheat Flour
2 Tablespoons Raw Sugar
3 Teaspoons Royal Baking Powder
1 Teaspoon Vegetized Salt
1 Cup Yellow Corn Meal
2 Eggs
1 Cup Raw Milk
1/4 Cup Olive Oil

Sift dry ingredients and combine with corn meal. Mix eggs and milk and add with oil. Beat until smooth. Pour in shallow baking pan and bake 20 minutes in oven 400 degrees F.

Soya Flour Bread

1 Cake compressed Yeast
4 Cup lukewarm Water
4 Tablespoons Raw Sugar
2 Tablespoons melted Butter or Olive Oil
1 Teaspoon Vegetized Salt
7-1/2 Cups Soya Flour

Dissolve yeast and sugar in lukewarm water and add shortening and vegetized salt. Sift and measure flour, adding gradually to the mixture. Knead thoroughly, keeping dough soft. Cover and set in warm place and let stand to rise for about 2 hours. When double in bulk, form into two loaves and place in well greased pans. Cover, let rise again about 1 hour, until dough is of a light consistency. Bake in moderate hot oven, 400 degrees F. 1 hour or until toothpick tester comes out clean.

One cup broken walnut meats added to this recipe makes it extra delicious.

CAKES AND COOKIES

Grace's Spice Cake

1/2 Cup Butter
1-1/2 Cup Raw Sugar   *(continued next page)*

281

2 Egg Yolks
1/2 Cup chopped Nuts
1 Cup seeded Raisins
2 Cup sifted Whole Wheat Pastry Flour
1 Teaspoon Royal Baking Powder
1/2 Teaspoon each Cloves, Nutmeg, Cinnamon
2 Egg Whites
1 Teaspoon Soda
1 Cup Sour Milk or Buttermilk

Cream butter and sugar together. Add egg yolks and beat well. Mix and sift dry ingredients. Add nuts and raisins to dry ingredients. Add to first mixture, alternating with buttermilk, mixed with soda. Mix well and fold in beaten egg whites. Pour into two well-oiled cake pans and bake in moderate oven 20 to 30 minutes. Cool and spread with caramel icing.

Carrot Cookies

1 Cup Soya Flour, sifted
1 Teaspoon Royal Baking Powder
1/2 Teaspoon Vegetized Salt
1/4 Cup Water
1 Teaspoon Lemon Juice
1 Cup grated Carrots

Mix well and drop on oiled baking sheet. Bake for 15 minutes.

HEALTH CANDIES

Natural Health Candy

1/2 lb. dried Apricots
1/2 lb. seedless Raisins
1/2 lb. Dates, pitted
1 lb. dried White Figs
1 Cup Walnuts

Put all ingredients through food grinder. Mix well. Press into buttered dish and cut into inch squares. Roll in sesame seeds or raw grated coconut.

Date Patties

Press 1 cup dates and 1 cup pecans through a food chopper. Mix thoroughly. Form into patties. Roll in freshly grated coconut or Mal-ba Nuts and serve.

Stuffed Dates

Remove the pits from dates and fill with cottage cheese or nut butter to which has been added chopped pecan meats.

Time Saving Suggestions in the Kitchen

It is brought to our consciousness today that we should get into the kitchen fast and get out of it as quickly as possible. We know that the fast food marketing program has set the pace that no time is wasted in the kitchen. This is the day of the career woman. This is the day of babysitters. This is the day when both Mother and Father are working. So, we don't want to spend the extra time in the kitchen.

TIPS TO HELP US

When using natural foods, they do not need extra time an effort as far as frying, cooking, boiling, baking, and so forth. So try to have more of the raw foods, which are better for you. When making some of your gelatin desserts, you can make enough for 2 or 3 days ahead. Try to see that what you prepare today will furnish something left for the basis of another meal on another day. It can be vegetables, washed and put away, ready to be used. If it is for soups or beans, this can be prepared ahead of time and frozen. If we don't have dishes that have a lot of greasy, fried material on it, we save time in washing the dishes and cleaning your stove. Frying pans take a lot of time to take care of. Shredded cabbage, shredded beets, shredded vegetables of any kind, can be prepared ahead of time. Many of these foods can be put in plastic a container and put in the refrigerator. If the food is going to be prepared fast or quickly to get our meals over with in a hurry, we probably have joined the demolition team of civilization, where we are destroying the health of our nation.

283

The liquefier and the juicer should be a great help, and a grinder in the kitchen can save a lot of time and gives us a variety of dishes. You don't have to be a gourmet cook to have variety and good looks on the table.

ELEVEN-DAY ELIMINATION REGIME

There are many eliminative regimes, and they all accomplish about the same results, through the fact that the body is given less food, simpler foods and simpler combinations, more water food -so a greater transition can take place in the cells of the body.

This Eleven-Day Elimination Regime can be used by most persons in health, and for those who want to overcome the average physical disorder. Those who are weak or feeble, however, should not follow the plan the full eleven days without supervision. Those with tuberculosis should have both supervision and assistance.

Variation, as to the length of time, and the manner in which the foods are to be taken, may be adjusted to suit the history of the patient, Examples: Fruits, vegetables and broths can be taken for 1 day; or 1 day of just fruit; or 1, 2 or 3 days of vegetables only.

Vegetables, taken in the form of broths, gently steamed vegetables and salads are a safer routine for the average beginner than citrus fruits.

A hot bath should be taken every night during this diet regime. Enemas may be used the first four or five days, then discontinued for natural movements. Nothing but water and fruit juices, preferably grapefruit, should be taken into the body for the first three days. Drink one glass of juice every four hours of the day. The next two days fruit only - such as grapes, melons, tomatoes, pears, peaches, plums; dried fruit such as prunes, figs, peaches, soaked overnight, and baked apple.

In the six following days breakfast should consist of citrus fruits. Between breakfast and lunch any other kind of fruit. For a lunch have a salad of three to six vegetables and two cups of vital broth. When hungry between meals, fruit or fruit juices may be taken. Dinner should consist of two or three steamed vegetables and two cups of vital broth. Fruit juices can be taken before retiring if wanted.

Rigid adherence to the diet is an absolute necessity for anyone attempting to regain good health. Eat plenty but not to satiety.

Let me give you the Vital Broth recipe here and now:

2 Cups Carrots tops
2 Cups Potato Peeling (1/2-inch thick)
2 Cups Beet tops
2 Cups Celery tops
3 Cups Celery stalk
2 Quarts Sparkletts distilled Water
1/2 Teaspoon Savita or Vegex
Add a carrot and onion to flavor if desired (grate or chop)

Ingredients should be finely chopped. Bring to a boil, slowly; simmer approximately 20 minutes. Use only the broth after straining.

When finished with the above regime, return to Dr. Jensen's Daily Food Regime.

The above elimination regime should be followed whenever a person changes from the old ways of living and begins to live right. As a rule, it is wise to follow the elimination regime in any and all of the following cases:

As a general cleanser two or three times a year.
At the time of crisis.
When reduction of weight is desired.
When hips get too large.
When joints get still.
When the skin breaks out.
When constipation is present.

ACID AND ALKALINE FOODS

There has been much talk in the last few years about acid and alkaline foods. It has been definetly determined that a body should be as nearly alkaline as possible. To have a perfect alkaline body would be impossible.

When one speaks of an acid body, he means that the body is no longer near the alkaline point. Health is determined by a good, acid-free body, while disease is always associated with an extremely acid body. Where one begins and the other ends is as problematical as the determination of hot and cold. Where does cold end? Where does heat begin?

We have found that certain foods tend to favor an acid condition in the body more than others. To keep the proper acid-alkaline balance in the body you should *theoretically eat four vegetables a day, two fruits a day, one protein a day and one starch a day.* But this acid-alkaline balance desired would actually be upset when you load your system with such complete combinations *each day.* We know that many people successfully achieve the correct balance on a *mono-diet* (one food at a time). *The idea is to approximate these proportions over a period of years.* Thus when you have nothing but fruits one day, and nothing but vegetables the next, you are in perfect balance. Eating the foods suggested keeps your diet about eighty percent alkaline and twenty percent acid.

ACIDITY AND ALKALINITY IN THE BODY

The following experiments illustrate the point: Balint and Weiss took a rabbit and alkalinized it. Then they slit the rabbit's leg and injected turpentine. The damage to the leg was very slight. When the rabbit was acidized, however, the injection of turpentine was followed by inflammation, tissue sluffing and death. In another experiment, this time with scarlet fever patients, it was discovered that when urinary acidity ranged high, there was an aftermath of nephritis in two-thirds of the cases. When the acidity was low, only three percent of the cases were thus complicated. Very defintely, a high alkaline balance is the body's first line of defense against illness and death.

ACID-ALKALINE CHART

The following table of foods is taken from
Ragnar Berg of Germany

Foods preceded by the letters AL are alkaline forming.
Foods preceded by the letters AC are acid forming.

Column No. 1 Non-Starch Foods		Column No. 2 Proteins and Fruits		Column No. 3 Starchy Foods	
AL	Alfalfa	AC	Beef	AL	Bananas
AL	Artichokes	AC	Buttermilk	AC	Barley
AL	Asparagus	AC	Chicken	AC	Beans (Lima)
AL	Beans (String)	AC	Clams	AC	Beans (White)
AL	Beans (Wax)	AC	Cottage	AC	Bread
AL	Beets (Whole)		Cheese	AC	Cereals
AL	Beet Leaves	AC	Crab	AC	Chestnuts
AL	Broccoli	AC	Duck	AC	Corn
AL	Cabbage (wh.)	AC	Eggs	AC	Corn Meal
AL	Cabbage (Red)	AC	Fish	AC	Crackers
AL	Carrots	AC	Goose	AC	Corn Starch
AL	Carrot Tops	AC	Honey (Pure)	AC	Grapenuts
AL	Cauliflower	AC	Jello	AC	Gluten Flour
AL	Celery Knobs	AC	Lamb	AC	Lentils
AL	Chicory	AC	Lobster	AC	Macaroni
AL	Coconut	AC	Mutton	AC	Maize
AL	Corn	AC	Nuts	AC	Millet Rye
AL	Cucumbers	AC	Oyster	AC	Oatmeal
AL	Dandelions	AC	Pork	AC	Peanuts
AL	Eggplant	AC	Rabbit	AC	Peanut Butter
AL	Endive	AC	Raw Sugar	AC	Peas (Dried)
AL	Garlic	AC	Turkey	AL	Potatoes
AL	Horse-radish	AC	Turtle		(Sweet)
AL	Kale	AC	Veal	AL	Potatoes
AL	Kohlrabi	AC	All Berries		(White)
AL	Leek	AC	Apples	AL	Pumpkin
AL	Lettuce	AC	Apricots	AC	Rice (Brown)
AL	Mushrooms	AC	Avocados	AC	Rice
AL	Okra	AC	Cataloupes		(Polished)
AL	Olives (Ripe)	AC	Cherries	AC	Roman Meal

287

ACID-ALKALINE CHART (Continued)

Column No. 1 *Non-Starch Foods*		Column No. 2 *Proteins and Fruits*		Column No. 3 *Starchy Foods*	
AL	Onions	AC	Cranberries	AC	Rye Flour
AL	Oysterplant	AC	Currants	AC	Sauerkraut
AL	Parsley	AL	Dates	AL	Squash
AL	Parsnips	AL	Figs		(Hub'd)
AL	Peas (Fresh)	AL	Grapes	AC	Tapioca
AL	Peppers	AL	Grapefruit		
	(Sweet)	AL	Lemons		
AL	Radishes	AL	Limes		
AL	Rutabagas	AL	Oranges		
AL	Savory	AL	Peaches		
AL	Sea Lettuce	AL	Pears		
AL	Sorrel	AL	Persimmons		
AL	Soybean	AL	Pineapple		
	(Products)	AL	Plums		
AL	Spinach	AL	Prunes		
AL	Sprouts	AL	Raisins		
AL	Summer	AL	Rhubarb		
	Squash	AL	Tomatoes		
AL	Swiss Chard				
AL	Turnips				
AL	Watercress				

For people with weak digestion it is best to make food combinations as simple as possible. Follow the suggestions on how to combine foods.

Combine foods found in Columns one and two; also Columns one and three.

Never combine Columns two and three.

All the foods in Column one will combine with all the foods in Column two.

FRUITS

Citrus fruits cause alkalinity. Citrus fruits, when broken down, release an alkaline ash which develops an alkaline condition in the body. Sometimes these acid fruits stir up the acids so rapidly that their effect is considered to be a bad one. This may be quite the reverse of the real truth! *Should the eating of fruit cause you distress, you may be sure you are misinterpreting your symptoms.* In any case like that, I would say you are VERY ILL and require the aid or advice of a specialist in NATURAL healing.

But, in general, remember that fruits should be eaten in a natural harmony; I mean, oranges and grapefruits and tangerines and lemons, as the ACID fruits mentioned, go very nicely with other acid fruits like cranberries, pineapple, strawberries. They do NOT combine well with the sweet fruits or the dried ones we mentioned, like prunes, figs, raisins, dates or grapes. And berries and melons should ALWAYS be eaten alone. There is no more disagreeable a surprise for your stomach, for example, than watermelon eaten in conjunction with another food!

The SUB-ACID fruits mentioned, such as apples, persimmons, pears, plums, peaches, apricots, combine fairly well with the ACID fruits, but I do not recommend the combinations, especially. The safest procedure is the SIMPLEST one, remember. You can use cream, if you must, but NEVER sugar. White sugar is actually a poison to your system, no matter how much energy you SEEM to get from it; and brown sugar is like gilding the lily: the fruit itself is plentiful with sugar - you do not need to PUT sugar on your sugar!

In general, too, remember that sweet milk goes best with the ACID fruits; while sour milk, like clabber, yogurt or even cottage cheese, goes best with the SUB-ACID fruits. In other words, a glass of milk at orange juice time is a permissible combination. Again, KEEP YOUR DIET SIMPLE.

KITCHEN HINTS

Cooking cabbage and cauliflower leaves an odor in the air. Burn a piece of cotton string and the carbon formed takes up the odor.

As a substitute for baking powder, use half as much cream of tartar.

When refrigeration is not obtainable, put wet sand around the butter bowl at night, or wrap in a wet cloth and newspaper. The butter will be cold and hard the next morning.

Two tablespoons of lemon juice added to a cup of sweet milk sours it immediately.

Dip knife in hot water before cutting meringue.

When grinding dry bread for crumbs, place a paper bag over the end of grinder, secure with a rubber band, and you will have no crumbs spilling on the floor.

Bread crumbs that are to be kept for any time should be placed in tightly lidded glass jars and bread to be used for crumbs should be dried in oven and then placed in paper bags until made into crumbs.

When buying grapefruit or oranges, weigh them in the hand. The heavier they are, the more juice they contain.

Cream swells to double its bulk. When a pint of whipping cream is beaten, it whips up to a quart.

Scissors are a great convenience for cutting celery, cucumbers, parsley, mint, lettuce, etc.; much quicker and better than using a knife.

The juice of a lemon added to a pan of water freshens wilted vegetables soaked therein for about an hour.

Buy vegetables and fruits in season when you are on a limited budget. Do not buy perishables in larger quantities than you can use immediately.

For economy, the method of cooking must be considered when planning meals. As nearly as possible have dishes that can all be cooked in the oven, or all on top of the stove.

Use wet or buttered scissors when cutting dates into small pieces. Wet or butter your grinder when grinding dried fruit.

To add flour to a mixture, either mix with cold water, sugar, or an equal amount of fat or oil. These substances separate the flour particles.

If you do not have a nut chopper use a small baking powder can. Punch some holes in the top.

Cover egg yolks with water before placing in refrigerator, and cover pimientos with oil. These foods remain usable much longer thus.

Slip a piece of wax paper over handle of beater and down around bowl in which cream is being whipped to prevent spattering.

Suit all meal planning to the season and think of the weather when planning your menus. Foods in season are an economical choice.

Do not guess at the amounts used in any recipe. Measure accurately for successful and uniform results and combine ingredients as instructed.

When butter proves too hard for spreading, turn a heated bowl or pan upside down over the butter dish for a few minutes. This softens butter without melting it. Heat the pan or bowl in the oven or by putting boiling water in it.

Mix nuts or raisins with dry ingredients to keep them from falling to the bottom of the bowl.

Use a simple garnish. Do not overcrowd the plate or platter of food, but rather use a simple garnish of parsley, ripe olives, sections of hard-cooked eggs, tomatoes or green pepper, or a dash of paprika or sea lettuce. Make an every day dish "supreme."

Before cooking rice, butter the pan to prevent sticking.

Do not use soda to keep vegetables green. It destroys Vitamin C.

Save all water in which vegetables have been cooked, except cabbage water. Use this water containing valuable minerals in soups and broths, and in vegetable cocktails.

When baking vegetables, always add just a little water to help vegetables cook more quickly.

Remember that grated vegetables cook quicker, therefore retaining their valuable nutrients.

All vegetables should be cooked according to their own tenderness and just to the point of cooking through.

When preparing vegetables, add a little onion juice, garlic, or parsley for flavor.

To give your body the best, use distilled water to drink and for all cooking purposes.

FREEZING AND DRYING FOODS

Freezing foods is the best way to keep them because it preserves most of the vitamin and mineral values.

Meat, fish and poultry should be frozen in plastic freezer bags. Some feel it is best to wrap them in freezer paper as well.

Berries should be frozen individually on trays, then put into plastic freezer bags. Otherwise they will stick together in a solid mass in the bag because they don't all freeze at the same rate.

Peaches, apricots and nectarines should have a little lemon juice added to the liquid you freeze them in to keep them from turning brown.

Corn, peas, beans and other vegetables should be blanched before freezing. Just dip them in boiling water and take them right out.

Drying can be done on boards and screens but they must be covered to keep flies, wasps and other insects out. Once, I took dates on a trip to India, but by the time we got there, they had maggots. You must be careful. The totally enclosed drying ovens are a good way of keeping out insect life. These dehydrate the fruits and vegetables at a low, constant electrical heat. A small fan blows the evaporating moisture out.

Lovely hot soups can be made from dried fruits in the winter time.

FOOD TIPS FOR THE WISE

Squash are among the easiest foods to digest, and they produce no gas or irritation. They are good for all bowel troubles.

Foods that cause the most gas are the sulphur foods such as cauliflower, broccoli, onions, leeks and garlic. Less gas is produced if you cook them in low heat, waterless stainless cookware. (Most people use a little water.) Many people can take raw sulphur vegetables without gas problems but not everyone. It may be best to steam them a little to break down the fiber structure.

I consider beets and broccoli the two finest vegetables. Beets cleanse the lilver and gently stimulate the bowel activity. Broccoli is made up of flowers and is one of our most mature plants in bringing all the vitamins and minerals to a finished stage. Broccoli, being green, carries a good deal of the sun energy and is one of the greatest foods for rebuilding the body and keeping it well.

Fruits and vegetables in the diet favor elimination. You can interfere with this elimination by adding a starch or protein. Starch and proteins inhibit the elimination activity. To get rid of catarrh, eliminate milk, wheat and sugar from the diet.

Start the day with a glass of water and a teaspoon of liquid chlorophyll. I think we should have two or three glasses of liquid before breakfast to clean out the kidneys and bladder from concentrated acidic urine accumulated during sleep.

Use a little dulse in your food every day to give iodine to the thyroid.

Use fish or chicken no more than three times a week, reduce or eliminate red meat from your diet. Dessert only once a week.

Drink enough liquid during the day to keep the urine colorless.

Everyone should take vitamin A every day. You may not need vitamin C tablets if you are not bringing toxins into the body. If you live in a smoggy city and drink chemically-treated water, you should take extra vitamin C.

For B vitamins, look to the silicon foods—sprouts, rice polishings, all foods that have shiny polishings. These are good for the hair, nails and skin. Rice bran syrup is good. If you get your B-complex from brewer's yeast, take a silicon supplement. The two go together in the body.

The foods in my **Health and Harmony Food Regimen** will provide most of your vitamins and minerals more than adequately.

Older people or younger persons beginning to have arthritis problems or memory problems should think of taking 500 mg to 1000 mg of niacin with every meal. Not niacinamide, but niacin, the vitamin that flushes the blood to the head, skin and organs. This might do more for you than anything else. Niacin is harmless even in large doses, but the flush makes some people feel very uncomfortable.

For insomnia, take a little warm milk at night, and find a way to warm your feet.

I believe in giving children cod liver oil, particularly where the winters are sunless much of the time, whether due to overcast, fog, rain or the very short days of the areas near the Poles in winter. If your child drinks a great deal of milk, you may want to add a teaspoon per day of blackstrap molasses for the iron. Milk has very little iron in it. Or add a teaspoon of liquid chlorophyll or green plant juice.

Women having a difficult time with menopause should take dulse (for the iodine), black cohosh and licorice. These have helped many women. Dong quai is also good for balancing the female glands and can be taken with the herbs previously mentioned.

For men, ginseng is a good sex gland tonic and fo-ti-tieng is an excellent rejuvenating herb, a tonic for the nerves and brain.

For liver troubles, take liquid chlorophyll, cherry juice or both together. For heart trouble, avoid red meat. The cure for alcoholism: Stop drinking. The cure for smoking: Stop smoking.

Ringing of the ears caused by hardening of the arteries may sometimes be eliminated by using lecithin and whey supplements in the diet. Also try chaparral tea or Pau D'Arco tea.

For high blood pressure, have brown rice and vegetables for two meals a day for two weeks.

Those interested in finding out more about foods and how foods can be our medicine should get my book *Nature Has A Remedy.*

BODY HINTS

Signs of a Good Chemically-Balanced Body

General appearance of good health.
Alert, active, vigorous
Skin clear, smooth, soft, slightly moist, and somewhat pink.
Weight proportionate to height and age, with pleasing carriage.
Hair plentiful, lustrous, having no indication of being brittle or excessively dry.
Eyes bright and clear with no dark rings or circles under them.
Muscles firm and strong.
Chest broad and deep.
Tongue pink and not coated. Breath sweet.
Posture straight and upright.
Nerves steady.
Joints limber, free from deposits and stiffness.

21

Herbs for Health and for Seasoning

Herbs are mentioned many times in the Good Book, and we find out that they are foods—not drugs—in their activity. Yet there is a concentrated activity in herbs that often goes beyond the effectiveness of ordinary foods in cleansing the body, promoting healing, balancing the glands and so forth. Everyone should at least be acquainted with what herbs can do. Some herbs make wonderful seasonings for foods, and we will describe some of those, too.

An herb tea is the best health drink you can have in your diet. I advise most patients to have 2-3 cups a day with or between meals.

HERBAL TEAS

Peppermint. Good for the nerves and for fermentation of gas from starches and sugars in the digestive tract.

Catnip. Rich in potassium, an effective gas driver. Stomach gas in children and old people after drinking milk is often relieved by this tea.

Sage. A good tonic, helpful for inflamed sinuses and colds, but a little binding to the bowel. Can be used with hot clam juice and a little lemon.

Spearmint, Mint or Dill. Soothing gas-driving teas.

Wintergreen. Eliminates catarrh, purifies the blood, aids digestion.

Juniper Berry. A diuretic, cleanses the liver and blood, tones the sexual system. Too much is hard on the kidneys. Father Kneipp

295

used to start with one or two berries, work up to 15 on the 10th day, then reverse his way back to 1 or 2.

Hawthorne Berry. To improve circulation and support the heart.

Comfrey. Soothing to the digestive system and bowel.

Oat Straw. High in silicon. Good for the nerves, skin, hair and lungs. Boil oat straw in water 10 minutes.

Parsley. A kidney cleanser. Rich in iron and manganese.

Fenugreek. Expels catarrh, can be used with comfrey for added benefit.

Blueberry. For low blood pressure.

Shavegrass. To supply silicon and cleanse the kidneys.

Cleaver. A diuretic.

KB-11. An herbal combination to cleanse the kidneys; a diuretic.

Licorice. Aids digestion; helps female troubles.

Valerian. A natural tranquilizer

Flaxseed. For the bowel.

Uva Ursi. For the kidneys.

All teas are made by pouring boiling water over leaves in a heated teapot, except for oat straw tea.

HEALING HERBS

Although many herbs can be taken as teas or infusions, capsules are sometimes necessary for various reasons. Most herbs can be purchased in health food stores.

Golden Seal. Stimulates gastric juices; aids digestion, good for all mucous membrane problems, colds, allergies, hay fever and colitis. Golden seal is also taken with other herbs to increase their effectiveness.

Echinacea. A cleanser of the lymph system, bacteriocide, active in eliminating toxic byproducts that contribute to degenerative disease.

Red Clover. For cleansing drug deposits and for diarrhea.

Yellow Dock. For acidity in the body and eczema.

Gotu Kola. A rejuvenator and brain function enhancer.

F o-Ti-Tieng. Strengthens digestion, stimulates metabolism; used also in cases of general debililty and decline. It is thought to energize the nerves of the body and brain.

Ginseng. Tonic for the male sexual system; for revitalizing the energy level and strengthening the natural immune system.

Valerian. Natural tranquilizer and nerve relaxant. Used for depression, coughs, insomnia, stress, nervous conditions and head congestion.

Dong Quai. Balances the female glands very effectively. One of the most widely-used herbs for female troubles.

Black Cohosh. Used for irregular menstrual periods, heavy flow and cramps.

Licorice. Supports adrenal glands; works together with black cohosh to normalize menstrual periods.

Dandelion. A good blood purifier.

Thyme. Bacteriocide, tonic, relaxant; helps stop itching.

HERBS FOR SEASONING FOODS

Basil. Tomatoes, eggs, fish.
Bay Leaves. Soups, stews, sauces.
Dill. Potatoes, vegetables, salads.
Mint. Lamb, vegetables, fruits.
Rosemary. All meats, vegetables.
Sage. Meats, cheeses (use sparingly).
Thyme. Meats, sauces, stocks, fish, vegetables.
Coriander. Meats, fish, soups, salads, vegetables.
Parsley. Soups, salads, garnishes.

SIMPLEST HERBS USED IN MY PRACTICE

The following are the herbs used most often in my practice. Many times I used more specific herbs for special conditions.

1. Hawthorne berry tea: heart.
2. Comfrey-fenugreek tea: catarrh, phlegm, mucus, sinus conditions, indigestion.
3. Blue violet tea: lymphatic congestion.
4. Dandelion tea: liver.
5. Black cohosh and licorice root: female gland balancing, change of life.
6. Oat straw tea: skin.

297

7. KB-11 (herbal combination): kidneys and bladder.
8. Ginseng and Fo ti tieng: male hormone balancing.
9. Red clover: blood purifier.
10. Papaya: digestion.
11. Peppermint tea: gas driver.
12. Pau D'Arco: blood purifier.

I use chlorophyll for alkalinizing acidic conditions, either liquid chlorophyll or chlorophyll as found in Sun Chlorella.

Instead of making herbal teas, many times I have used herbal extracts so there is not too much liquid intake during the day.

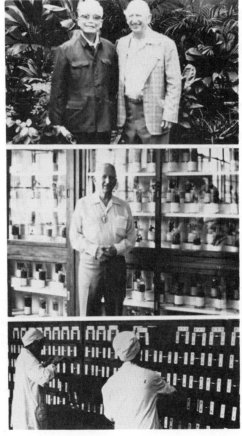

There were 250 doctors in Canton studying acupuncture and herbalism. In the hospital, a patient can choose herbal therapy, acupuncture or Western medicine, as he wishes. Middle: A Chinese herb museum. Bottom: Herb storeroom with thousands of herbs for out patients.

Ailments and Herbs Indicated

TO AID CIRCULATION
Basil, raspberry, spearmint, peppermint, dwarf elder, hawthorne berries, oatstraw, cayenne, prickly nettle.

NERVOUSNESS
Alfalfa, black cohosh, chamomile, skullcap, catnip, thyme, mistletoe, hops, lady's slipper, lavender, passion flower, valerian, lobelia.

TO AID HEART PROBLEMS
Hawthorne berries, anise seed, cayenne, garlic, horehound, mistletoe, sage, basil, marjoram.

NEURALGIA & NEURITIS
Motherwort.

LYMPH GLAND & CONGESTION
Cayenne, golden seal, poke root, echineacea, myrrh, onion pods, blue violet, blue flag.

TO ENERGIZE THE NERVES AND BRAIN CELLS
Fo ti tieng, black cohosh, ginseng, dong quai, gotu kola.

ADRENAL GLANDS
Borage, parsley, licorice, juniper berries, blood root, gotu kola, kelp, ginseng, lobelia, ginger.

LONGEVITY
Gotu kola, ginseng, dong quai.

DIABETES (ISLETS OF LANGERHANS/PANCREAS)
Huckleberry, parsley, burdock, nettle, licorice, elecampane, dandelion, juniper berries.

ASTHMA, BRONCHIAL PROBLEMS, LUNGS
Angelica, fenugreek, black cohosh, garlic, onions, licorice, pleurisy root, comfrey, lungwort, sage, mullein, marshmallow, eucalyptus, thyme, elecampane, buchu, cayenne, elderflowers, peppermint, yarrow.

HYPOGLYCEMIA
Blueberry, licorice, dandelion.

PINEAL—PITUITARY
Sage, mistletoe, veronica, ginseng, dong quai, cayenne, licorice, golden seal.

COUGHING
Blue violet, thyme, licorice, garlic, onions, coltsfoot, mullein, sage.

THYROID
Dulse, horseradish, parsley, pokeweed, radish, kelp, burdock root, ginseng.

CONGESTION IN LUNGS—HEAD
Rue, garlic, onions, comfrey, elderflowers, peppermint, yarrow.

FATIGUE
Gotu kola, ginseng, cayenne, dulse, licorice.

NASAL DRIP
Golden seal.

FEVER
Cayenne, fenugreek, ginseng, catnip, parsley, sorrel, feverwort, nettle, hysop.

ANEMIA
Parsley, wheatgrass, dandelion, yellow dock.

COLD HANDS AND FEET
Sage, parsley, cayenne, hawthorne berries.

TO REGULATE BLOOD PRESSURE
Hawthorne berries, capsicum.

TO AID KIDNEY—BLADDER
Alfalfa, comfrey, golden seal, cornsilk, yarrow, uvi ursi, oatstraw, shavegrass, sage, slippery elm, buchu, dandelion, elderberry, juniper berries, red raspberry, parsley.

BLOOD PURIFIER
Burdock, sage, dandelion, juniper berries, comfrey, sarsaparilla, sasafras, strawberry leaves, red clover, yellow dock, golden seal, licorice, cayenne, echinacea, chapparal.

ARTHRITIS—RHEUMATISM
Comfrey, parsley, nettles, alfalfa, dandelion, black cohosh, sarsaparilla, aloe vera.

URINARY—PROSTATE TRACT CLEANSER
Kelp, black cohosh, gotu kola, ginger, golden seal, licorice, cayenne, juniper berries, buchu leaves, gravel root.

DIGESTIVE HERBS
Chamomile, fenugreek, golden seal, peppermint, spearmint, thyme, sassafras, savory, huckleberry, fennel, papaya.

FOR FERTILITY AND FOR SEXUAL IMPOTENCY
Saw palmetto, damiana, kila nut, sarsparilla, false unicorn, licorice.

EAR INFECTIONS
Golden seal, echinacea, poke root, cayenne, chamomile, mullein, garlic oil.

MALE REJUVENATING AND MALE HORMONES
Sarsaparilla, garlic, ginseng, damiana, echinacea, white willow, gotu kola, saw palmetto, cayenne, golden seal, chickweed.

EPILEPSY
Black cohosh, blue cohosh, vervain.

OVARIES—GONADS
Elderberry, Catnip, raspberry, black cohosh, damiana, dong quai, ginseng, licorice, uva ursi, chickweed, saw palmetto.

299

HYDROCHLORIC ACID, A LACK OF
Papaya.

INDIGESTION—ANTACIDS
Catnip, angelica, cayenne, chamomile, dandelion, boneset, lovage, ginger, golden seal, papaya, peppermint, spearmint, yarrow, anise, juniper berries.

BOILS
Onion pack, aloe vera, cayenne, comfrey, golden seal.

TO CLEAR THE COMPLEXION
Sage, scurvy grass, garlic.

PERSPIRATION—TO BRING ON, DIAPHORETICS
Blue cohosh, boneset, chamomile, ginger, thyme, kava kava, marigold, pennyroyal, sassafras, elder flowers, hyssop, catnip.

SLEEPLESSNESS
Catnip, chamomile, passion flower, sage, skullcap, linden, balm, lavender, valerian, lobelia.

GALLSTONES
Cornsilk, slippery elm, parsley, white oak bark, wild yam.

TO INCREASE THE FLOW OF BILE
Dandelion.

TO AID THE LIVER
Yellow dock, alfalfa, dandelion, golden seal, blue violet, boldo, cascara sagrada, marigold, white oak bark, oatstraw, nettle, mullein, archangelica, artichoke sage, juniper berries, parsley, horsetail, gentian, blessed thistle, goldenrod, liverworth, strawberry, turkey rhubarb.

MUSCLES
Juniper berries, rosemary, tansy, black walnut.

JOINTS
Elderflowers, chicory root, juniper berries, arnica flowers.

ACIDITY
Yellow dock, dandelion.

ALLERGIES—HAYFEVER
Ginseng, gentian root, blessed thistle.

ANEMIA
Dandelion, pau D'arco.

SMOKING—TO STOP
Chamomile (chew), gentian (chew).

MENSTURATION—TO INCREASE FLOW
Chamomile, parsley, yarrow, red sage, basil, ginger, gentian, lemon balm, rosemary, saffron, red clover, rue.

TO DECREASE FLOW
Red sage, barberry bark, yarrow, uva ursi, black hawthorne, raspberry, shepherd's purse, white oak bark,ginger, blue cohosh.

CRAMPS
Raspberry, cramp bark, peach bark, dill.

TO AID IN PREMENSTRUAL TENSION
Chamomile, comfrey, lavender, mugwort, horsetail grass, spearmint, peppermint, valerian, licorice.

MENOPAUSE—TO STIMULATE; NATURAL ESTROGEN
Black cohosh, elder, licorice, sassafras, sarsaparilla, lady slipper, sage, passion flower, Mexican wild yam, false unicorn root, cramp bark, holy thistle, vervain, raspberry.

BOWEL POCKETS
Alfalfa, psyllium seed, cascara sagrada, golden seal, garlic.

COLITIS—ULCERS OF BOWEL AND STOMACH
Agar, fenugreek, shavegrass, comfrey, golden seal, flaxseed, slippery elm, woodruff, cayenne, arrowroot (nouroishes), aloe vera.

COLON
Flaxseed, psyllium seed, alfalfa, slippery elm, comfrey, aloe vera.

CONSTIPATION
Flaxseed, senna, aloe vera, yellow dock, castor oil, dandelion, cascara sagrada, agar agar.

DYSENTERY—DIARRHEA
Elderberry, huckleberry, red clover, slippery elm, white oak, yarrow, cayenne, flaxseed, golden seal, raspberry, licorice, aloe vera, blackberry.

ENEMAS FOR BLEEDING BOWEL
Flaxseed, golden seal, slippery elm, white oak bark, aloe vera, yarrow.

GENERAL, SOOTHING ENEMAS
White oak, flaxseed, slippery elm, comfrey root.

GAS—FLATULENCE
Balsam, ginger, catnip, chamomile, fennel, pennyroyal, peppermint, spearmint, shavegrass, savory, rue, caraway, angelica, anise, juniper berries, papaya.

300

22

Specialty Foods
and
Food Supplements

Nature has provided some foods that are exceptional in their overall record of preventing disease or getting rid of symptoms of disease. Many of these foods react differently with different people, and we can't tell if they will work with a particular person. Whether you use these foods or not, you should know about them.

Whenever we find that we are feeling below par and fatigue settles in or we have a problem in the body, we can suspect some vitamin/mineral deficiency in our body. Usually we find that any adverse physical condition in the body is a sign of some vitamin or mineral missing. Many times the most effective way to deal with the problem immediately is to use the specialty foods. But you should realize that changing your daily eating regimen is often the key to building a better body and better health. It is also possible that the deficiency is due to fatigue, overwork or stress, all of which can burn out nutrients faster than we can replace them with foods.

Carotene. Carotene is pro-vitamin A, found in carrots, all yellow fruits and vegetables, all green vegetables (very high in parsley and chlorella), eggs, milk and butter.

Malva (Mallow). Used as a tea or enema, malva soothes the bowel. Root infusions are said to be good for urinary tract infections.

Bee Pollen. Full of natural sugars, enzymes, vitamins and protein. Builds the red blood count, balances the glands, soothes the nerves.

Royal Jelly. This is the nutrient fed by nurse bees to their queen. It is believed to build up the glands and restore vitality faster than any other food. It is a *whole body food.*

Propolis. The dark substance used by bees to coat the interior of their hives, used to treat allergies, kidney problems and other conditions. It is a health builder.

Aloe Vera. Good externally for burns, sunburn, insect bites, rashes, etc. Taken internally, aloe vera is said to have a tonic effect on the vital organs. The skin of the aloe has a powerful laxative effect.

Garlic. A wonderful resistance builder and natural antibiotic, may be eaten to get rid of intestinal parasites. Can be chopped fine and put in capsules to avoid bad taste.

Ginseng. Sustains vitality, tones the male sexual system, strengthens the natural immune system and revitalizes the body's energy system. One Chinese emperor paid $3,200 a pound. It is said to be helpful as an antidote for narcotics.

Chlorophyll. The green substance in the leaves of plants. This is one of the most powerful and effective cleansers found in nature. Liquid chlorophyll is available in many health food stores.

Colloidal Sulphur. An effective detoxifier of the body, according to studies at Harvard University, eliminating chemical and bacterial toxins.

Dulse. An excellent natural source of iodine. May be taken in tablets with meals or purchased in flakes to sprinkle on foods. Dulse is a type of kelp, and other edible types of kelp are also good sources of iodine.

Soybean Flour. Can be made into soymilk to substitute for cow's milk or formula. Usually non-allergenic. Can be added to soups, casseroles and other foods to increase food value.

Alfalfa Tablets. For cleansing and toning the bowel. Four to six tablets taken with meals, cracked and swallowed with water.

Protomorphogens. These dried extracts of animal glands or organs used in extreme depletion of one or more glands to help rebuild and revitalize that tissue. This is a way to get the specific vitamins, minerals and cell-building nutrients we need to build up specific glands. They are available for the adrenal glands, ovaries, thyroid and so forth.

Rice Bran Syrup. A high source of organic silicon; also rich in B vitamins.

Auxins. Plant hormones in sprouts and young plants brought out by Dr. Brown Landone.

Colostrum. Colostrum is a choline-rich substance found in mother's milk in both humans and animals the first three days when feeding the young. This substance starts the bowel activity, the bowel movements, and helps to develop the friendly bacteria in the bowel. There is now a colostrum product to be used with the acidophilus culture in restoring the proper balance of friendly bacteria in the bowel, for those who have bowel problems.

Lactobacillus Acidophilus. This is a beneficial bacteria for the bowel, sold in tablet, powder or liquid form. The acidophilus bacteria produce B vitamins, inhibit the multiplication of undesirable putrefactive bacteria, helps reduce overgrowth of candida albicans, and are reported to reduce cholesterol.

Digest Aids. Digestive aids help the digestion. Most contain animal derivatives (protomorphogens). There is also an herbal digestant for vegetarians.

Yogurt, Kefir, Clabbered Milk. Easy-to-digest fermented milk, semi-solid or liquid.

Beet Tablets. These stimulate the bowel and help cleanse the liver and gallbladder.

Egg Yolk in Black Cherry Juice. My best nerve tonic.

Fiber. This is undigestible fiber needed by the bowel for proper muscle tone and efficiency of elimination.

Brewer's Yeast. High in B vitamins, protein, RNA.

Blackstrap Molasses. An excellent iron source, also good for B vitamins, potassium and various other minerals.

Dessicated Liver. High in iron; helps build the bloodstream and overcome anemia.

Lecithin. This is an important brain and nerve food and is needed to balance cholesterol in the body.

Cod Liver Oil. A vitamin A and D supplement. Vitamin A protects the mucous membranes and eye tissues, while vitamin D helps control calcium in the body.

Chlorella. This is a dried, edible algae, in powder, tablet or capsule form, high in protein, pro-vitamin A, chlorophyll, iron

and a growth factor that stimulates healing. It also has a considerable amount of potassium and phosphorus. Because it is a
single whole cell algae, it is a whole natural food with the components that sustain life. Excellent for cleansing and building the
blood and repairing and rebuilding tissues.

Whey. Goat whey is the best source of biochemical sodium
and helps bring undesirable calcium deposits in the body back
into solution. Whey is a very good food for restoring electrolytes
in the bowel. The best is a dried goat whey product called Whex,
available from Briar Hills Dairies, P.O. Box 1007, Chehalis, WA
98532.

NOTE ON SEEDS

Seeds have the next generation principle, and because of this,
nature has concentrated her best nutritional values in them. The
life of the next generation of any species is found in its seeds.
Everything in a plant was first in its seed. The power and ability to
regenerate, the material for the development of our glands, is
found in seeds. Seeds are glandular support foods, needed to
support and build the male and female principles in our bodies. We
should be eating all the seeds possible as found in our foods.

Female sex hormone is said to be highest in citrus seeds,
male sex hormone highest in date pits. Pumpkin seeds are high
in zinc. Sunflower seeds are very high in potassium, phosphorus
and have considerable vitamin A. Alfalfa seeds are best for overall mineral values. Berry seeds are high in vitamin F, needed by
the bowel. Sesame seeds resist rancidity better than most seeds,
are high in calcium and are good sources of protein. Pomegranate seeds are good for the genito-urinary system. Most seeds
have iron, and two of the highest are pumpkin seeds and sunflower seeds. Fluorine is found on the outside of most seeds.
Cantaloupe and cucumber seeds are high in mineral values.
Most seeds are low in sodium, have a high potassium-to-sodium
ratio and contain lecithin which builds the glands, nerves and
brain. All seeds have vitamin A and a few of the B vitamins. Fenugreek seeds made into a tea reduce catarrh and mucus in the
body. The oils in seeds are good for the body and have no cholesterol. It is claimed that nutrients from tahini, made from

sesame seeds, are so easily digested that they begin entering the bloodstream in 15 minutes. While we may not eat date seeds or citrus seeds, there are many others we can and should eat. Hard-hulled seeds should be put in a blender with vegetable juice and strained after blending to remove hull fragments.

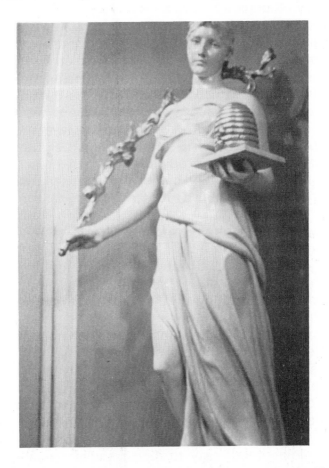

Mr. Royden Brown, C. C. Pollen Company, Scottsdale, AZ, says, "As far as I know, bee pollen is one of the few foods containing all of the essential nutrients needed for perfect health. As you and I know, the bee collects the strongest part, the reproductive part of every herb and every flower and converts it into bee pollen. Since there are from 500,000 to 6,000,000 pollen spores in every granule of bee pollen, bee pollen must represent the closest we can come to totally eating that life force or that whole food you (Dr. Jensen) so scholarly discuss."

This statue in Czechoslovakia holds a bee hive and celebrates the goodness of honey.

THE WONDERFUL BENEFITS OF POLLEN

Pythagoras, the great 5th century B.C. Greek philosopher and mathematician, taught that honey in the diet promoted longevity. In those days, honey was not refined, and it contained a good deal of pollen. Although honey is a healthy sweet, it doesn't compare, nutritionally speaking, with the healthful and rejuvenating qualities of bee pollen, and it is bee pollen that should be given the credit for the life-extending ability mentioned by Pythagoras.

Bee pollen was used both as a medicine and food in ancient civilizations such as China, Egypt and the Persian empire, as archeologists have discovered from ancient writings. Roman centurions carried pollen cakes, alternate layers of honey and pollen, pressed and dried. Some historians believe this is one of the reasons the Roman legions had such great stamina and endurance in marching and battle. Similar pollen cakes have been discovered among primitive tribes in the Far East in modern times.

A TREAT OR A TREATMENT?

We find in the past 30 years or so, pollen has been extensively researched both for its food value and for its value in treating a variety of health problems. Pollen grains, the male fertilization factor in plants, have been analyzed in modern research laboratories and found to be one of the most balanced and complete foods known to man. Protein, carbohydrates, fats, enzymes, vitamins, minerals and a few mysterious compounds not yet understood by science are found in pollen in such quality and proportion that this wonderful food tends to correct imbalances in the blood chemistry as it feeds and restores tissues deficient in the various vitamin and mineral factors. It is a blood-building food, a tissue-building food, easy to digest and assimilate, with great rejuvenating power and no known undesirable side effects. Used as a food, bee pollen has not been known to trigger any allergic reactions in any of the people who have used it.

In one experiment, subjects fed only bee pollen and water under controlled fasting conditions were actually in better health at the end of the experiment than at the beginning. Bee pollen may be a potentially excellent survival food as well as a food supplement.

THE ULTIMATE NATURAL FOOD

Pollen is entirely a natural food from vegetable sources. An average hive of bees may gather 80 pounds of it over the flower blooming season. Natives in some areas of the world use nets to scoop pollen from the surface of creeks, rivers, lakes and ponds, drying the pollen cakes for later use. In recent years, Swedish researchers have developed a machine for harvesting pollen directly from flowering plants. Pollen grains are easily as small as grains of fine flour and are different in each plant, as can be seen under a microscope. About the 1950s, pollen directly gathered from flowers began to receive attention as a food supplement.

Athletes use bee pollen tablets to increase endurance and stamina and to speed up recovery time. Teams in football and ice hockey, weightlifters, long distance runners, wrestlers and champion boxers such as Mohammed Ali have used bee pollen tablets to improve their performance.

Finnish long distance runners, taking bee pollen supplements, won several gold medals at the 1972 Olympics and again in the 1976 Olympics.

The Russian Olympic coach, Remi Korchemny, tested bee pollen on his athletes, proving that regular use speeds up the recovery time of runners. Those using the bee pollen, after running a race, were able to run again and were able to equal or better their running time for the same distance after a brief rest break. A control group of equally fast runners who had been taking placebos remained fatigued after a brief rest break following their first race and did poorly on their second run.

Some experts believe that pollen, like chlorophyll in green plants, stores up the life force from sunlight and makes it available to the body after assimilation. A teaspoon a day is the usual amount recommended as a supplement to those without health problems.

HEALTH RESEARCH ON POLLEN

In the 1950s, a French physician named Chauvin, performed extensive studies of pollen used as a food supplement by considerable numbers of people, from the very young to the very old. Effective results were found in anemia, constipation, relief of gas, colon infections, diarrhea, normalizing body weight, restoring appetite and general improvement of vitality among the elderly. Pollen showed bacteriocidal properties in killing harmful bacteria in the bowel. More recently, University of Arizona researchers have found natural antibiotics in pollen.

Children in a French tuberculosis sanitarium were given a teaspoon of bee pollen in a glass of juice at breakfast, and in a month, their red blood cell counts increased up to 800,000 more than previously. Pollen is considered of great value in overcoming anemia.

Bee pollen was shown to help many bowel conditions. In many cases, constipation, diarrhea and spastic bowel problems disappeared when pollen was taken every day. Many cases of colitis were helped. One patient with a severe case of diverticulosis had fever, alternating diarrhea and constipation, bloody mucus in his stools, and had been losing weight for eight months. Taking two teaspoons of pollen a day ended nearly all these problems within two weeks. In a month, he gained two pounds in weight. Several cases of chronic constipation that were not helped by laxatives were completely restored to natural regularity and movements.

A teenager placed in a sanitarium for recovery from a severe and painful case of rheumatism in the joints and neck vertebrae developed catarrh problems, fatigue, loss of appetite, and failed to grow in weight or height for eight months. He had been given cortisone, without notable improvement. When he was given a tablespoon of bee pollen a day, his appetite came back, and in the following six months, he gained 15 pounds and 2 inches in height.

Acne problems were treated with bee pollen with great success. Some health researchers believe that acne, in many cases, is linked to bowel disorders or an underactive bowel. It is significant that one of pollen's most effective results is in improving bowel health and regularity.

Another use for bee pollen is weight normalization. Among overweight subjects, weight loss was stimulated by taking a teaspoon of pollen half an hour before meals. With underweight people who experienced great difficulty trying to gain weight, taking a teaspoon of pollen after meals provided good results. Again, we find that the normalization of the bowel probably plays some part in weight normalization.

German researchers tried bee pollen on patients taking radiation therapy, starting 3 days before the radiation treatments and continuing during and after the treatments. Expected side effects such as hair loss did not occur. Another group of patients who took the same radiation therapy without taking pollen supplements had the usual radiation side effects.

Russian researchers have reported success in treating nerve disturbances and endocrine disorders with pollen. In these cases, three factors concerning pollen are possibly at the heart of this success. First, pollen is about 15% lecithin, which feeds the nerves and sex glands in the endocrine system. Secondly, pollen tends to normalize the blood chemistry, helping correct vitamin and mineral deficiencies which are often found in nerve and endocrine problems. Thirdly, the normalization of the bowel by pollen would reduce any toxic accumulations in the body which could have been irritating the nerves and upsetting glandular balance.

In the U.S., allergy specialist Dr. Leo Conway of Denver, Colorado, treated 6,200 allergy patients with directly harvested (non-bee) pollen taken orally, and 94% became symptom-free. Dr. Conway later compiled 60,000 documented cases of allergies being relieved by pollen supplements, at 1/3 to 1/2 the cost of the usual allergy shots.

German and Swedish urology teams tested pollen on men with prostate conditions, with good results. Pollen is believed to contain a chemical compound similar to the pituitary hormone that is needed by the sex glands. In fact, there have been many reports of pollen restoring sexual potency in men, including some in their 70s and 80s.

Research at Harvard University medical school has indicated that diets high in the amino acid methionine and low in vitamin B-6 may initiate heart disease. Researchers feel that diets and foods high in B-6 and low in methionine could help prevent heart disease. Carrots have a 6-to-1 ratio, bananas are 40-to-1, but bee pollen is 400-to-1, the highest ratio of B-6-to-methionine yet discovered.

Because of its beneficial fats and oils, pollen also helps keep the skin young, according to Swedish dermatologist Dr. Lars-Eric Essen.

Dr. Alois Schusta of Vienna, Austria, treated 9 women with menopausal or premenopausal disorders, ranging in age from 40 to 59, and one 29-year-old. Previous treatments had given only temporary relief until bee pollen was tried. All 9 women responded favorably to the bee pollen, and their symptoms disappeared without further problems.

In addition to the results published by the German and Swedish urology teams, Dr. Yutaka Saito of the Nagasaki School of Medicine in Japan reported an 80% cure rate of chronic prostatitis in men using bee pollen.

Pollen has been found to provide relief or eliminate symptoms completely in premature aging, rickets, anemia, bowel troubles, prostatitis, menopausal troubles, nervous problems, insomnia and lack of appetite. It reduces the incidence of colds and flu and increases strength and energy so people feel better if they do get a cold or flu virus.

We find that bee pollen has such a broad and balanced array of nutrients that are so easily digested and assimilated that it is no wonder it has proved to be such an effective health builder. In the analysis of basic pollen ingredients to follow, you will see that you would have to take 5 or 6 different foods to get all the nutrients found together in pollen. Of all natural foods now known, bee pollen is claimed to have the most complete, complex and balanced combination of nutrients known to man. Its normalizing effect on the bowel plus its nutritional value make it both a cleansing and building food.

ANALYSIS OF BEE POLLENS

Keeping in mind that bee pollens differ from area to area, the following analysis of the main ingredients of bee pollen made from clover gives some idea of its nutritional power.

Moisture	23.9%	Protein	20.2%
Solids	76.1%	Ash	2.7%

Enzymes and Coenzymes

Diastase	Phosphatase	**Carbohydrates**
Amylase	Catalase	Sucrose
Saccharase	Diaphorase	Levulose/Fructose
Pectase (and others)	Cozymase	Glucose

Fatty Acids	**Minerals**
Caproic	Calcium
Capric	Phosphorus
Myristic	Iron
Palmitoleic	Copper
Linoleic (and others)	Sulphur
Caprylic	Zinc (and others)
Lauric	Potassium
Palmitic	Magnesium
Stearic	Manganese
Oleic	Silicon
	Sodium
	Iodine

Vitamins

All of B-Complex, C, D, E, K, biotin, choline, inositol, rutin.

Amino Acids (percent)

Arginine	5.3	Methionine	1.9
Histidine	2.5	Phenylalanine	4.1
Isoleucine	5.1	Threonine	4.1
Leucine	7.1	Tryptophan	1.4
Lysine	6.4	Valine	5.8

Plus Cystine, Tyrosine, Glutamic Acid, Glycine, Serine, Proline, Alanine, Aspartic Acid and others.

Miscellaneous

Fats and oils 5%.

Carotenoids and other pigments.

Waxes, resins, steroids, growth factors, guanine, lecithin (about 15%), nucleic acids, flavonoids, various amines, phenolic acids and many more.

GETTING THE BEST FROM POLLEN

Bee pollen is best, like most other natural foods, when it is fresh. It can lose up to 76% of its nutritional value in a year. The best known method of preserving the nutritional value of pollen is flash freezing at zero degrees. It is not advisable to use pollen in cooked, baked or heated foods, as enzymes and lecithin are destroyed by heat. Pollen should be stored in the refrigerator or freezer to protect its potency.

PROPOLIS

Honeybees make propolis from a resin gathered from the buds of trees, forming the resin into a kind of antiseptic "varnish" used to coat the interior of the hive and close all cracks from the weather. Its composition is about 5% pollen, 30% wax, 55% resins and balms and 10% oils. German beekeepers in the 1800s were said to have discovered its health-enhancing properties, but no doubt other beekeepers and honey gatherers through the ages knew of its usefulness. Propolis is high in vitamins, minerals, amino acids and flavonoids, and has been found to have a natural antibiotic as pollen does.

Bee propolis or some ingredient in it, kills bacteria, viruses and fungus. In the U.S., it has been used for hay fever, infections unresponsive to antibiotics, mononucleosis and stress reduction. Russians have been using propolis for almost 20 years for bowel and kidney problems, allergies, hypertension and vascular problems. The Chinese claim propolis reduces blood lipids. Yugoslavian doctors have found propolis effective in periodontal problems, in staph infections and flu viruses. An Austrian doctor who gave bee propolis to 150 patients with gastric and duodenal ulcers, and the usual medication to another 150 with the same ailments, found that 70% of the propolis-takers obtained relief in 3 days, as compared with 10% of the others.

A European symposium on bee propolis drew doctors from the USSR, Czechoslovakia, Yugoslavia, Poland, Rumania, West Germany and France. Papers were given showing evidence that bee propolis stimulates cell growth, reduces inflammation of the mucous membranes, lowers high blood pressure and alleviates catarrhal problems. The natural antibiotic effect of propolis is of interest to doctors all over the world because of increasing problems with strains of bacteria that have developed immunity to man-made antibiotics.

ROYAL JELLY

Royal jelly, another honeybee product, is the substance fed to the queen bee in the hive who may lay up to 10,000 eggs a day, eating only this food. The queen also lives 5 or 6 years, as compared to the average worker bee who lives from 28 to 42 days. Royal jelly is said to prolong life, build the sex glands and restore vitality faster than any other food.

In practice, royal jelly has been found to be the most help to people with heart problems. It was found to provide relief in cases of angina and infarction, to normalize blood pressure—whether high or low—and to reduce blood cholesterol levels. Patients reported taking 100 mg of royal jelly daily with honey for at least a month.

Britain's Royal Family has discovered the benefits of royal jelly. Princess Di has used it for morning sickness, while Prince Charles has taken it for arthritis. Royal jelly is high in B vitamins, lecithin and has anti-bacterial properties. Iron, calcium, copper, potassium, sulphur, phosphorus and silicon are among the minerals found in it.

Anorectics, post-operative patients and premature babies have all benefitted from the use of royal jelly. This special food is reportedly beneficial for skin problems, depression, asthma, change of life problems in women and insomnia. It is known to increase vitality, stimulate the appetite and aid the digestion.

BROMELIN (BROMELAIN)

We find that pineapple contains a digestive enzyme called bromelin, similar to the activity of papain as found in papayas. The difference between the two has not been investigated, but we know that papain is taken from green papayas and is destroyed in the ripening process, while bromelin is found in ripe pineapples. After extraction from the pineapple, the bromelin is freeze-dried to protect and preserve its vital principles.

As an aid to digestion, the bromelin enzyme splits proteins. As a health supplement, bromelin has been used to treat internal inflammation and swelling, soothe the digestive system and speed up tissue repair. It has reportedly helped sore throats, ulcers, gastritis, enteritis, colitis and catarrhal conditions. Fresh pineapple juice, taken daily for a week during menstruation, helped relieve painful periods.

In tropical areas where pineapple is grown, the fresh juice is taken for indigestion and sore throats. For the latter, it may be used as a gargle. People with inherently weak stomachs eat a few slices of pineapple at the end of the meal. Crushed pineapple pulp is put on external swellings and bruises or on corns or troublesome calluses. Pineapple has been used as a beauty aid, rubbed on to freshen, tone, vitalize and soften the skin.

VITAMIN B-3—NIACIN

Vitamin B-3, niacin, produces a warmth to the skin and a flush to the head in most people after it is taken. This vitamin increases circulation to the extremities and to the organs of the body. In all my years of practice, I have never found anyone who experienced abnormal, bad or ill effects from this vitamin, except for the flushing.

Vitamin B-3 may be indicated to improve circulation. Symptoms such as a short concentration span, poor memory, mental dullness, poor circulation in extremities such as skin, legs, hands, etc., usually mean B-3 is indicated. When symptoms indicate this need, a patient may start by taking 150 mg per day, dividing it into 50 mg per dose, 3 times a day. Niacin may be gradually increased to any level that does not cause extreme discomfort. (Suggested limit: 3 gm/day.)

IMPORTANT
Vitamin B-3 should be taken 3/4 of the way through a meal or at the end of a meal. It must not be taken on an empty stomach. This will prevent or reduce the hot flush to the head—in most cases.

The reason for increasing the dose slowly, over a period of days, is because the flushing in the head will usually diminish over 3 or 4 days. If the flush does not go away, take more time before increasing dosage or take the amount you can stand, maintaining that over a period of time.

────────────23────────────

Stress

There is much that can be said about stress today as it appears to be silently developing in person after person, and there are very few who actually realize that there are actual changes in body chemistry and immune system function when we add our emotional and mental troubles to other physical problems that come from an unhealthy lifestyle. We've gotten to the place where we realize that this body can take only so much stress, which affects the nervous system more than any other system in the body. We find that nerve stress deals with the responses that the nerves have and what is going on in our own realm of nerve responses. Previously, scientists have found that disturbances of the nervous system often contribute to imbalances and problems in the endocrine system. More recently, researchers have found out that depression, grief and other emotional states depress the body's immune system and lower resistance to disease.

Many people go through a lifestyle and are able to take a certain amount of stress and strain from the home, children, money fluctuations, job conditions and so forth, and we feel we're getting along with it all right. However, we do not realize that we do not actually get along with it at all. Sometimes we think we are setting our problems aside, and yet they are silently festering on the inside, and with the addition of a few more problems, stress symptoms begin to come out to the place where stress interferes with the nerve supply to the various organs in the body.

Stress is a brain-originated condition, and we find that it deals with the brain and nerve supply in the body. If we were like jellyfish and had no responses to our environment, we would possibly have no stress at all. However, stress affects everyone quite differently simply because we are all experiencing different feelings toward what is happening on the inside of the body. We have found that stress effects are not usually recognized until many years after this silent disease has developed to the place where we're no longer handling situations properly. In other words, we get to the place where we cannot handle a particular situation properly because we do not have the nerve function, the mental activity, the brain force, the vital energies in the nervous system in order to take care of the events happening on the outside of our body.

Possibly the first body system (after the nervous system) to respond to stress is the digestive system. When the nerves are tense, the hydrochloric acid doesn't secrete properly in the stomach, the digestive juices do not flow sufficiently, and the appetite is usually dull or lacking. We may be unable to enjoy food properly, and nausea after meals can be one of the symptoms of stress. Ulcers and inflammation in the digestive system are common in cases of chronic stress.

Many conditions can be built up from the effects of stress or physical conditions in the body. Personally, I look at stress as something which hasn't been taken care of properly, such as an unresolved problem. There are many people who develop high blood pressure and are unaware that they are developing it. But it comes from internal stress.

First of all, we find that that stress, over a period of time, is handled according to the inherent conditions of the various organs in the body. Many people have a strong mental drive. Many people can tolerate a lot of stress and strain, but this is because they have inherited a good body which doesn't break down easily. But how about those who did not inherit a good body? A weak organ in the body can be likened to a bridge. We find that it can only take so much strain, and then it gives way. When an engineer builds a bridge over a harbor, he's got to know how much strain that bridge can actually take. The same principles go for people.

If we could only realize, in analyzing a person, just how much stress or strain that person could take, we could advise him to stay within certain work and lifestyle limits. As our stresses are developed from an emotional standpoint, a mental standpoint, we find that the stress itself produces another disease and this comes about because of the way we look at life, the way we handle it, and we get to the place where fears and anxieties take over. Or, we get to the place where we develop dislikes and we start feeling resentments; we build up resistance until we find that we are fighting a "thief in the dark," so to speak. This has come over us and is taking our nerve energies away from us. We don't know exactly what the enemy looks like or how to get a handle on the problem, and we do not know how to take care of it properly. I'm saying problems should be taken care of in our lifestyle as they come up.

No one can live without a good philosophy. It was Professor Hans Selye who spent so much time on the effect of mental responses on the body, and he has defined stress as "the response of the organism to the demands which are placed upon it." In other words, the stress itself is not exactly the problem, but it is how we handle it (or fail to handle it). We often add to this stress by wrong ways of dealing with it. We may try to dismiss our troubles or set them aside instead of taking care of them.

Stress today is probably causing more digestive and bowel problems, blood pressure problems, heart attacks and strokes than anything else I can tell you.

Many problems come from the kidney structure, from adrenal gland breakdowns, from liver disturbances, and there are probably many more organs which contribute stress-related problems when they show inherent weaknesses. Yet, we have more trouble taking care of distress from the acids which are produced as this silent disease gets a hold on us. The worst part of stress is its similarity to cancer — we find that the American Cancer Society tells us that it takes 20 years to develop a cancer, and then, again, we wonder where the doctor was 20 years ago. The same can be said of this silent disease stress. Where did it actually begin? Why didn't you take care of it at that time? Where was your philosophy? Where was your emotional control? Where was your health in the very beginning? As time goes on, these things tear you to pieces.

There are no two people alike. There are no two bodies alike. We all have different ways of responding mentally. However, it is *how* we respond which determines what this strain is going to do to us.

Many people do not realize that when a person has a dull mind, as in the case of a drunk person, he can fall down and not get hurt. Often he doesn't understand why he hasn't hurt himself as the average person would in a similar situation. I believe that in a shock of any kind, a tragic event or great distress, we may almost have to go mentally "limp," like a drunk person, to keep from hurting ourselves. Otherwise, the effects of stress may be slowly growing in this body that we have to take care of. Prevention is a great deal better than treating the disease when symptoms have taken over.

Stress is a universal thing today, and there are over 30 million people with high blood pressure in this country. We have many heart and blood pressure disturbances which could be eliminated if we would take better care of the stress in the individual. Millions of people have ulcers, irritable bowel syndrome, colitis and other digestive system disturbances.

I believe stress could have a genetic background. However, we must do much more research on this problem. We have a brain center which controls blood pressure, and a genetic weakness in this center may not allow us to take as much stress as another person can take.

We must consider that there are many things which can cause all of these problems. First of all, I believe when we get entangled in people's problems which we are seeing today, we start to develop stress. In a family, the father's, mother's or child's problems can begin to cause stress and strain. There are many things we have to consider and, above all, our personality, our character building and our training as a child, and how these may help us to handle a good deal of these emotional stresses.

There are differing levels to this stress, and we find that it starts out as an acute condition. If we can handle it at the acute stage — we can generally get over it fairly well. In other words, we get up, we go on, we don't think about it anymore. However, many times stress memories are held in our subconcious mind,

318

and we find that many people have these unseen problems come up later on in life, and preventing this is precisely what we must consider.

We find that we may encounter one big emotional strain, and all the small problems which have built up to this moment come in and help to break us down and bring in more stress and strain. Guilt and anger can bring out these things more than anything else I can tell you. In short, we have to learn how to handle these stresses, and we should be aware of these things right from the very beginning.

Most of us do not have our life put together so that we know how important a good philosophy is in helping to take care of all the different problems that come up.

Our attitudes, our thinking and our beliefs are often a strain on our nervous system, and we find that the nervous system is the first thing which must be taken care of in order to keep our body well. I consider the nerves first because without the proper nerve supply, we find that no organ can work properly. This is the path I feel stress takes in getting to the heart, the liver, the kidneys, the adrenal glands, the thyroid and so forth.

In order to reconstruct the body, we must consider the part the mind plays and we also have to consider that stress is a mental thing. However, if we overwork any system in our body, whether it is the respiratory system, digestive system, cardiovascular system or skeletal system, we've got to consider that we are actually burning out certain chemical elements that must be fed back to the body. Then, of course, we must begin to improve our lifestyle, and by doing both things we finally get to the place where we are lowering our level of nerve tension.

I believe the average person has a very difficult time in this day and age of television, not to mention the newspapers or what they call the scandal sheets. News of the stock market, politics, prices, crimes, terrorist highjackings and nuclear disarmament talks make it very difficult to keep a normal mind. As a result, I feel we must rearrange many things in our life. Sometimes we find that noise can be an excessive problem in our life and yet most of us have never realized that noise creates a good deal of stress.

In the graduates from our universities, we find that 30% of

them have hearing problems which are going to affect them for the rest of their lives. It is claimed this is coming about because of the harsh, loud music that these young people have been listening to. Many of the disc jockeys, and there are large numbers of them, have stress problems and nervous system problems because of the high level of stress produced by the type of music which they are playing so much.

Of course, we do have to consider that the body must initially be clean. We have to take care of all the elimination channels. And we must recognize that the circulation is built up in the body from a good nervous system. If we have depleted the nervous system, then we find we are adding more stress simply because we do not have a normal nervous system to work with. Often, good health habits are learned, not inherited. They come through education, and we find that there are many things that we must realize. There is a natural essence to our internal self, and we live on what we pour out. If this essence is interfered with at any time from a normal and natural standpoint, then we are already headed for stress.

I don't particularly like to say this, but I feel that during the last 30 years, I have been unlearning many of the things which I've learned about before that. I have learned some new things about fears. And I realize that fears can be controlled now better than they ever were when I was a younger person. I feel we've gotten to the place where we have begun to realize that resentment and resistance produce nerve tension in the body that can bring in a disease 20 years later. We find that all of these mental things must be cared for as soon as we can and as young as we can. One way of coping with stress is meditation. Another is biofeedback. Still another is regular physical exercise.

Many times, we find that the thyroid itself has to be built up in order to take care of our emotional system. This can possibly be done by taking dulse or seaweed supplements to increase iodine availability. We find that the brain and nervous system need lecithin. Phosphorus for the brain is essential, and we find that an egg yolk is probably one of the finest of the brain and nerve foods and cod roe is another. I realize that there are many people who wouldn't particularly care to use these foods, but if we are developing a stressful life then we have to consider how to overcome it in the very best way we can.

Many people would like to change their lifestyle. Usually, every one of my patients wants to do the right thing, but they don't know what to do, and we find that we have to give them a program to follow. There are those who improve through mind healing and even the spiritual touch many times has changed a person's life, so that stress has been eliminated almost entirely. There are many things we can do to help, but the most important thing is motivation — to actually want to make changes in our life. And if we can just do that, then we find that a stress management program can be brought out which will give us even a greater self-confidence. We find that many things do not belong to us and we get to the place where we do what the Good Book has to say, "What is that to thee . . . follow thou me." We get to the place also where we see the spiritual way which can "put your mind and heart on the higher talents and even higher paths I will go on to show you." So, it is just a matter of awareness, and I believe those people who are giving these awareness programs today are doing a great job in helping people to reduce the stress which is producing so much nerve tension within the body.

We must come to realize that we must have a certain amount of rest. This is extremely important and necessary. It isn't just a matter of resting from thinking, but a matter of resting and having a hobby, going in another direction or even taking up another job. If you have an active mind, it's perfectly all right to keep it busy. However, we have to realize that monotony is one of the things we feel should be avoided, as this alone can cause tension in the body. In other words, we have to find time to do some of the things we love to do.

In fact, we cannot get along without doing the things we really love to do. Anyone working 6 hours on a job that he hates is bound to develop an ulcer. It's bound to bring on some stomach troubles. So we have to manage our life and our lifestyle, and we have to know what projects we should take on in life. We've got to realize that enjoyment, happiness, harmony and joy are all mental responses which help reduce tension or stress. However, just like one woman said to me, "My husband has a heart of gold . . . and just as hard!" There are times when we do have to put our thoughts on money, but we have to see that we're not overdoing it. The stress comes in hard on the debt-ridden person and the executive with so much responsibility. He is the one trying to achieve and to get ahead, and the extreme achiever today is often troubled with stress and nerve tension.

I have been one of those who have lived in that stress and strain. Somehow or other, I like it. It seems to be my natural way, and I love to handle things under pressure. In other words, for me to rest is very difficult, but, on the other hand, I have to watch my limits like everyone else. So I leave you with the thought expressed by a sign I keep on my desk. The sign reads: "Let it go . . . let it flow."

It may be strange to talk about stress in a food book, but I don't think there is one thing that disturbs digestion more than a disturbed mind. It is in the mind that we deplete or build our nervous system. It takes a good nerve reserve and nerve power to digest our foods well. I feel that no one can digest his foods well and keep his digestion right unless he lives most of the time with a good philosophy. Over a period of years, I have found that it is not what we eat that counts, but what we digest.

LOVE, SEX AND NUTRITION

BREAKING DOWN THE SEXUAL SYSTEM

How do we influence the breakdown of this important system for our well-being and overall health? Generally, anything that uses up the red corpuscles, decreases hemoglobin, diminishes the body's iron or depletes glandular functions, nerve force and the will power eventually leads to troubles with the sexual system.

BUILDING THE SYSTEM

Iron and sulphur foods are particularly called for, as in vitellin — found in egg yolk. One of the best nerve and brain tonics is black cherry juice with egg yolk, taken once daily, and it is also very good for the liver. Raw, well-whipped egg yolk with milk and clover honey; parsley and parsley soup; dark cherries, strawberries, blackberries — all are helpful.

Sulphur foods help to stimulate the brain and sexual system when more activity is needed, and brain biochemicals such as silicon, calcium and phosphorus are very important. We must have iodine foods for the thyroid, the "emotional gland." Eucalyptus honey is extremely good along with elderberry juice.

Sometimes cod liver oil is necessary, and fish roe is the best food obtainable for the sexual system and the brain. It can be mixed in the blender with a little tomato or vegetable juice.

In the teas, watermelon seed tea and sage tea are very good. Avena sativa (oat straw tea) contains avenin, helping the system very much, and this ingredient is also found in rice polishings in heavy amounts. Another tincture of avena sativa, half a teaspoon twice a day, tones the system. Burdock, damiana, ginseng, dong quai, fo-ti-tieng and gotu kola are herbs considered as important aids to the female sexual system.

SPECIFIC PROBLEMS

Excess Desire. With this problem, it is advisable to eat from the vegetable kingdom, cutting out white sugar and white flour products and using grains to emphasize a left-side, negative diet for the body. Avoid excessive use of protein and heavy meats such as beef. Foods high in sulphur, fats and even at times, iron (due to overabundance) should be avoided. Use more foods high in potassium, foods that are sour, bitter or pungent, such as tops of vegetables, greens, chlorophyll and citrus fruits. Stimulants must be avoided.

Self Abuse. The problem with sex activity taken to extremes, including excessive masturbation, should be obvious. Any activity that is seriously depleting the glands is also depleting the nervous system. Taking care of the nervous system with sodium, silicon, magnesium and phospholipid-containing foods is important. It is necessary to be sure that indican is not developing in the urine. Lecithin foods are needed more than anything else. Seminal fluid is 80% lecithin.

A brain and nerve phospholipid used in the glandular systems, lecithin is destroyed when the nervous system is overworked. It is found in eggs, wheat germ and vitamin E, which is not to be considered only for sex purposes. Vitamin E builds a stout heart, helps varicose veins and generally tones up the tissues.

Change of Life. Here again, lack of that important food, lecithin, plays a major role. A woman may come to this moment due to chronic lack of vitamin E foods.

For the daily intake, I particularly recommend 3 to 6 dulse tablets and 800-1200 I.U. of vitamin E to women with lumps in their breasts and to persons with extremely high blood pressure. In most cases, however, vitamin E greatly aids in the change of life time. Herbs are useful for these problems. I recommend 2 or 3 cups a day of licorice and black cohosh tea, about half and half.

Prostate Troubles. Caution should be taken in eating too much red meat, particularly by men. Most long-lived people do not eat beef, but lamb. They cook broths and make bone soups that do not have uric acid which can become very irritating to the genito-urinary system and the prostate gland. Cold sitz baths will help, or hot and cold sitz baths — alternating one minute hot, one-half minute cold, one minute hot, etc. Bee pollen has been successfully used to treat 170 prostate cases by a Swedish/German urology team.

Impotence. A nerve-building diet is particularly called for with this problem, although more serious causes of deficient erectile power are sometimes traced to injuries of the cerebellum or to locomotor ataxia. More often we find sexual blocks and neurasthenia, fears, bashfulness, overexcitement or deep grief to be the essential causes.

A good nerve-building diet will consist of silicon, iron, sulphur, lecithin, cholesterol and essential fatty acids. Tonics such as prune juice with egg yolk are effective. Additionally good are parsley soup, onions, garlic, beets, leeks, celery, blackberries and wild cherry essence.

Sterility. In the man, sterility originates from many of the same causes—the breaking down of the nervous system from various activities, excess drinking, drugs, wrong diet, catarrh and pus formation—all lead to weak or damaged spermatozoa.

For sterility, once again the diet should consist of foods high in iron and supplements high in calcium, phosphorus, plus some sulphur foods. Avena sativa is indicated and the black cherry juice tonic with egg yolk in it. Fish broth and cod roe are needed, and fresh air, sleep, exercise, a genial climate, etc.

The Turks, who have an active sex life until their latter years, eat differently than people in most other countries. At the base of their halva and tahini foods is the sesame seed, which is essential to their strength, their sex life and their longevity. The sesame seed is one of the champions of all seeds, and in Turkey, they grind it and add concentrated grape juice to make candy. Grape juice contains the quickest sugar to be absorbed by the body and to aid in heart health. The sesame seed has the most vitamin E of any seed—it is the smallest but most powerful seed we have. Take a glass of raw goat milk (if that is not available, use soy milk powder), put in a tablespoon of sesame seed butter, a sliver of avocado and a teaspoon of honey and mix in a blender. Few tonics will give you greater energy or better care for the glandular system.

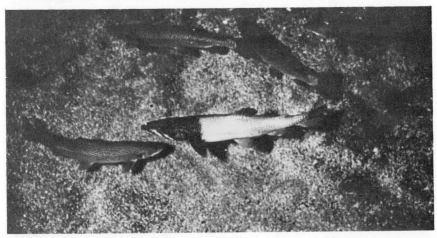

Harvey the New Zealand trout (center), was naturally half yellow and half brown. During feeding, extreme anxiety, Harvey changed his color completely to brown. This is where we see how the mind influences our digestion and our bodies.

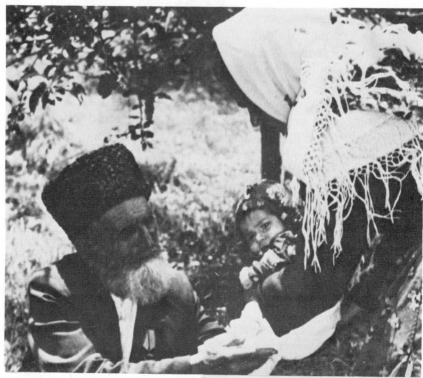

Shirali Mislilmov, at 168, was the oldest living man in the USSR and the world before his death a few years ago. He was a shepherd most of his life. He didn't smoke or drink, used clabbered milk and walked half a mile in his native Caucasus mountains every day.

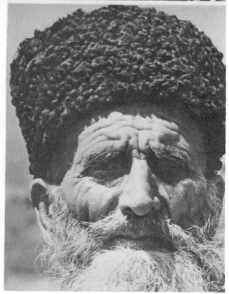

24

Brain and Nerve Feeding— Lecithin

Many will wonder why we talk about the brain along with our foods. There is food for our mind, for our nerves and there is thinking food. The brain is the symphony director of all activities in the various organs of the body. To have harmony throughout the whole body, let us take out a moment to see how we can keep our brain in the best order possible. This is done through our associations with people, how we handle problems, a polluted bloodstream, take care of panics, how we look at things that could be harsh on our body and to know how to release it. To wear out our brain and nervous system will affect every organ in the body. If we do not feed the brain and the nervous system every organ will also be affected. We must take care of the body through four ways; first, through the nerves; second, we must have a good well-mineral-balanced bloodstream; third, a good circulation; and, fourth, is eliminating fatigue, tiredness and enervation.

Often, we find that nutrient deficiencies, overwork, excess mental work, emotional depletion, exposure to cold or weather extremes, stress and various other causes result in abnormal acidity in the body. This irritates the nerves to such an extent that nerve pain is encountered, and we have to take care of the problem.

NERVE PAIN

Nerve pain has received different names in different parts of the body, such as:

Angina pectoris is nerve pain in the heart.

Neuralgia is nerve pain, in general.

Sciatica is nerve pain in the hip and leg.

Hemicranis (when half the head aches) is a nerve pain of the scalp or meninges.

Neuralgiac toothache, when the pain occurs in the jaw nerves.

Otalgia, when the pain occurs in the ear.

Neuralgia of the eye, or photophobia, when the pain is in the eye.

Tic douloureaux, when it occurs in the face.

Nephralgia, if it takes place in the urinary organs.

Gastralgia, nerve pain in the stomach.

Causes may include anything that uses up the cerebellar force, such as exposure to cold, heavy lifting, excessive sex, great excitement, mechanical injuries, psychosomatic conditions, severe disease, acids, gases, bacterial poisons generated by germlife in the system which irritate the nerves, toxic or depressed states of the system, lack of nourishing nerve food, nerve salts and fats, anemia, visceral congestion of the blood causing pressure of the nerves, sleeplessness, changes of the electricity in the atmosphere or electromagnetic imbalance acting upon and irritating the nerves, gastric catarrh, growth of a bone causing pressure upon a nerve, ulcer, tumor, abscess, curvature of the spine, decay of a tooth, excessive cold and wind, moisture, excessive tea-drinking, late hours, loss of sleep the first part of the night, dissipation, drunkenness, excessive brain labor or use of the nerves, excitement, gout, rheumatism and tobacco. A highly alkaline diet overcomes nerve pain.

Those subject to nerve pain include mental temperament people, nervous people, emotional-esthetic people and very lean people.

To get rid of nerve pain, we should consider the following.

Magnesium foods, myristic acid found in coconut and nutmeg, warmth, feeding the nerves, sleep and rest, wet compresses, hot baths, sand applications, warm salt baths, forceful massage and an alkaline diet.

SUPPORTIVE FOODS FOR THE NERVES AND BRAIN

Foods that carry silicon, chlorine, phosphorus, iron and iodine. Fish broth, southern (yellow) corn, apples, whey (contains salts of great importance for the nerves) and spinach (contains nerve salts, sodium and acid). Spinach is excellent in times of constipation caused by lack of nerve force. Celery is a tonic for the nerves. Grapes strengthen and cool the nerves. Prunes are of the greatest importance because of the nerve salts they contain. Dill is soothing to the nerves, especially to the pneumogastric nerve. Nutmeg and coconut soothe the nerves because of myristic acid they contain. Red cabbage, fish, oat and barley preparations, black cherries, strawberries, blackberries, beets, leaf lettuce, dried figs, carrots, asparagus, lentils, German prunes and sage tea.

To improve the liver and sexual system, sleep between sundown and 12 o'clock at night when the cerebellum recuperates. Tepid baths soothe the nerves and cool packs are good for nerve aches.

Avoid overusing the cerebellum. Black pepper destroys the nerve ends and the nerves themselves. Tea increases tissue waste in nervous people suffering from palpitation of the heart and sleeplessness. Uric acid in the system will lead to nerve pain. Sunstroke affects the nervous system, especially in the axis-cylinder cells of the spinal cord. Cold coagulates the white nerve substances (cholesterol/lecithin) surrounding the axis-cylinder cells in the brain and spinal cord. If reaction takes place, inflammatory changes may set up in the nervous substance which leads to neuritis or weakness of the nerve function. Tomatoes, strawberries, raw cabbage are good if the nervous system is weak and the digestion poor.

NERVE SALTS

Lack of nerve salts and phosphorus lead to disturbances of the nervous system, nervousness, nervous prostration, lack of vitality and sexuality, early decay, mental and bodily weariness, headache, noise in the ears, hay fever, nervous dyspepsia, gas or flatus, dizziness, belching, sleeplessness, exhaustion, general debility, brain fever, sunstroke, hysteria, disturbances of the sexual system.

DISEASE CONDITIONS AND THE NERVES

In nervous diseases, the breathing is usually rapid and the

pulse is changeable. (In lack of nerve energy, the pulse is sluggish.)

Causes may include drinking habits, sexual inflammation and narcotics. Excessive mental work leads to nervous indigestion.

To prevent or reverse nerve diseases, improve the liver and sexual system, supply the food needed for the liver, sexual system and brain. Use dill, coconut, spinach, nutmeg, nerve salts and sea air.

For nervous prostration, nervous indigestion or nervous irritability, use lecithin, sulphur and phosphorus foods, fish, cucumbers, spinach, cauliflower, meat, milk, eggs, beans, asparagus, lettuce, almonds, radishes, lentils, peas, grapes, cabbage, onions, gooseberries, chestnuts, cherries, plums, strawberries, blueberries, rice, corn, oats, barley, rye, wheat, walnuts, figs, apples, horseradish, raw whipped egg yolk. Fish roe is a wonderful food for the starved nerves.

For nervous exhaustion (mental debility), we find the condition not benefitted by any diet at times, even if the foods are the best of everything. Phosphorized fat, or lecithin, provides the vitality of the nervous system. Bran bread, sweet cream, fresh milk, clover honey, fresh homemade butter, cod liver oil, oily fish, bran tea, physical work and brain rest are all excellent for this condition.

NERVOUSNESS AND HOW TO GET RID OF IT

Use magnesium foods and drinks, tonic diet, soothing food, boiled onions, garlic, parsley, nutmeg, spinach, roasted lean mutton, turkey, duck, grouse, whey, baked fish with lemon juice, bran tea, celery, celery juice, garlic tea, parsley soup, raisin juice, fish broth, fresh raw cow or goat milk with lemon juice.

NEURALGIA

Neuralgia is characterized by alternating, sharp, darting, benumbing, burning, pulsating, stitching, crawling, tingling, aching, boring, excruciating, creeping, severe pain coming and going and not situated in one spot. Restless nerves may make the sufferer feel as though he is falling apart, as though needles are thrust into his very nerve substance. The person may feel cold, and the skin may be moist or dry and hot.

Causes are anemia, gout, rheumatism, acidity, syphilis, gonorrhea.

A favorable diet would include laxative foods, nerve-building foods, iron, mgnesium, potash, silica, phosphorus and chlorine foods. Lecithin, alkaline foods, cod liver oil, fish and fish broth, white clover honey, sweet cream, strawberries, spinach and bran bread. We can also use sand applications, warm salt baths, forceful soothing massage. This will draw out the acids that cause the pain.

We can use hot salt applications, mud baths, nerve stretching, change of environment, static electricity, hot douches, steam vapors, fresh air, rest and recreation. Cold ice bags applied to the aching nerve helps some. Try warm baths and gentle friction with a soft hand after pain is over. Use natural laxatives.

If a person believes a certain thing will cure the problem, whatever that may be, they should be encouraged, but other agents should be applied at the same time. This is very effective. Use stretching exercises and dry heat applied as hot as possible and persistently. Wet compresses and, in some instances, moist heat or even excessive cold may help some people. Changing hot and cold applications may help others. A cool, dry, bracing climate, free from wind will help a mental temperament personality type. Neuralgia caused by anemia is helped by an iron diet or a trip to the mountains.

NEURASTHENIA

In cases of neurasthenia, we find restless nerves making the person feel as though he is falling apart, as though needles are thrust through the very nerve substance. It is generally caused by anything that uses up cerebellar force such as exposure to cold, excessive sex, heavy lifting, great excitement Neurasthenia is often caused by a type of iron deficiency anemia, but also by a bad emotionalism, overwork of the brain, lack of brain food, too much use of the tongue and a vegetarian diet low in the brain feeding elements. Silicon foods such as sprouts and rice bran should bring relief. A vegetable diet may lead to neurasthenia because of lack of lecithin and phosphorus.

NEURITIS

Neuritis or nerve inflammation, with the same causes as previously-described nerve conditions, is helped by magnesium foods (such as green vegetables and yellow cornmeal).

THE BRAIN OF MAN

Chemicals of the brain include cholesterol, lecithin, water, amino acids, calcium, phosphorus, magnesium, iron, iodine, potassium, sodium, acetylcholine, hormones and various nerve salts.

Two percent of the nourishment for the brain should consist of phosphates, to keep the brain and nerves healthy. If the brain is used a great deal, five percent or more of phosphate is needed.

Each brain center needs a different food. The phosphorus needed by one brain center is different from the phosphorus needed by another brain center. The chemist may not be able to distinguish between phosphorus and phosphorus and lime and lime, but the brain centers and the organs of the body are the most skillful chemists of all. The difference between the lime of a lime bed and the lime of a bone is an evolutionary difference. *The brain requires animal phosphorus.* Vegetable phosphorus feeds the bones and other physical organs mainly, but the brain is a highly evolved organ and requires a highly evolved phosphorus. This is important to remember in feeding and building the brain, also in treating cerebral neurasthenia, brain fag and brain anemia.

What feeds one brain center does not feed another. What strengthens the chest brain does not strengthen the muscle brain, and so on.

The pneumogastric nerve is centered in the medulla. This nerve has branches that centralize in the gray cortex of the cerebrum. When the cortical cells in those faculties are excited by sight or smell of food, they act upon the pneumogastric nerve ends that are distributed in the mouth and in and around the stomach, so that the various salivary, gastric, hepatic, pancreatic and intestinal glands may secrete the digestive juices, and so that the motor nerve ends may act upon the muscular coats throughout the alimentary tract and produce those peristaltic movements so necessary for the transportation and conversion of foods and juices.

Brain foods include silicon, phosphorus, sodium, easily-handled fats, oat muffins, fish broth, bran tea between meals, southern corn because of its high percentage of magnesium, tea made of wild wheat seeds (cough grass), green wheat or kernels of ordinary wheat (1 cup at a time reduces heat in the brain). Use fish roe, raw egg yolk, barley porridge cooked in milk and water.

Brain congestion can be caused by the arteries pumping blood while the veins are contracted so that the drainage of the brain is defective and the brain becomes congested. Use vitamin E, fluorine and iodine foods, prickly cucumbers and grapes.

Brain fever is characterized by singing in the ears, a rush of blood to the head, wild red eyes, flushes of the face, nosebleed, pain in the base of the brain, headache, constipation, disturbance of the mental functions is helped by magnesium foods, soothing classical music and soft nonstimulating colors.

Brain workers should use silicon foods and tonics; phosphorus and lecithin, a combination of phosphorus, sulphur and oil.

CEREBELLUM

The cerebellum is a musculo-electrical dynamo, generating an electrical force similar to electricity itself, different in nature, not in kind. The following conditions are unfavorable to the cerebellum: Colds in the head because they charge the cerebellum with too much blood. Whooping cough because it weakens the cerebellum like malaria. Exposure to cold. Heavy lifting. Excessive sex. Great excitement. Great sexual passion exhausts the brain. Sunstroke affects the brain, also fretting, studies, worry, sleeplessness and pain. Persistent work night and day when the system is exhausted and long hours weaken the cerebellum beyond recuperation. Neurasthenia. Typhus fever. Sicknesses that use up motor force.

Cerebral trouble may produce great fear of the opposite sex, strong inclinations for solitude, fear of society, periodic headache and listlessness. Also loss of ambition, inclination for nunnery or for the life of a hermit. The systolic murmur of the heart is caused by cerebellar weakness and a feverish sex brain. The cerebellum can be drained of its force, and the myelin in the spinal cord may undergo disintegration because of sexual taints.

Foods favorable to the cerebellum include calcium foods, iron salts from the vegetable kingdom, honeybee pollen, phosphorus, vitellin (a nucleoprotein from egg yolk), nerve salts, bile salts, sulphur foods, oils, nerve fats, parsley, leeks, garlic, oat oil, sage tea.

MEDULLA (CHEST BRAIN)

The chest brain takes care of the chest function, the lungs and their function, the diaphragm function, the heart function, the vasomotor system, the circulation, the oxidation of the blood and tissues.

So long as the medulla is in a good state of health, the heart beats, the lungs work, the blood is active everywhere. The medulla keeps the heart beating before birth and keeps it going until the thread of life is spun and the eyes close in death. When the medulla is weak, the heart is weak and the lungs are feeble. When the medulla dies, the heart stops and no human invention can put it into motion. From injuries of the medulla, millions of people have died simply because the heart stopped.

Weakness of the medulla is indicated by a changeable pulse. A diet favorable to the medulla contains iron sulphide foods, sulphur foods, lemon juice, garlic, onions, radishes, coconut, watermelon seed tea, sage tea, parsley, easily-digested fish, fish broth. Nutmeg calms the medulla.

SEX CENTER (IN THE HYPOTHALAMUS)

The sex brain needs iron foods and sulphur foods. Parsley and watermelon seed tea are good for the sex brain. In times of fevers of a sexual nature, when the life force is low or sluggish, phlegmatic people use onions, garlic, radishes and other sulphur foods such as leeks and cauliflower.

Cold weakens the myelin of the brain and spinal cord, which weakens the sexuality. Excessive heat weakens the axis-cylinder

334

cells of the brain and spinal cord and has a weakening effect on sexuality. Anything that uses up the myelin, the nerve and brain fat will weaken the sexual system and prevent the formation of red corpuscles of the blood. Anything that uses up iron salts in the system interferes with the aeration of the blood, hence causes sexual neurasthenia, cerebral neurasthenia, dropsy, hysteria, etc., according to the nature of the sexual draining and the parts most affected.

LECITHIN

Lecithin is a very important nerve and brain food found in all nerve and brain tissue, and it is abundant in egg yolk. It is formed by the union of glycophosphoric acid with two fatty acids and with choline. The most common fatty acid in lecithin is stearic acid.

When the system lacks lecithin, the nerves lack strength, the brain vitality and individuals become weak and feeble, even irritable.

The blood serum contains double the sulphuric acid salts as phosphoric acid salts. The body has, however, about 20% of phosphates to 2% of sulphates. Sulphur holds the balance against the phosphorus in the blood, so that lecithin is kept under control.

It is important in times of nervous indigestion, irritabililty, nervous prostration, weakness of the nerves or brain, to remember that one important fact, that sulphur holds the balance against phosphorus, so that that important nerve substance lecithin may be manufactured and held in the system.

In treating people, I observe the person from four different angles. The first thing I check is to see if the nerves have been taken care of properly. Without nerve suppy no organ can work properly. This is why chiropractic has become so popular. There has been a tremendous growth in the number of psychiatrists and psychologists practicing these days. Secondly, the blood must be clean and chemically balanced. Circulation is necessary to get the blood where it is needed, and of course we do this through exercise, water treatments, acupuncture and many of the special healing arts within the healing regimen. Enervation or tiredness is the beginning of every disease. A tired body cannot repair, rebuild or rejuvenate properly. Remember these four different things so necessary in taking care of every organ in the body.

LECITHIN—WONDER FOOD FOR THE BRAIN AND GLANDS

Over the past 50 years of my sanitarium work, I have found that the sex life and mentality are linked to the well-being of the whole body, to the proper functioning of every system of the body. For this reason, it is necessary to make sure that the brain, nerves and glands are fed with the right foods. Lecithin is one of the most important of these foods.

The brain, nerve and glandular system nutrients can be depleted by excess—by excess mental work and activity, late nights, fatigue, financial worries, marriage and family problems, excessive study and the kind of mental stress faced by corporate executives, businessmen and administrators. A fast lifestyle can cause depletion. We find that excessive drinking of alcohol, smoking, using stimulant drugs, dancing, partying, overindulging in sex, exposure to extremes of climate and weather—all of these things can burn up the chemical elements needed by the brain, nerves and glands.

Poor food habits can result in nutrient deficiencies. The brain needs protein, fats, water, glucose, oxygen, phosphorus, iron, magnesium, sulphur, silicon, cholesterol and lecithin, as well as a variety of vitamins and trace elements. Without these, the brain becomes restless and the nerves uneasy.

We find that it is necessary to realize how important the relationship between the sexual system and proper brain function really is. The liver manufactures cholesterol and lecithin and stores a certain amount for future needs of the body, while a good deal of cholesterol, lecithin and nerve salts are stored in the sex glands. The male sexual fluid is about 80% lecithin. When we deplete the sexual system by excessive sexual activity, we not only use up its supply of nutrients, but we draw on lecithin needed by the brain to carry out its functions. When we deplete the brain by excessive mental activity, we also deplete the sexual system. As we find in so many of the body structures, functions and activities, balance is very important here.

I want to especially emphasize the importance of the medulla in the brain, because most people don't realize that nerves from the medulla or "chest brain" as we call it, take care of the lungs, diaphragm, heart, vasomotor system, the circulation of the blood and the oxidation of the blood and tissues. When we deplete nutrients and energy in the brain or sexual system, it isn't just a matter of slower thinking, impeded memory and loss of sexual enthusiasm that we're talking about. We're talking about interfering with the proper activity and function of the heart, lungs and blood circulation, processes that keep you alive and healthy when you live right.

FEEDING THE BRAIN, NERVES AND GLANDS

We find that lecithin works in combination with cholesterol in the body, and both are found in every cell, but they are especially important in the brain and sexual system. The brain is about 20% lecithin with about 13% cholesterol, making up the white matter, the myelin coatings of the nerve cells. Many of the sex hormones are made up of cholesterol, and the male sex fluid, as I have previously said, is 80% lecithin. So, we see that these are extremely valuable brain, nerve and sexual system foods.

The problem of excess cholesterol in the diet, resulting in hardening of the arteries and certain brain tissues, is caused, in my opinion, by using heated oils and fats in cooking. Heating foods over 212 degrees—the boiling point of water—destroys the lecithin and leaves the cholesterol. Fatty meat and pork should be eliminated from the diet. If you want to use cream and oils with your foods, add them *after* the foods are cooked.

Lecithin is more important to consider in the diet because it is more often lacking than cholesterol, and it is needed to balance cholesterol. Lecithin is possibly the most needed food in taking care of the brain, glands and nerves. We find lecithin in egg yolk, soybeans, whole cereal grains, seeds, nuts and pollen. Another source is codfish roe. Frying or scrambling eggs destroys most of the lecithin. Boiling or poaching is the best way to prepare eggs. Roasting soybeans, seeds or nuts destroys the lecithin, and so does using them in baked goods at oven temperatures over 212 degrees. Baking bread or any other bakery goods destroys the lecithin in whole grain cereals. It can be preserved only by preparing in boiling water. Nuts and seeds should be taken raw, either in butters, pulverized or used in a blender to make nut and seed milk drinks.

When we break lecithin down to its chemical ingredients, we find it is made up of glycerol, fatty acids, phosphoric acid, inositol and choline. We need lecithin foods, but we also find that lecithin is made in the body when we have an adequate supply of magnesium, vitamin B-6, choline and inositol. (We nearly always have enough fatty acids and phosphorus.)

ANALYSIS OF SOY LECITHIN (1 Tbsp, 7.5 gm)

Protein	0 gm	Cholesterol	0 gm
Carbohydrate	0.5 gm	Sodium	2 mg
Fat	7 gm	Potassium	60 mg
Unsaturated	5 gm		
Saturated	2 gm		

Some lecithin is used whole in the brain and elsewhere in the body, and some is broken down to be used as food for the cells. The phosphorus from egg yolk lecithin meets the brain's need for highly evolved phosphorus, the "light bearing element." Glycerol is used to prevent hardening due to excess cholesterol deposits. The fatty acids are used for energy or for carrying the fat-soluble vitamins. Choline aids in the transmission of nerve messages after it is transformed into acetylcholine. Inositol is used in fat metabolism, usually together with choline.

MODERN EXPERIMENTS WITH LECITHIN

Egg yolk lecithin may help restore impaired memory and reduce withdrawal symptoms in drug and alcohol addicts, according to Dr. David Samuel of the Weizmann Institute in Israel. Brain cell membranes hardened by cholesterol deposits become softer in the presence of lecithin, and nerve message transmission improves. Dr. Samuel feels egg yolk lecithin is better than soybean lecithin.

Scientists at the Massachusetts Institute of Technology in 1978 gave choline, one of the components of lecithin, to 20 people with tardive dyskinesia, brain dysfunction caused by long-term

338

use of tranquilizing drugs. Nine of them improved, even though the disease is said to be permanent and incurable.

Does lecithin help dissolve cholesterol deposits from the arteries? Some scientists say it does. Liquid lecithin was found to dissolve cholesterol in test tubes. In the bloodstream, fatty particles called high-density lipoproteins, 30% lecithin, work with vitamin C to remove cholesterol from artery walls and eliminate it from the body.

Doctors from the University of Alabama believe that some of the problems of memory loss and brain function loss in the elderly may be reversed by lecithin if caught in the early stages. Canadian scientists feel lecithin may help persons with Alzheimer's disease. Choline, one of the ingredients from lecithin, has already been shown to help Alzheimer's disease patients.

One type of lecithin is used in the lungs to prevent tissue adhesions. Some types of impotence are believed due to lack of choline, as found in lecithin. All cell membranes in the body use lecithin to some extent.

Experiments in 1976 showed that lecithin and cholic acid dissolved gallstones in some patients and reduced their size in others. Gallstones are made primarily of cholesterol. It enhances absorption of vitamin A, helps metabolize fats, protects the liver and assists in keeping the skin healthy, according to Dr. Philip S. Chen.

WE NEED MORE LECITHIN FOODS

The average person in the U.S. uses too many foods that have been fried, broiled or baked until the lecithin is destroyed, which makes you wonder whether people are getting the lecithin they need. When we consider that a large part of the average diet is made up of packaged foods, refined foods, junk foods and fast foods, we find it is very likely that most persons lack sufficient lecithin. Cardiovascular disease, hardening of the arteries and hypertension are often associated with high blood cholesterol, indicating a lack of lecithin.

Most people can have two eggs a day, poached or softboiled, without any problems. It isn't necessary to eat the whites of the eggs. The best nerve tonic I know is an egg yolk with black cherry juice. Codfish roe, high in lecithin, can be blended with a little tomato juice to make it easier to take. Whole grain cereals—brown rice, millet, rye, yellow cornmeal and buckwheat—should be eaten at least once a day, prepared by bringing to a boil in water and soaking overnight or cooking in a double boiler. Nuts and seeds can be blended raw as nut and seed milk drinks or as ingredients in blenderized health cocktails. Sesame butter and almond butter are the best seed and nut butters. Bee pollen, which contains lecithin, is available at many health food stores, and can be taken by the teaspoonful or blended with fruit juice.

It is interesting that health and nutrition researchers have never discovered any problems with *excess* lecithin, but many problems have been discovered where taking lecithin brings healing or improvement. This is another reason why I feel lecithin is short in most persons and why most people need to use more lecithin foods in the diet.

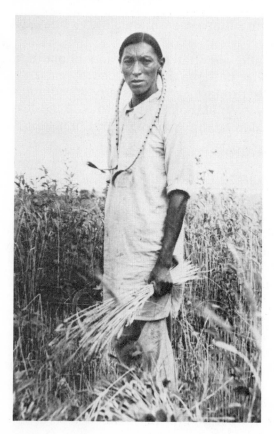

Our Native Americans, living on natural grains received all the lecithin, brain and nerve food elements.

340

AN EXTRA BRAIN FOR MAN'S USE

Dr. Jensen's analyses are now going into the computer.

Computerized Neural-Optic analysis can be valuable in several ways. It can be used as an index of your present health potential since the collective condition of the elimination organs and lymph system is one of the most important indicators of overall health. Perhaps most importantly, the extreme accuracy, reliability and memory storage capacity of the computer can be used to whether you are going forward or backward in health at the basic tissue level, to demonstrate whether your present diet and lifestyle are making you healthier or whether changes need to be made. Repeated analyses at six-month intervals, each compared to the previous analysis, provides an objective measure of progress (or lack of it) in your health. Neural-Optic analysis is the most sensitive method we are aware of in determining whether a particular health program is working, and how well it is working.

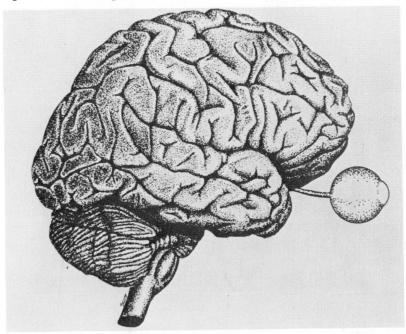

The eye is an extention of the brain, and by means of Neural-Optic Analysis we can tell the inherent weakness, mineral deficiencies, toxic-laden organs and activity level of various tissues in the body.

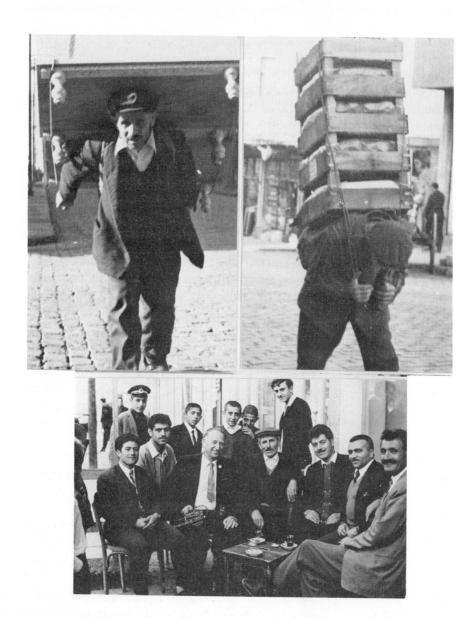

In Turkey, I saw strong old men carry unbelievable loads. The Good Book says our lives will be 3-score and 10 (70), but if we have strength, our years will be 4-score (80). Health and strength go together.

25

The
Candida Albicans
Yeast Problem

An estimated 80% of the American people are said to be infected with candida albicans, a yeast growth known to exist in small quantities in the body, but which has in recent years gotten out of control, according to health researchers.

In past years, candida was recognized as the cause of thrush in infants and a good deal of the vaginitis in women, but now candida is known to be able to expand and colonize throughout the body, causing symptoms ranging from "feeling bad all over," to allergy-like symptoms and symptoms mimicking those of hypothyroidism and hypoglycemia.

We find that the introduction of broad-spectrum antibiotics in 1947, steroid drugs and the later emergence of the birth control pill set up ideal conditions for a candida epidemic in later years. Antibiotics kill the bacteria in the bowel and everywhere else in the body, including the beneficial bacteria—but they do not kill yeast. Taking antibiotics over a period of weeks allows the normally minute colonies of candida to expand like a vast army into territory formerly controlled by bacteria. This may start in the bowel or vaginal tract, then travel throughout the body.

Birth control pills, steroid drugs and drugs that suppress the immune response assist in the rapid reproduction and expansion of candida in the body. The candida feed on sugars and yeast-containing foods like bread, cake, cheese, candy, soft drinks, beer, wine, syrup, honey, root beer, cider, catsup, processed meats, canned or frozen fruit and fruit juices, smoked meat, dried fruit, coffee, tea, melons, buttermilk, sour cream and most processed foods.

I feel strongly that cumulative effects over the years of too

343

much milk and wheat have made the average bowel an ideal breeding ground for candida albicans, after the "native" bacteria are eliminated from competition for food and space. Most baked goods require yeast to make the dough rise, and candida thrives on yeast foods. A government report said 29% of the average American diet is wheat products, which means that the average American body is a feast for the candida. Milk sugars are a favored food of yeast organisms.

Symptoms generally include some combination of the following:

Abdominal discomfort	Insomnia
Anal itch	Irritability
Anxiety	Joint pain
Arthritis pain	Loss of sex interest
Bloating	Menstrual problems
Canker sores	Muscle pain
Colitis	Nasal congestion
Constipation	Numbness
Coughs	Pelvic pain
Depression	Poor memory
Diarrhea	Premenstrual tension
Dizzy spells	Prostatitis
Enteritis	Sensitivity to fumes,
Fatigue	odors, tobacco smoke, etc.
Food intolerance	Sinusitis
Headaches	Sterility
Heartburn	Tingling
Hiatial hernia	Urinary infection
Impotence	Vaginitis

Yeast problems are found in both sexes and all ages. They are not usually identified by standard laboratory tests. Children who are hypoactive, have learning disorders, show delinquent behavior, do badly in school work or abuse drugs and alcohol may have candida problems.

HOW TO IMPROVE CANDIDA

The first thing in getting rid of candida is to cleanse and normalize the bowel, as described in my book *Tissue Cleansing Through Bowel Management.* The drug Nystatin, along with a strict diet, eliminating foods that feed candida, is being used with success. Avoid using antibiotics, steroids and birth control pills; see your doctor if you feel you have candida and are using these drugs. Take supplements of lactobacillus acidophilus, bulgaris or bifidus to restore beneficial bacteria in the colon, and use raw "live" yogurt to feed these bacteria. Take garlic—raw or the odorless Kyolic tablets, which help remove candida. Fast on fresh juices only a couple days a week. Try these things for 2 to 3 months, then see your doctor for a review of your condition.

Pau D'Arco tea, an herbal tea, has been reported to help get rid of candida. Chlorella, partly because of its powerful tissue and bowel cleansing activity, may be one of the greatest natural supplements for eliminating candida from the body.

HOMEOPATHIC REMEDY FOR CANDIDA?

At least one case has been reported where the use of drugs to treat candida was followed by a powerful return of the yeast in a more painful form, which was treated successfully with homeo-pathic remedies. Homeopathic remedies are minute doses that interact with the electromagnetic properties and energy fields of cells and tissues in the body. One idea about the spread of candida throughout the body is that immune system breakdown comes first and allows the spread. There are homeopathic and dietary approaches to strengthening the immune system.

TO REDUCE YEAST ON FOODS

Because yeasts are present on many foods, a Massachusetts doctor advises cleaning fresh fruits, vegetables, meat and fish by soaking them 15 minutes in 2 gallons of water with a teaspoon of Clorox added. (No other bleach is recommended.) After 15 minutes, remove food and soak it in clean water for 15 minutes. Then drain and use or store in refrigerator. There will be some food value loss in the case of meat and fish, but we have to consider this a worthwhile trade in getting rid of candida.

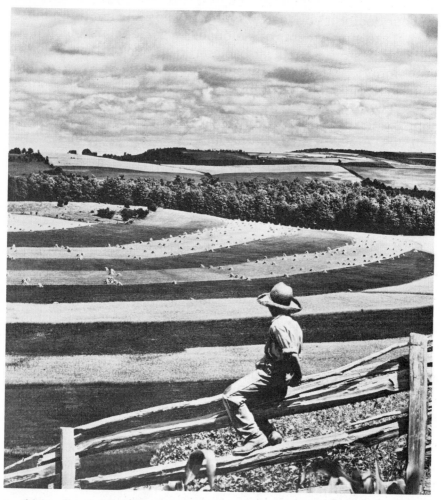

Living the natural lifestyle, close to nature, allows the nervous system to replenish itself through rest, proper foods and keeping the body active while at work. We found in reports that the average farmer died at 79, while the average doctor died at 49. We should all seek a balance and include a more natural life in our daily living habits.

26

Acidophilus: Feeding the Friendly Bowel Bacteria

For over 50 years I have emphasized the importance of a clean,healthy bowel to promote good health, well-being and long life. My studies with Dr. John Harvey Kellogg at his famous Battle Creek Sanitarium showed that the bowel was often the most neglected factor in health care, and that about 80% of the people have an imbalance of bowel bacteria favoring the undesirable bacteria.

Over 400 microorganisms live in the bowel, including bacteria, yeasts and viruses. These organisms may assist in breaking down bowel waste, keeping the bowel wall clean and producing B-vitamins for the body. Some are useful in small quantities, but harmful if allowed to grow beyond certain limits.

We find out that a proper balance of bowel flora is necessary to health and to maintaining a strong natural defense against disease in the body. In the dark, warm, moist climate of the bowel, disease-producing germlife can multiply to dangerous proportions if not held in check by the "friendly" bowel flora. The bowel is like a garden. If we ignore it, the weeds (undesirable flora) can choke out the flowers and vegetables (beneficial flora). If we take proper care of our garden, it is a wonderful help in promoting good health and preventing disease.

There are several ways that disease can be promoted in the bowel. An underactive bowel has been linked to high blood cholesterol and triglycerides, formation of cancerous and precancerous substances multiplication of disease-producing bacteria such as salmonella, shigella, pseudomonus and staphylococcus, and increased levels of toxins in the blood due to excessive production of toxic wastes by certain bacteria in the bowel. Poor food habits contribute to an underactive bowel in the first place, then provide the kind of food on which the undesirable bacteria thrive, displace the desirable bacteria, then produce bowel disturbances, putrefaction, toxic wastes and gas. A diet high in meat and refined foods favors the putrefactive, disease-producing bacteria.

In my world travels in search of the secrets of good health and longevity, I have found that many of the long-lived people used clabbered milk products, such as kumiss in Turkey, matzoni in Russia, and yogurt in Bulgaria. We find that these foods not only contain lactobacillus bacteria which is one of the most desirable bowel flora, but they also promote the growth and reproduction of existing lactobacillus bacteria in the bowel.

In fact, it was Bulgaria where the Nobel-prize winning biologist, Elie Metchnikoff, found out that the lactobacillus in yogurt was responsible for the unusually long lives of so many of the elderly in that country around the turn of the century. He considered lactobacillus to be the long-life factor. In his research, Metchnikoff discovered bowel bacteria that fed on incompletely digested meat protein, producing toxic amino wastes in the bowel and creating putrefaction and gas. On an imbalanced diet, these putrefactive bacteria multiply so fast that they drive out the beneficial bacteria. With a balanced diet, using yogurt or lactobacillus supplements, the process can be reversed, favoring the friendly bacteria and driving out the undesirable bacteria.

When we look at the research done over the past ten years or so, we find that over 200 strains of lactobacillus acidophilus bacteria are known, but there is a great deal of difference among them. Some are much better than others in helping normalize bowel conditions.

Studies of newborn babies show an interesting contrast. Doctors have known for some time that breast-fed babies are generally stronger and have fewer colds and infections than bottle-fed babies, but until recently they didn't know why. Breast-fed babies develop a bowel flora which is 99% lactobacillus bifidus within 3 or 4 days, which is stimulated by the colostrum the baby takes in. Bottle-fed babies, in contrast, tend to develop a weaker lactobacillus acidophilus flora. The bifidus predominates in the bowels of children until about age 7, when a shift to the acidophilus flora takes place and remains throughout adult life. Only a few adults have a predominant bifidus bacteria in the bowel. Nearly all favor the lactobacillus acidophilus.

There are 9 types of lactobacillus organisms that can live in the adult bowel. When taken in the form of yogurt, the milk product is tolerated better by milk-sensitive persons because it is partly predigested by the lactobacillus. Both the protein and fats are partially broken down to increase ease of digestion. A study of Massai tribesmen in Africa showed that blood cholesterol was lowered by lactobacillus. After two days straight of meat eating, 24 Massai tribesmen, ages 16-23, ate nothing for 3 weeks but milk fermented with lactobacillus. Their cholesterol levels dropped over that period by an average of 28 mg/dl, for reasons not completely understood.

The best strains of lactobacillus show antibacterial properties against undesirable colon bacteria such as E-Coli, types of salmonella, clostridium and staphylococcus and others. One strain of lactobacillus has antibiotic activity against 27 known bacteria, 11 of them harmful.

Several studies have been done on the anticarcinogenic effects of lactobacillus, one of them reported in the *Journal of the National Cancer Institute* (1973). In one case, tumor cells were reduced from 28 to 35%, while in another case the reduction was from 16 to 41%. The studies were done with mice.

Other research suggests that lactobacillus acidophilus increases food absorption, stimulates the immune system, inhibits growth of non-bacterial flora such as candida albicans and produces significant amounts of B vitamins.

Lactobacillus-rich products like yogurt, buttermilk and acidophilus milk have been successfully used to treat gastroenteritis and other bowel disturbances.

A number of lactobacillus acidophilus and lactobacillus bifidus supplements are carried in health food stores. These vary from liquid mixtures to powders, capsules and pills. Some are more potent than others. One of the powdered products claims on its label that one teaspoon is equal to 1,000 capsules of other available lactobacillus acidophilus supplements or 6 bottles of liquid-containing acidophilus. I feel that these supplements can be very helpful to those with bowel problems and disturbances.

Constipation, bad breath and a gassy bowel are signs that putrefactive bacteria have probably gained the upper hand in the bowel. When oral antibiotics have been taken for a week or two, you can be certain that the great majority of all bowel bacteria have been destroyed. Under these conditions, taking acidophilus supplements is advisable.

Acidophilus can be taken orally and suppositories in the form of gelatin capsules can be inserted at the same time to speed up bowel repopulation. Research by the Japanese has shown that taking chlorella along with the acidophilus may greatly speed up multiplication in the bowel. Also, we find that foods such as yogurt, sugar of milk, kefir, chlorophyll-rich vegetables, pectin, fruits and vegetables, vitamin C and fiber-rich foods encourage the rapid multiplication of lactobacillus acidophilus. It is best to cut out red meat for a while and use chicken and fish instead.

I feel that the proper bowel flora contributes to health and long life while helping to prevent disease and to strengthen the natural immune system. This can be a great advantage, in particular, to those who have problems with bowel regularity or constipation.

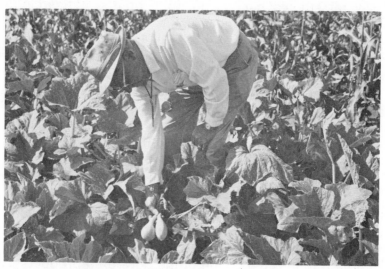

Fresh squash just picked from the garden are excellent foods for the eliminative system, especially the bowel.

350

────27────

Chlorella—
My Latest Discovery

Over the past 50 years, I have traveled to dozens of countries all over the world, searching for the secrets of health and longevity, looking for foods that would bring out the best in health and well-being for everyone. In Rumania and Russia, I found all the old people using yogurt or clabbered milk as some call it. In the Orient, I found brown rice, a wonderful whole grain cereal. In Latin America, the people used a good deal of the yellow cornmeal, high in magnesium. In Turkey, where we find some of the strongest people in the world, I found sesame seeds in wide use and tahini, a sesame seed butter, rich in the glandular factors. In the Hunza Valley, I found people well over a hundred years old still working in the fields, weighing the same as they did in their 20s and with every tooth still in their heads. They used a good deal of millet, one of the least fattening grains. These and many other discoveries helped me develop one of the finest possible food regimens—my Health and Harmony Food Regimen—for building strong tissues, preventing disease and keeping the best of health when used with the proper exercise and lifestyle.

I call my latest discovery **green magic**, because it has so many wonderful health benefits that it is hard to believe so much good can come out of a food.

CHLORELLA: A TWO-BILLION-YEAR-OLD DISCOVERY

For over two years now, I have been recommending a two-billion-year-old discovery to my students and patients, a green microalga named chlorella. Scientists have found this single-celled alga in fossils dated at about two billion years ago, but it is

351

CHLORELLA: A MAGIC GREEN FOOD

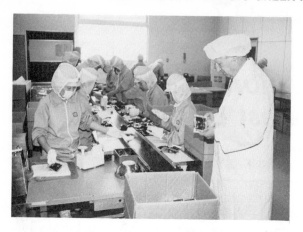

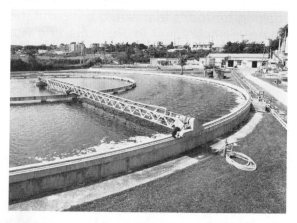

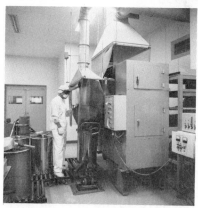

These photos were taken at various Sun Chlorella plants in Japan and Okinawa. They have also developed a method of breaking down the cell wall, which improves chlorella's digestability some 48%. The live-giving property from the nucleus of this algae is considered the greatest adjunct in building our immunity and developing greater resistance to disease.

only in the past 70 years that it was discovered to be one of the most nutritious health-building foods known to man. It is only in the past 20 years or so that the technology has been available to grow, harvest and process this alga for human consumption.

Chlorella is over 50% protein, high in nucleic acids (the long-life factor), chlorophyll, vitamins, minerals and trace elements. It is high in iron, needed to build the blood; in phosphorus, needed by the brain and nerves; in calcium, needed to repair tissue and to build a strong bone structure; and in magnesium, needed to relax the nerves and for proper bowel function. The trace elements and general balance of vitamins help to control and balance the coarse elements. The rich content of chlorophyll, about 2 or 3%, is higher than any other known plant source, and we find that chlorophyll is nature's most effective cleanser of the human body and bloodstream.

For the past 20 years, thousands of Japanese have been using chlorella tablets and powder as a food supplement, with verified beneficial results. Scientific researchers from the U.S., Russia, Germany, France, Japan, China, Israel and other countries have investigated chlorella and its properties, finding out many useful and health-enhancing qualities. Space program researchers in the U.S. and Russia have shown interest in chlorella as a possible space food. I will share some of these interesting findings a little later in this chapter, but first I want to tell what it is about chlorella that caught my attention in the first place.

GREEN VEGETABLES AND THE SUNSHINE FACTOR

Many years ago, I discovered that calcium, called "the knitter," for its role in healing, is controlled by sunshine. I found out that green leafy vegetables concentrate sunshine during the process of photosynthesis, so when we eat enough green vegetables, the body is assisted in balancing the blood calcium for repair and maintenance of strong tissues. Sunshine has healing properties of its own when we are not overexposed or underexposed to it, and I feel these healing properties are passed along to the plant chlorophyll which uses the sun energy to transform chemical elements into food for man. I have seen these healing properties at work in my sanitarium patients over the years, as they changed from imbalanced diets and poor food habits into a right way of eating and living. At the Ranch, patients would eat two green salads a day along with other vegetables, two fruits, a starch and a protein each day.

THE HEALING POWER OF SUNSHINE GREENS

One of my most important cases concerned a woman who came to me over 30 years ago with 13 open leg ulcers that refused to heal. She had been to the best doctors and clinics, who gave her "chalk" calcium to try to stimulate healing, but nothing happened. While I considered what I could do for this woman, I thought of the Hunza Valley and the calcium-type people who lived there, people with strong bones and teeth, hardly ever sick a day in their lives, with no pigeon chests or pronated ankles. They worked outside in the sun every day, but how could I get the sunshine energy into this woman to control the calcium? Then I thought of trying the greens—the "concentrated sunshine" vegetables.

We took half a dozen different kinds of green leafy vegetables and green tops of vegetables, chopped them up fine and let them "bleed" their green chlorophyll magic into a pint of water for an hour or so. Then, we strained out the chopped vegetables, and the lady would take the chlorophyll drink. This process was repeated several times a day. In three weeks, the leg ulcers this lady had for three years were healed. This was the first time I had encountered the healing power of green plants, and it was one of my greatest discoveries.

In working with other patients, I found out that green vegetables bring down the bile from the liver and gallbladder, aiding in the digestion of fats. A poached egg on a nest of steamed spinach was more easily digested than the egg alone would be. I found out that greens helped cleanse and deodorize the bowel, the chlorophyll helped by the fiber that toned the bowel wall and moved things along more quickly. I found out that chlorophyll-rich vegetables helped build the red blood cell count, getting rid of anemia.

HELPING ANEMIA WITH CHLOROPHYLL

One year a family from Canada sent a young lady to me with a severe case of anemia. Ordinarily, anemia can be taken care of with a good balanced diet and supplements of bone marrow or dessicated liver, but this young lady was a vegetarian. What could I do for a vegetarian with anemia? I knew that greens had an affinity for iron (chlorophyll only develops in the presence of iron) and I also knew that the chlorophyll molecule was almost identical with the hemoglobin molecule in red blood cells. So I put this vegetarian lady on a chlorophyll-rich diet, plenty of green salads, spinach, broccoli and liquid chlorophyll added to her juice or water several times a day. In three months, her red blood cell count was normal, and it was hard to tell whether she was happier than I. I feel wonderful whenever I see a patient getting better, but I feel twice as wonderful if the improvement is due to a new discovery on my part that I can apply to other patients. Not all my discoveries are original, but many have been new to me—things I have found out in the course of working with patients.

One of the things I found out about chlorophyll is that most green plants have less than half of 1% of it by weight. Alfalfa, the crop from which most chlorophyll is commercially extracted, has about 0.7% of chlorophyll, but not more than about 0.4% can be extracted. One of the things that attracted my attention immediately when I heard about the chlorella alga was its high chlorophyll content, from 2 to 5% by weight. I knew right away that chlorella would help speed up healing, even if the only biochemically useful substance in it was chlorophyll. (There is much more to chlorella.)

My experience with chlorophyll and greens in healing several hundred patients with various physical conditions prepared me to recognize the potential of chlorella when I knew about the high chlorophyll content. But I soon found out there were other beneficial factors in this magic green alga.

A MAGIC GREEN FROM THE SEA

The term *alga* refers to a large number of plants, from single cells a few thousandths of an inch in diameter, to giant sea kelp several hundred feet in length. These primitive plants are found everywhere on earth, and green algae are extremely important to life on this planet because of the oxygen-carbon dioxide exchange that takes place in photosynthesis. Green plants take in carbon dioxide and give off oxygen, while animals take in oxygen and give off carbon dioxide. Chlorella is a microscopic, single-cell green alga that grows in water in the presence of certain nutrients and chemicals. It has its own nucleus and is roughly spherical in shape.

Commercially, chlorella is grown in concrete mass culture pools where the nutrient medium and temperature are controlled and where stirring encourages as much exposure to sunlight as possible. These alga cells multiply so rapidly that about 40 tons per year can be grown on a single acre, under ideal conditions.

When the chlorella is harvested, it is cleaned, centrifuged, then spray-dried in a manner similar to the making of dried milk powder. The dried powder is either packaged or pressed into tablets for sale. We find out that the outer cell wall is so hard that chlorella is only 40 to 50% digestible, which is very nice for protecting the nutrients inside but not so nice for human assimilation. However, one chlorella company has developed a way of breaking down the cell wall mechanically to increase digestibility to 80%, and this is very good.

In the early days of chlorella investigation, researchers were surprised to notice that animals with supplementary chlorella in their food gained in size and weight much faster than animals on a normal balanced diet. This was one of the factors that triggered widespread research on this unusual food.

GREEN MAGIC FOR BETTER HEALTH

Analysis of the magic, mysterious "growth factor" in chlorella showed that it consisted of nucleic extract which had healing properties as well as growth-stimulating effects. Its early name stuck, and it continues to be called Chlorella Growth Factor or CGF for short. CGF is sold in liquid form. It is more highly concentrated in nucleic acids than chlorella.

Hospital tests showed that ulcers and nonhealing wounds responded very well when patients took chlorella tablets, CGF or both. The ulcers healed more quickly than by conventional treatment, and nonhealing wounds showed granulation of tissue in response to the use of chlorella. Doctors in Japan found out that chlorella stimulated the bowel, so they tried it on chronically constipated patients, some with spinal nerve damage. Regularity was restored in nearly all cases. Later it was found that chlorella stimulated rapid multiplication of the beneficial bowel bacteria, lactobacillus acidophilus, which is so important to bowel health.

MORE EXPERIMENTS WITH CHLORELLA

Further tests, first with animals in laboratories, then with people, showed that chlorella cured anemia and lowered abnormally high blood pressure. Chlorella was shown to protect the liver from toxic chemicals and to increase its rate of healing. Chlorella given to over a thousand Japanese sailors at sea reduced the incidence of colds and flu as compared to a control group not taking chlorella. School children given chlorella supplements grew taller and weighed more, on the average, than those who did not receive chlorella.

Chlorella given to patients receiving radiation or chemotherapy for cancer supported the natural immune system and helped prevent the usual drop in resistance.

In many cases, the beneficial results from chlorella occurred even though the people whose conditions were healed or improved did not change the eating habits or lifestyle habits that contributed to the problem in the first place. Many were taking prescription drugs as well, and I feel that the chlorella probably helped prevent the undesirable side effects from the drugs. We must recognize that although the drugs may have contributed something, the healings cannot be credited to them because chlorella was generally taken *only* when the drug itself was not bringing any improvement.

At this time, the healing effects of chlorella have not been fully examined, and I feel we have much more to learn, much more to discover about this wonderful food. What we do know is impressive. It detoxifies the body, cleanses and regularizes the bowel, feeds the beneficial bowel flora, supports the immune system, protects the liver, builds the blood and normalizes the blood pressure, among other things. *It builds the whole body.*

I have always taught that *only food can build the new tissue* needed for complete healing of any disease or damaged tissue, because only food can supply the chemical elements needed to make up for past chemical deficiencies, strengthen tissue to throw off old catarrh and toxic settlements and increase the activity level of underactive tissue to create the conditions which allow the formation of new tissue.

I do not say that chlorella is a panacea, but I feel it is one of the finest all-around food supplements I have encountered in years. Many of our foods and food supplements are derived from plant or animal sources grown or raised on nutrient-depleted land exposed to toxic chemical sprays, pollution and chemical fertilizers that do more harm than good to the soil. The amount of good we are getting out of such foods and food supplements seems to be less and less, and I feel it is wise to begin looking for foods and food supplements that come from less contaminated, less depleted sources.

When we consider the range of health benefits associated with chlorella, we find it fits nicely with any health building program or any program in which food and supplements are used as a remedy to bring recovery to tissues rather than suppression of symptoms. It can be used during weight loss diets, tissue cleansing programs and limited fasting. However, I want to say that it is absolutely necessary to adopt a healthy lifestyle, proper diet and a regular exercise program to stay well and avoid disease.

Good health is not a supplementary program or freedom from disease—it is a right way of life.

HEALTH, LONG LIFE AND THE NUCLEIC ACIDS

Researchers have found out that DNA and RNA in the cells of the human body may have a great deal to do with health and longevity. As we age, or if we do not eat and live properly, more and more of the DNA is broken down and not repaired. Less and less RNA is manufactured. There is less energy in the body for tissue repair and rebuilding. As a result, we find out that organs are weakened, tissues are weakened, and we become vulnerable to disease and signs of aging such as wrinkles, fatigue and loss of memory.

The interesting thing about this process is that we can do something to reverse it. We can use foods high in DNA and RNA to provide the repair material for DNA and the building materials for RNA. That is, the DNA and RNA in the foods we eat help repair and manufacture DNA and RNA in our own bodies. I want to say that we can't **replace** one with the other, but since they are made of the same basic substances, nucleic acids in foods provide what we need to repair or form nucleic acids in the human body.

I feel that foods high in nucleic acids and the glandular building foods such as lecithin may hold the key to long life. Many dietiticans and nutritionists of the past have talked about foods that fill the body, foods that repair, foods that provide the chemical elements we need, yet we find there has to be some way all these things come together to provide energy and a long life. I am particularly interested in helping the elderly people live a long and healthy life through proper foods and living habits.

ENERGY IS LIFE

Some scientists feel that foods high in nucleic acids may supply more energy at faster rates than other foods. This, in turn, speeds up cell repair and rebuilding, healing and slows down aging. Of course, we find that several of the B vitamins are needed in this process, but we see this is something that lifts the whole body.

Old age can only be slowed by taking care of every organ, gland and tissue in the body. The thyroid gland controls the metabolic rate of the whole body, but unless we take in foods that provide sufficient energy and tissue repair, the thyroid can't do the job by itself. It takes proper cell function, proper support at the cell level that can finally build to good health. This is what we are looking for. The value of chlorella will be understood when we get into energy medicine.

WE MUST CONSIDER THE WHOLE BODY

Over the years, we have seen many nutritional supplements or diets claimed to be the best thing for the heart, the best thing for the liver or the best thing for the glands. But we can't build a good body by lifting up only the heart or some other organ or system. What good does it do to support one organ while everything else in the body is breaking down?

When we consider the results of the diet high in nucleic acids, we see it works on the whole body, and this is what I believe in. One of the food laws I teach my patients and students is that we should eat only **whole** foods, because whole foods have a greater tendency to build a **whole body.**

In taking any supplement to build up the body, we must consider several factors. It must not stimulate or sedate any part of the body. It must not have any toxic effects or undesirable side effects as we find in drugs. There has to be a building effect on every part of the body. This is the path to wellness, the path to prevention or reversal of disease.

Many people still seem to think we "catch" diseases. They haven't yet learned that we actually build our chronic diseases— we eat and drink our way into them. We work for them in our poor lifestyle habits by smoking, drinking, overeating, worrying, living too fast and exercising too little. We *earn* our chronic diseases. Since we live in a country where there is plenty of food, we cannot say we are not getting enough to eat. It is more likely that we are neglecting something. There are reasons for believing that we are creating nutritional imbalances and deficiencies in the body by eating too much of the wrong foods and not enough of the right foods.

WHAT DOES THE SKIN TELL US?

One of the first things we see when we have been using a diet high in nucleic acids is that it has quite an effect on the skin. Most of us pay little attention to the skin because it doesn't seem to do much for us. On the other hand, it does tell some things that are going on inside the body. If the liver is not working right we may see signs on the skin. If the lungs and bronchials are not working right, skin problems often appear. If the liver and gallbladder are not taking care of oils and fats in the digestive system, the skin will often reflect that condition.

Foods high in RNA often clear up the skin in young people who have problems with acne. In older people, we find dry, wrinkled skin becoming tighter, moister, with the wrinkles gradually disappearing. This tells us that healthy changes are going on inside the body.

FOODS HIGH IN NUCLEIC ACIDS

Canned sardines are highest in the RNA factors in foods. Next are fresh sardines. Other foods high in RNA are chicken liver, calf liver, organ meats, nearly all seafoods, beans and lentils. We find that chlorella is also very high in nucleic material, and liquid chlorella growth factor (CGF) is a concentrated extract of nucleic factors.

The chlorella alga is a spherical single-celled plant with a tough outer shell and a nucleus at the center. In the nucleus, the activities of the cell are determined. The nucleus is like the brain of the cell, controlling the manufacture of food from sunlight and the disposal of wastes. The chlorella cell has everything needed to support life in it, including the healing and long life factors in the nucleus. The best CGF factor is manufactured by Sun Chlorella Company.

CGF and its nucleic factors, when taken into the body, stimulate repair and rebuilding of damaged tissue and raise the health level of the entire body. It stimulates cell division, not in healthy normal tissue, but in tissue that needs repair. When we realize that the "signal" for cell division comes from the nucleus of the cell, then we will understand that factors in CGF are able to reach inside the nuclei of cells surrounding damaged tissue and are able to repair that tissue.

REVERSAL OF THE AGING PROCESS

In persons who have used a high RNA diet or who have taken chlorella for some time, we see a higher level of energy, changes in attitude, quickened mental responses and a stronger, healthier body. These people have more energy, more power to do things. They become more youthful in their appearance and outlook. When we consider all these things together, we find there seems to be a reversal of the aging process.

I believe the primary role in the reversal of the aging process is a catalytic activity brought about by the nucleic factors in foods. This has been brought out a great deal in the work of Dr. Benjamin Frank. The importance of the nucleic factors in chlorella is also emphasized in the work of Dr. Liang-Ping Lin at Taiwan National University in the Republic of China. Medical institutions in Japan have demonstrated the catalytic activity of chlorella and liquid CGF in accelerating healing, even in some of the most difficult cases. When we have more energy, when we are able to build a better cell structure, we can expect to develop a stronger immune

361

system, a greater resistance to disease, and these are the essential requirements for living a longer life.

Possibly the most interesting thing about the nucleic acid foods is that they don't force the cells of the human body to do anything different, they only stimulate them to carry out their functions more efficiently. Of course, along with this process, waste materials are being eliminated faster than before. This explains why a number of chronic diseases such as diabetes, asthma, arthritis, high blood pressure, acne and others simply disappear as foods or supplements high in nucleic acids are used. When the whole body is taken care of, the pathway to disease is reversed. Stronger organs help weaker ones, old toxin settlements and catarrh are thrown off, new tissue grows in place of the old. This is the way nature heals.

THE IMPORTANCE OF OXYGEN IN THE BODY

The brain is a relatively small organ averaging two and three-quarters pounds in the adult, yet it rules the whole body and requires 20% of the oxygen used by the body. So we see that oxygen is one of the most important elements we should have.

Researchers claim that cancer cells do not grow in the parts of the body in which oxygen is being used. Instead, they tend to grow in oxygen-poor tissues, such as those between the brain cells. It has been claimed that one way to increase the resistance of the body to cancer is to increase the amount of oxygen available to the cell structure.

When I stop and think about the photosynthesis in green plants from which oxygen is developed, and how chlorophyll is always found together with iron, the great oxygen-carrier in the bloodstream, I wonder if we realize the importance of the chlorophyll-rich foods in the diet. I wonder if the high chlorophyll in the chlorella alga, together with the nucleic factors and iron, would increase the oxygenation of tissues enough to prevent many types of cancers from forming. We have to consider that our bodies are designed to be self-building, self-eliminating, self-repairing and self-rejuvenating, but it needs the opportunity to do these things. Sometimes we have to help it by changing our diet, lifestyle and exercise routines. I have found that adding various nutritional supplements to the diet has brought some of the best results for my patients.

THE PROOF IS IN THE SEEING

Dr. Frank feels that sardines are the greatest of the nucleic acid foods we can take into the body. I agree.

Sardines, of course, live in the sea, feeding on plankton that are probably very rich sources of nucleic acids themselves. Some of the plankton are algae, like chlorella. The genetically flawed or weak sardines are eaten by the larger fish such as tuna that follow the sardine schools. This means that only the strongest, fastest and most fit sardines survive. These are the ones caught in nets for human consumption. We must also consider that the **whole sardine** is usually eaten, which brings in more of the health-building food factors.

In general, most ocean fish are high in nucleic acids and low in cholesterol. A recent scientific study showed that people who eat fish twice a week or more have a significantly lower rate of heart disease than people who eat fish less often than that. Muscle meats like steak and hamburger are much lower in nucleic acids and are high in cholesterol.

HEALTH IS A WARM FEELING

I have often wondered about those people who have cold hands and cold feet, those who complain about feeling cold all the time. We cannot digest our foods properly if we don't have a warm body, and poor digestion can lead to other problems. What can be done?

People who used the high nucleic acid diets frequently reported an increase in body heat and far less sensitivity to cold. They wore lighter clothing than others when the weather was cool to cold. The greater body heat allowed them to digest their foods better, to get more good out of their foods. We especially need body warmth and strong digestion for the cold proteins such as beans and lentils.

Both high RNA foods and CGF lower the cholesterol in the bloodstream. When cholesterol is lowered, the blood is able to circulate more freely through the arteries and bring more oxygen to the cells. Oxygen helps prevent disease and helps burn away toxic wastes that can settle in the tissues if they are not taken care of. I think that improved circulation and better oxygenation help account for the greater feeling of warmth in people who are on the high nucleic acid diets.

MORE HIGH RNA FOODS

Beside organ meats and seafoods, the next highest RNA foods are dried legumes: pinto beans, lentils, garbanzos, blackeyed peas, small white beans, large lima beans, great northern beans, cranberry beans, baby lima beans, split peas and red beans. Nuts have some nucleic acids, as do wheat germ, asparagus and onions.

In addition to possibly being very high in nucleic acids, codfish roe is high in calcium and lecithin.

Calcium is nicknamed "the knitter" because of its role in healing the body. Lecithin is a brain and nerve food. Cod roe has been called the poor man's caviar, and it is most easily taken when blended with a little tomato juice.

SOME FINAL THOUGHTS ON NUCLEIC FACTORS

When I consider the effects of the nucleic factors on the body, I feel that it is most encouraging to see that the whole body benefits from them. Chlorella works in exactly the same way. This is working *with* nature in the prevention and reversal of disease, as demonstrated by the fact that there are no undesirable side effects. This is the way I believe we should go, the way of well-being and long life.

TECHNIQUES ADVANCING PROPERTIES OF CHLORELLA

Sun Chlorella is a whole, pure, natural food, meeting the requirements of the most important of all food laws.
We will have a book on Chlorella out in the latter part of 1986.

I recommend Sun Chlorella in particular, because I have toured 5 Sun Chlorella plants in Japan, and found the cleanliness standards and production standards were absolutely impeccable. I am impressed that Sun Chlorella has developed a process for breaking down the cell wall and increasing the digestibility to 75-80%, nearly 40% more than chlorella was previously. I was able to observe the processing and development of Chlorella Growth Factor, a liquid extract from the chlorella nucleus which stimulates the immune response and speeds up rejuvenation and regeneration. I feel that Sun Chlorella cares a great deal about the quality of its products and the consumers who use them.

Sun Chlorella is:

Whole: Not subjected to any refining process. The *whole cell* with all the nutrients necessary to support life is available.

Pure: Not exposed to chemical pesticides or agricultural chemicals. No preservatives, artificial coloring or flavoring—no chemical additives.

Natural: As nature made it, including the long-life and healing factors from the cell nucleus.

Digestible: The cell wall disintegration process used exclusively by Sun Chlorella Company has increased digestibility to 80%, 20% to 40% higher than chlorella used in the past.

High Chlorophyll: Chlorella content is 2-3% chlorophyll, higher than any other known plant source. Chlorophyll is the most effective natural tissue-cleansing agent known.

Nutrients: Protein 55-65%, carbohydrates 20-25%, fats 5-15%. Contains 19 amino acids, including all the essential amino acids needed by the body. Fats are 82% unsaturated, 18% saturated.

Vitamins: Includes pro-vitamin A, B-1 (thiamine), B-2 (riboflavin), B-3 (niacin), B-6 (pyridoxine), B-12, pantothenic acid, folic acid, biotin, PABA, inositol and vitamin C.

Minerals: Iron, phosphorus, magnesium, calcium, iodine, zinc, potassium, sulphur and trace amounts of manganese, sodium and chlorine.

Bowel Normalization: Chlorella helps restore the underactive bowel to regularity; it cleans and deodorizes the bowel.

Cleansing: Chlorella has an affinity for drugs, herbicides, pesticides and heavy metals, and carries them out through the elimination channels.

Lactobacillus Acidophilus: Chlorella *greatly multiplies* the friendly bowel flora such as lactobacillus acidophilus and increases levels of the B-vitamins in the bowel.

Bowel Cleansing and Building: The chlorophyll in chlorella helps cleanse the blood while the iron, B-12 and folic acid aid in building new red blood cells.

Liver Protection: Animal experiments show that chlorella helps protect the liver from some toxic materials.

Hypertension: High blood pressure is reduced, in many cases, after chlorella has been taken for several months. Blood cholesterol and triglycerides are also lowered.

Growth Factor: Nucleic material of chlorella stimulates cell division, tissue repair and healing, as shown in Japanese hospital reports and studies.

Acid/Alkaline Balance: Chlorella neutralizes the excess acids and heavy acidic materials in the body, restoring the acid/alkaline balance.

Immunity: The latest research shows that chlorella increases the immune response and strengthens the body's natural defenses against disease by increasing at least five important factors in the immune system.

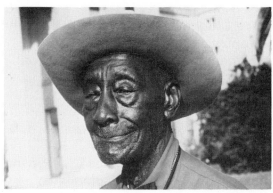

Charlie Smith, 136 years old when I met him, ate sardines every day for the last 30 years of his life. Sardines are high in RNA, the longevity-promoting nucleic acid.

28

Nutrition
and
Tissue Cleansing

When I opened my first office practice, I knew a little about nutrition and hygiene, but not as much as I know today. Experience, of course, is the best teacher for the student who is ready, and since nutrition had saved my life when the doctors had given up on me, I was wide awake and ready to learn. I was ready.

One of my most eye-opening experiences came while I was working with a doctor named Glen Sipes in San Francisco. He was a good deal older and more experienced than I. One day we received an emergency call from Walnut Creek, and after we arrived, we found a young man in his 20s, lying on a couch, his body bloated and feverish, his face red as a beet. His skin was so sensitive that the slightest touch caused considerable pain. The young man's mother stood by the couch.

The first thing Dr. Sipes asked the man was when he had his last bowel movement. He couldn't remember. So Dr. Sipes asked the mother to prepare an enema. She didn't know what an enema was and had no enema apparatus in the house. After asking the woman to warm some water, Dr. Sipes went outside by the creek, cut a section of reed with his pocket knife and hollowed it out with a piece of baling wire.

For an hour or so, I saw Dr. Sipes repeatedly blow water through the reed into the patient's rectum, then help him to the bathroom to relieve himself and return to continue the process. By the time we left, the man's fever was gone, his skin color had gone from red to normal, and he was no longer in pain. The change was dramatic and made quite an impression on me. I was surprised that constipation could have such an effect on the whole body, and just as surprised that a series of enemas could bring such relief.

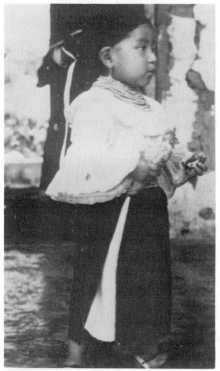

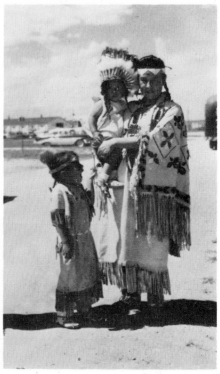

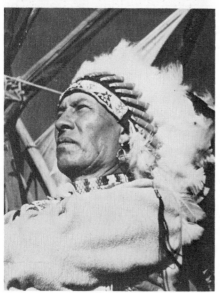

Corn, or maize, considered the staff of life in all the ancient cultures of the Americas, has been a staple food of Indians in the Southwest U.S., as well as in Mexico, Central and South America. Notice what is in the little girl's hand, upper left.

A DIFFICULT CASE COMES MY WAY

My college training was in chiropractic, and I began my practice specializing in mechanical manipulation. When a lady came into my office one day with a wry neck, a condition where the neck vertebrae are quite malaligned. I was sure I could take care of her. "Can you help me with this condition?" she asked. "I'm sure an adjustment will help," I told her. "I don't want you to touch my neck," she said. "I've been to several chiropractors and it hasn't helped. There has to be some other way." Nearly all my training was in chiropractic. What else could I do? Well, doctors are supposed to know what to do. "Well, then," I said, "I believe it would be best to start out with a couple of enemas." I made a physical examination and a tremendous abnormal bowel presented itself with bloating and extreme tenderness. She had no movement in the past two weeks and had been constipated as long as she could remember. We worked with enemas taking four or five until we had a complete cleanout.

When finished, the lady came to me and said, "Look at me!" I could hardly believe my eyes. She was holding her neck and head perfectly straight, without apparent pain. Yet, I hadn't touched her neck. I had only taken care of the bowel and her neck problem was relieved on its own!

WHAT I LEARNED FROM THESE CASES

From the earliest days of my work, I learned the importance of the elimination channels, especially the bowel. I learned that bowel toxemia could bring troubles to the entire body, and I found out it could cause particular problems in specific places remote from the bowel. And, I knew enough about nutrition to realize that the basic cause of constipation and bowel underactivity was in the diet, in taking too many of the wrong foods and not enough of the right foods.

The basic lesson, of course, is that when the elimination channels (the lungs and bronchials, the skin, the kidneys and the bowel) are underactive, toxic wastes are not eliminated as fast as they are built up in the body. I am talking not only about food wastes, but chemical additives in foods, pesticide spray residues on foods, chemical pollutants in the air and water, chemicals assimilated on the job and sometimes in the home, drug residues and metabolic wastes developed even by the cells and tissues of the body during normal activities. All of these things are meant to be eliminated regularly from the body at the same rate as they are accumulated. We find that even overwork, stress and fatigue can build up excess acids in the body. The average person is capable of tearing down the body faster than it can be built up.

When toxins accumulate in the body, they settle in what we call the inherently weak organs. Everyone is born with some organs, glands and tissues somewhat weaker than others. The actual weakness is in the function, and these organs cannot hold nutrients as well as normal tissues or get rid of their own wastes as rapidly as they should. They are more subject to mineral deficiencies, and they are less able to get rid of outside toxic materials when an excess of toxins is carried to them by the bloodstream. When this toxic accumulation goes on constantly, day after day, underfunction develops and a foundation for a future disease is created.

NEW DISCOVERIES IN MY SANITARIUM WORK

After starting my sanitarium work, I had the wonderful advantage of working with patients on a daily basis, sometimes over a considerable period of time. A sanitarium is a place where people live on the same grounds with their doctor, who designs an individual health program for each patient and checks with patients regularly to see how they are progressing. Often a patient is able to recuperate and get well much faster away from home, in a beautiful relaxing environment where only nourishing food is served and regular exercise is encouraged. Poor lifestyle habits are more easily broken this way, replaced by new, more healthful habits.

With my sanitarium patients, I tried various ways of improving the function of the elimination channels, while making sure they followed a food regimen that was half building, half eliminating. When I emphasized skin brushing, sun baths and exercise to the point of perspiration, I could see benefits not only to the skin but the whole body. Improving skin elimination was helpful, but I found that it was very slow in bringing results. To bring out better elimination from the lungs and bronchials, I taught patients sniff-breathing exercises and had them take long vigorous walks in the fresh air and sunshine. Again, this brought good results, but not as fast as I hoped. I tried improving the kidney function in several ways, starting with having certain patients take 8 glasses of water a day or more while on a regular balanced diet, with herbal teas three times per day to stimulate mild diuretic activity. I fasted some patients, others were put on vegetable juices only or watermelon only. We were able to increase kidney activity very nicely in many cases, and we saw good resulte. But the greatest, most dramatic results came from working with the bowel.

I believe at least 90% of my sanitarium patients had underactive bowels. What do I mean by underactive bowels? Well, we find that healthy babies have a bowel movement after every meal of solid food. The movements of the stomach in digestion stimulate muscle contractions in the bowel which move wastes along for elimination. This is nature's way, and in nature, we see that animals always eliminate shortly after they eat. Most children, however, are trained to have only one bowel movement a day, and they grow up that way. If they are busy playing with friends, children may suppress the urge to eliminate and miss a day or even two. I have many patients who average a bowel movement once a week. A poor diet with a good deal of refined foods can slow down the bowel. So can chronic fatigue. The thing to keep in mind, however, is that nature designed the body to have a bowel movement after every meal, and when we develop a bowel to move less often, there are consequences in the body.

When I began to find out that most of my patients used excessive amounts of wheat and milk in their daily food routines, I could see another problem coming in. Allergists were beginning to find out back then that milk and wheat were two of the foremost causes of allergies, and I knew that my patients with allergies had more problems with constipation than almost anyone else. I could tell, even then, that milk and wheat were causing bowel underactivity and bowel troubles. Later, when I visited England and found out about celiac disease, I knew that people could become "bowel-sensitive" to wheat and milk simply by using large amounts of them. The body was not designed to take so much wheat and so much milk as the average person was taking.

371

One of the first things I cound out in taking care of the bowel, increasing the bowel activity through the addition of more fiber, was that other elimination organs improved in their function without doing anything special for them. Skin conditions would clear up, bronchial problems would disappear, kidney troubles would greatly improve, simply by increasing the rate of bowel activity. I became convinced that bowel care was more important than most people in the health arts realized.

DEVELOPING THE ART OF TISSUE CLEANSING

I decided to make a project of the bowel, to understand its relation to other elimination channels, to the various organs and tissues of the body, to nutrition, to health and disease. I studied the work of Sir Arbuthnot Lane, physician to the Royal family of Great Britain, whose surgical removal of sections of the bowel in various patients caused the disappearance of diseases such as bronchial asthma and chronic arthritis. I studied with Dr. John Harvey Kellogg of Battle Creek Sanitarium fame, who taught me the importance of maintaining the proper balance of friendly bowel flora. I studied colonics with a colonic specialist in New York and could hardly believe some of the things that were eliminated. We found out that people who ate mostly refined foods had the most bowel problems, while those who used the high fiber foods—fruit, vegetables and whole cereal grains, had the least trouble. From a report prepared by the Royal Society of Medicine in Great Britain, I found that over 36 toxins may be found in the bowel, some of which are able to get into the bloodstream in cases of constipation and bowel underactivity. Examples include indol, skatol, phenol, indican and methylmercaptan.

Working with my sanitarium patients, I found that the most frequent cause of troubles with the skin, kidneys, lungs and bronchials was due to the toxic overload forced upon them by an underactive bowel. (Single foods such as milk and wheat, when taken too much, could also cause toxic reactions.) When the bowel was taken care of, problems with other elimination channels usually cleared up quickly. Often problems elsewhere in the body cleared up as well, leading me to believe there was a neural-reflex connection between the bowel and other organs and tissues in the body which was somehow able to selectively direct toxic materials to specific tissues, whether near to or remote from the bowel.

I made a discovery which has been taught to many doctors that a neuralreflex exists in the bowel affecting definite organs. I could tell by the symptoms or problems that existed what part of the bowel was responsible. This discovery had a great advantage in finding where bowel pockets existed and sources of infection began in the body. These sources of infection were usually in the form of diverticula.

The relation between nutrition and the bowel became abundantly clear over my years of sanitarium experience. Those who followed my recommended food regimen, now called the Health and Harmony Food Regimen, which emphasizes *pure, whole, natural foods, 60% raw and 80% vegetables and fruits,* developed greatly improved bowel activity. Dr. Dennis Burkitt's study of the diets and bowel health of rural East African natives has confirmed the value and practicality of my diet. Among these rural villagers using a high fiber diet, Dr. Burkett found no colon cancer, appendicitis, colitis, polyps or hemorrhoids, and very few instances of the "diseases of civilization" such as diabetes, cardiovascular disease, arthritis and so forth.

Elsewhere in this book, I have discussed at length how the average person who uses an excessive amount of milk, wheat and sugar (63% of the average diet), and how these foods often contribute to a sluggish, underactive bowel, as well as to allergy reactions and, more rarely, celiac disease (in the case of wheat). The best thing you can do for yourself is to cut these down to a minimum or eliminate them from your diet. I did this with all my patients in my sanitarium and got my best results.

SOME FOODS ARE NATURAL LAXATIVES
"Alfalfa Tablets Are Best"

I found that yellow fruits and vegetables worked nicely as natural laxatives, and that alfalfa tablets were a wonderful aid in keeping the bowel clean and well toned. I always advise cracking them before swallowing. Five tablets with each meal are generally

373

enough. Liquid chlorophyll, as found in health food stores, and also chlorophyll-rich green, leafy vegetables help keep the bowel clean and free of putrefactive odors, in part by helping feed the friendly bowel flora. Yogurt, kefir and clabber milk, in general, help to feed and increase the friendly bowel flora. Fiber from fruits, vegetables and whole grains tones the bowel and helps keep it regular.

SODIUM, POTASSIUM AND ACIDOPHILUS ARE NEEDED

I believe that sodium and potassium will help to balance the electrolytes more than any other elements. The intestinal wall needs these two elements. The intestinal flora develops best with the introduction of these two elements.

Biochemical sodium, as found in foods, is often deficient in those with gastrointestinal problems. These chemicals are needed to neutralize acid wastes in the bowel and to assist in the transport of nutrients through the small intestinal wall. The best sources are whey, okra, celery and green leafy vegetables. If constipation has been present for some time, it is very likely that the friendly bowel bacteria need replenishing and this can be done by taking acidophilus supplement as found in the health food stores. Concentrated acidophilus supplements are available. One brand claims to be able to destroy several types of undesirable bacteria. While taking the acidophilus, I recommend also taking Sun Chlorella tablets (5 with each meal). The chlorella will help to feed and multiply the lactobacillus acidophilus a great deal. Avoid coffee, even decaffeinated, soft drinks, chocolate, excessive proteins and too much wheat and milk products, which can be destructive to the acidophilus bacteria.

Proper use of foods and supplements, along with at least half an hour of regular exercise every day, will slowly cleanse and restore the bowel, encouraging the release of any catarrh and toxic settlements dammed up in the tissues due to inadequate elimination. When the elimination channels are open and clean, tissue cleansing takes place throughout the whole body, followed by replacement of the old tissue by new tissue in a natural rejuvenation process. All tissues in the body are affected by the state of health of the bowel. Tissues cannot be rebuilt while toxins are present, and the toxins cannot be released until the elimination channels are open and active.

LAXATIVES CONTRIBUTE TO BOWEL PROBLEMS

I do not recommend using laxatives to increase bowel activity, for the reason that habitual laxative use weakens the natural bowel activity and compounds the problem of underactivity and constipation in the long run. The proper way to improve bowel regularity is through correct diet. Two beet tablets per meal or raw shredded beet the size of a golf ball once a day in a salad, act as a natural laxative. I feel it is all right to use an enema once in a while to overcome constipation, but I do not recommend daily enemas, unless in a temporary program supervised by a doctor.

While I have used various fasting techniques and enemas to stimulate faster tissue cleansing in patients from time to time, I have found a more effective means of rapid tissue cleansing in recent years. Tissue cleansing by means of proper diet and exercise works very well, but it may take several months or as much as a year. For those whose body systems are extremely underactive or toxic laden or whose bowels are toxic and loaded with mucus, there is a fast way.

THE ULTIMATE TISSUE CLEANSING PROGRAM

In the 1970s, I began experimenting with a 7-day tissue cleansing program with several unique and perfectly safe features. Mr. V. E. Irons, a health product developer, had been using this method very successfully and I adapted it to my patients' needs. The program involves having no solid foods for 7 days but having instead a variety of supplements, a bulk drink and clay water to clean the old mucous lining from the bowel wall. Several hundred patients have now gone through this program, with dramatic results that I will describe a little later.

This tissue cleansing program involves use of the colema, so-named because it resembles colonics in a way and the enema in a way, while avoiding the pressure of colonics and the inadequate cleansing of the enema. The patient lies comfortably on his or her back on the colema board, head on a pillow, knees raised, buttocks braced against curved wooden or plastic supports on either side of a hole in the colema board, through which elimination takes place. The "hole" end of the colema board goes over the toilet, while the other end is supported on a chair.

A five-gallon bucket of lukewarm water is hung on a sturdy support about 3 feet above the colema board. A hose of surgical rubber tubing goes from the water bucket to the splashboard backing the colema board opening, and connects with a pencil-thin, clear plastic tube with several holes near the tip. The plastic tube, lubricated with K-Y jelly, is inserted about 3 inches into the anus; and, when ready, the patient releases the valve holding the rubber tubing closed. The warm water enters the rectum by gravity flow, and waste is gently washed out from time to time *around* the plastic tube, without removing it, and down into the toilet.

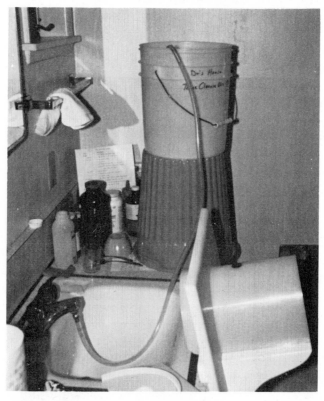

This home equipment is used in giving this cleansing treatment. This is not a colonic, but an improved style of taking an enema.

The person taking the colema simply lies comfortably on the board for 30-45 minutes while the cleansing procedures takes place. The process is clean, comfortable and effortless.

The 7-day program consists of colemas twice a day (morning and evening) and taking supplements, bulk and clay water at regular intervals during the day. The old mucous lining of the bowel wall is removed and eliminated and toxins are absorbed and eliminated by the clay water.

What happens when people go through this 7-day cleansing program? Have a look at the following case histories and testimonials for a sample of results. I want to say here that tissue cleansing through the colema method is not considered a treatment or therapy, and we do not claim that it treats any disease or abnormal condition. It is simply a very effective means of detoxifying the bowel. I present full details on this method in my book *Tissue Cleansing Through Bowel Management.*

CASE HISTORIES AND TESTIMONIALS

Case 1: R.M. (Male). Patient came in with advanced ulcers of the feet, ankles and lower legs; ulcers running yellow-green purulent matter and feet and ankles too swollen to wear shoes. Condition previously treated by several physicans without success. Blood pressure 80/58. Patient complained of cold hands and feet. History included 7-1/2 years of diarrhea, 7 or 8 bowel movements per day, not helped by any medication. Foot ulcers began 2 years prior to examination. Patient's grandfather had hardening of the arteries, low blood pressure and diabetes prior to gangrene developing on the right foot. Grandfather's right leg amputated, then gangrene appeared on other leg and it also was amputated. Grangrene returned and patient's grandfather died. Patient wondered if the same pattern was happening to him.

Patient was placed on 7-day tissue cleansing program. Clay packs and aloe vera were applied externally to the legs. On the 4th day of program, swelling in right ankle went away. Incrustations on feet, ankles, insteps and heels dried and began to come off. At end of 7-day program, feet, ankles and legs had almost completely cleared up. No drainage from ulcers. New skin developing. Patient reported, "It is almost miraculous!"

BEFORE   AFTER

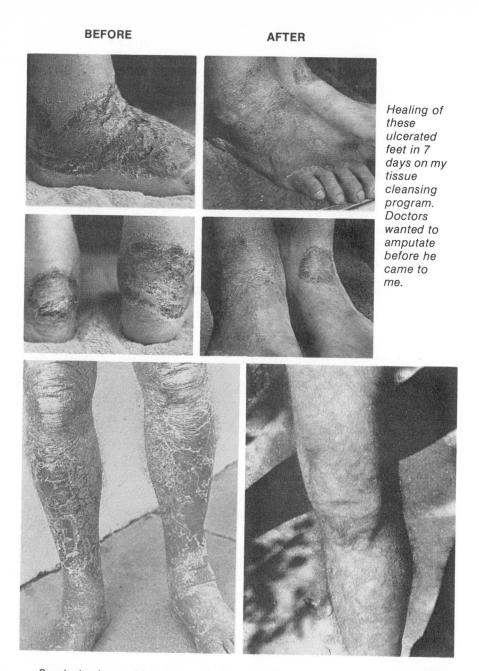

Healing of these ulcerated feet in 7 days on my tissue cleansing program. Doctors wanted to amputate before he came to me.

Psoriasis changed by proper nutrition. All therapies must have nutrition at their base, because food is necessary for new tissue.

BEFORE AFTER

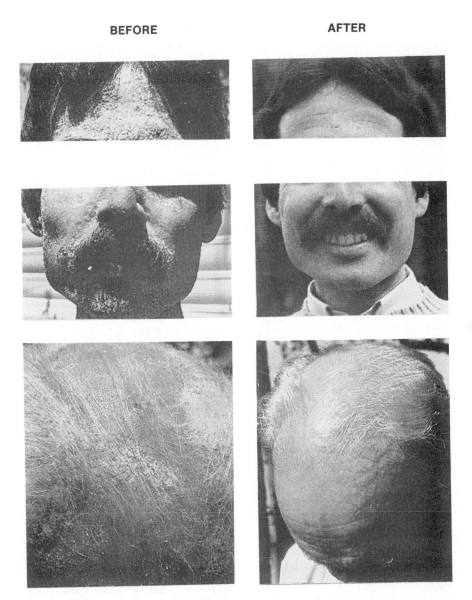

Upper: Skin problems are especially troublesome when they involve the face. This is a bad case of psoriasis that responded to a good diet. Lower: Scalp problems can be very hard to take care of, but nutrition did wonders for this man. These are a few of hundreds of case histories I have collected.

Case 2: B.F. (female). "I am dropping this note to let you know that the Tissue Cleansing Regimen I took the first week in April cleared up the cysts in the breast which had troubled me."

Case 3: A.W. (female). Patient had been found by her physician to have uterine growths. Pap test showed 4+. Patient went through tissue cleansing program and three months later, went for another Pap test and examination. Everything was normal, with no sign of uterine growths.

Case 4: S.D. (female). Patient complained of fatigue, low energy, neck pains, lower back pains. Lab blood test showed red blood cell count of 3.84 (normal is 4.8) and hemoglobin of 10.7 (normal is 14.0). Patient reported, "A month after my first blood test, a second blood test showed my red blood cell count was up to 4.47 and my hemoglobin was 12.8. My energy is much better now, and my back and neck have been better since I took the cleansing program."

Case 5: S.B. (female). Before going through her first tissue cleansing program, patient's lab blood test showed triglyceride reading of 1938 (normal is 50-200 mg/dl). At the end of the 7-day program it dropped to 253. Patient reported, "Nearly 3 years later, after a year of living under high stress conditions, my triglycerides shot up to 1403 mg/dl. I went through the tissue cleansing program again, and the level dropped to 325."

Many people have reported good results with this program. We believe people can expect the best results if we start our program of rejuvenation with an elimination program. The whole body benefits from this kind of elimination.

For those interested in more information on tissue cleansing, please refer to my book *Tissue Cleansing Through Bowel Management.*

Cleansing is only one part of rejuvenating the body; there must be a building and maintenance program. This is discussed in my book to work toward a good health lifestyle.

These cases and the work brought out in the book were done in my own practice, working with individuals who desired to work for the best possible health. It does take a certain amount of counseling and knowledge of the natural healing art and nutrition to accomplish these results. Therefore, we advise a person to seek good counsel to work out their individual problems and illnesses.

─────29─────
The Natural
Reversal Process—
A Remedy with Correction

There is more to good health than eating the right foods, as we must realize. Every person is unique, made up of body, mind and spirit. Both health and disease involve all three levels.

Peace of mind comes from peace with the Creator, which is a spiritual thing. If you know you are not living right, the best doctor cannot keep you well or help you feel good about yourself. You need to take care of these things and live a lifestyle approved by nature.

At the mental level, we find it is hard to stay healthy and feel good when the marriage is not doing well or we are not happy with our job or we let money troubles get us down. We have to confront and overcome these problems to be fully well. All mental problems and all thinking have an effect on every cell and all body systems.

Physically, in addition to proper foods, we must have adequate rest, fresh air, sunshine, physical exercise, recreation, companionship and exposure to beauty and music, *BUT ONLY FOODS CAN BUILD NEW TISSUE*. Remember, whatever you do, *FOOD AND NUTRITION ARE FUNDAMENTAL IN REBUILDING AND REPAIRING ALL LIFE IN THE BODY.*

I can't think of a better way to start a day than to take a walk in a beautiful garden, then do 10 minutes of exercise to happy music with a good beat. But your world will fall if good nourishment isn't there to support you.

If you think that you can live with hate on one side of your living and joy on the other, you become a mixed-up person. If you think you can live on a healthy meal once a day and on junk food the rest of the day, you are going to have a body so mixed up that you will not be able to live the kind of life you would appreciate. We become a double-minded creature, living with faith in one hand and doubt in the other. We have to recognize that we have to live right seven days of the week, not just Sunday. We have to do the right thing most of the time. It is not a once-in-a-while job.

This chapter is one of the most important chapters you will read. It is a very fundamental chapter. You will have to make a decision now as to what kind of tomorrow you are going to have. Your future is going to be made up of the kind of thinking you have today, with the kind of foods that you eat today, with the associations you have, the drugs you take, the amount of alcohol you use and the habits you have. Don't let the negative things determine the biggest part of your future.

You are going to have to take **POSITIVE** action in a **POSITIVE** way with things that are **POSITIVELY** good for you to have the good life that we promise or that has been promised by other health teachers.

Now there is a **REVERSAL** process that we would like to talk about and that is how we can go in one direction with our habits: junk food, junk thoughts and so forth, and then we can reverse the process. A path of greater living habits, finer living habits and a more healthful attitude with better nourishment is going to start a reversal process.

In other words, we go back over the path that we have followed and we make good in our body, mind and spirit those things that we took on that were not of the highest value. When we put in better values than we had before and break up the old habits, we live a better lifestyle than we ever had. We find that our body responds to environment and polluted thinking, polluted foods and polluted water and so forth. Our body molds to the food we eat and the environment in which we live. The body is the one that repairs and rebuilds and does it beautifully when we give it the opportunity. *THAT IS WHY WE SAY THAT NATURE CURES, BUT SHE NEEDS THE OPPORTUNITY.*

Now the decision is yours. For a more complete discussion of the path of health and the reversal process, see my book *Doctor-Patient Handbook.*

NATURAL REMEDIES LEAD TO A RECOVERY— TO A CORRECTION OF OUR ILLS

When we are on the path to right living, an interesting process begins. As the body increases in strength and level of health, the old catarrhal and toxic settlements in the body (long dried and isolated in various tissues and organs) begin to liquefy. What does this mean?

We find that most people live in such a way that whenever they get a disease or illness, they use drugs or other therapies to suppress their symptoms. Every disease, every illness, is accompanied by the body's effort to rid itself of catarrh, mucus and toxins that we ourselves have built up in the body through inadequate nutrition and a poor lifestyle. When we suppress these discharges, they are driven back into the body where they settle in the tissues least able to resist. (We call such areas inherent weaknesses.) There they stay, causing low-level inflammation at first and eventually contributing to the development of a chronic or degenerative disease. On the other hand, right eating and living can reverse this process.

NUTRITION OF GREATEST VALUE

We find it is *chemical imbalance in tissue that expresses itself as a disease,* and it is often refined foods, wrongly cooked foods, abnormal foods that create the chemical imbalance in the first place. It is not only what you eat but what you don't eat that counts in tissue activity.

If you violate the food laws, *the law of variety, the law of excess, the law of whole, pure and natural foods, the law of proportions,* you cannot build a normal-functioning body. Foods were made by the Creator with a certain chemical structure, and they have stored solar vibrations and fine essences that man is only beginning to understand. We need to realize that nature—not man—determines what is normal. It is our job to operate close to the laws laid down by nature. We must learn to select the mode of living that will develop a healthier body.

While we have talked about the mineral balance and the nutritional needs for the body, we must also recognize that when we speak of a lifestyle, there are many things that can lead us into poor health such as enervation, tiredness, fatigue. A body subjected to these conditions cannot digest foods properly even when we have learned to use healthy foods, and we find that a new law can come in. *It is not what we eat that counts. It is what we digest.* It takes a rested body to digest and assimilate foods well. Balance is important in making up your menu for the day, as brought out in our food healing laws.

SUPPRESSION CONTRIBUTES TO CHRONIC CONDITIONS

Suppression is the process of stopping and drying up the discharge of catarrh, phlegm and mucus through drugs, fatigue, overwork, disharmony and other improper living habits. The more energy we have, the cleaner the body. The more energy we have, the more power we have to work with. The closer we live to nature, free of environmental pollution, the more we are able to automatically eliminate this catarrh, phlegm and mucus. An ill body is unclean, unable to repair and rebuild itself to the highest state of well-being. When we drive this debris back into the body, we create a more chronic condition.

Catarrh is a natural elimination that takes place in the body when we are trying to establish good health. A healthy body does not have these discharges. And we learn that catarrh is something that we have to stop from coming out, or so we have been taught. This is just the opposite of what should be done. Catarrh does not belong in our body. As long as we have an unclean body and there is material to be eliminated, such as drugs, toxins, chemical food additives, pesticide residues, tar, nicotine, cadmium and other chemicals; it is only through catarrh, phlegm and mucus that we will rid the body of debris. The secret is to never stop catarrh in its discharge. The secret is to stop making it.

Catarrh becomes trapped in inherently weak tissues where it becomes a constant tissue irritant, lowering the activity level of tissue and providing a breeding ground for disease. For this reason, I don't believe in stopping a catarrhal discharge, which is usually a natural elimination.

Abnormal foods create abnormal bodies. Fried foods produce one kind of body. Coffee and donuts produce another kind of body. **Soft** drinks are **hard** on the body. All abnormal tissues in abnormal bodies invite and build the abnormal condition we call disease.

Drugs can suppress discharges and symptoms, but they don't do it by restoring abnormal tissue to normal. They do not allow a natural elimination to take place. Drugs change or control tissue function by stimulation, paralysis or sedation, not by building or rejuvenating body tissue. Side effects appear as the body tries to detoxify or isolate drug residues it can't use. Drug residues, metabolic acid wastes and catarrh are forced into storage in the tissues and cell structures of the body as a result of taking suppressive drugs.

When we start living right, this process automatically begins to reverse and this is where Western medicine and nutritional science differ. **Nutritional science believes in natural methods of cleansing, detoxifying, rebuilding, renewing and repairing, so there can be tissue recovery without side effects.** We do not store catarrh in the body; we get rid of it.

Western medicine advocates the use of drugs which suppress symptoms and which seldom encourage the elimination of catarrh, phlegm and mucus. In the long run and sometimes the short run, this leaves side effects. All drugs have side effects; some have genetic effects and time-bomb effects. Eventually as body tissues develop an abnormal accumulation of catarrh and a lower state of health, they begin to show the side effects. In most cases, we have to take care of these conditions years after we have taken the drugs.

We have found that we don't have to deal with side effects when we use proper nutrition. A balanced diet, together with a healthy lifestyle do not produce undesirable side effects, genetic effects, long-term effects or time-bomb effects. Excessive catarrh is not produced. Tissue building and elimination of metabolic and other wastes are balanced, as is necessary in a healthy body. **Nutrition is a better alternative to use when we can get it to do the work. Most times it will.**

What we have to realize is that it is necessary to be careful in our use of foods and nutrition. Perhaps because of inherited genetic conditions or improper past food habits, we may have allergic reactions to certain foods, and these should be eliminated from our diet. Chemical sprays used on fruits, vegetables and grains, chemical additives in canned or packaged foods, and chemical fertilizers may also cause allergic reactions. We have to find ways of dealing with these things, avoiding chemically-contaminated foods as much as possible. We also have to watch out for imbalanced proportions of certain foods in our diet. We need variety to meet all the nutritional requirements of the body. The average person cannot handle a diet which is 29% wheat and 25% milk, as shown by government figures, because this will overload the body tissues, imbalance the body chemistry and crowd out other foods needed in an adequately balanced nutritional regimen.

We need substitute foods for milk and wheat, and these are discussed elsewhere in this chapter and other chapters. We replace wheat with millet, brown rice and corn. We replace milk with the seed and nut milk drinks, such as sesame seed milk or almond milk or we can use soy milk powder to make a soy milk. Use only natural sweets. No refined sugars.

THE REVERSAL PROCESS—NATURE'S WAY

In nutrition, as we develop new tissue in place of the old, we have to go through the reversal process, which is nature's way of cleansing and restoring the body. We call this replacement therapy—new tissue in place of the old that is not satisfactory. When we reverse the process that brought on a disturbance or disease, we will eventually liquefy and eliminate the old toxic material and catarrh from the body, and the conditions which brought on the problem will be eliminated. *New tissue grows in place of the old.* This, I feel, is true healing, and it is nature's way because tissue is restored with full recovery of function and activity.

WISDOM IS THE ABILITY TO DISCOVER AN ALTERNATIVE

It is not that we object to all the different treatments that are given today, but there is an alternative that many more people could use to be well and have a healthier body. It is yet to be discovered by most people. It is yet to be recognized by many of the various professions in the healing arts. It is in this alternative way of living that we come closer to nature, building a superb body. We can build toward well-being by just living closer to natural principles, closer to natural foods. Of course, we must have a good philosophy. We must know how to relax, to let go.

We need to find a lifestyle that is going to provide us with the healthy body we are all seeking. It is much better for a doctor to work on a patient who has been living a healthy lifestyle, if some health problem arises. The patient's chance of recovery is greater. His recovery time is shorter. The hospital expense would be less, and his doctor bill could be minimum. We have to learn how to take care of ourselves. This is what I mean by an alternative way of life.

There is a growing number of people who have been turned on to this alternative way of living and they should be encouraged by the doctors. We recognize that health extremists have developed out of this alternative philosophy, but the various health professions have driven these people to extremes. Doctors should respond to the search for a better way of life by teaching a healthy, balanced, natural way of living. There is usually some good in every extreme approach to health. Many of the extreme approaches are out of balance, however. Now, a balanced life, a balanced way of living, staying away from the edges, is in order. Extremes may show a lack of balance. An extreme way is an alternative, but it is not the best alternative for the great majority of people. The alternative we are speaking about calls for coming to a balance. *A balanced person shouldn't have to seek the extremes in life in order to be well.* Some people try to be well with exercise alone. Some people will try a peanut-and-grapefruit diet. But, we find the extreme always creates an imbalance.

CATARRH, PHLEGM AND MUCUS— FOUND AT THE BEGINNING OF MOST DISEASES

My food regimen and my entire approach to health care are aimed at getting rid of catarrh, drug residues and toxic wastes in the tissues and in restoring chemical balance through proper nutrition so tissues can repair and rebuild themselves.

The term *catarrh* comes from the Greek words *cata* (down) and *rhein* (flow)—to flow down, and it refers to the mucus flow produced as a consequence of tissue inflammation and a cleansing taking place.

Catarrh precedes the onset of any disease, and it seems as though everyone has it during their growing years. It is a universal symptom, but it is also a condition that people can take care of by themselves through their lifestyle and nutrition. However, the standard response to catarrhal conditions tends to be suppression—*stop that flow*—which drives it back into the body and prevents it from being expelled.

Acidity and catarrh appear during any elimination process. Our body is always eliminating and building. It is perfectly natural for a person to have catarrh to excess when not well or whenever any of the elimination channels is not working properly, but we should never suppress a catarrhal discharge.

Catarrh is developed when the kidneys are not working well; when the skin is not eliminating to its fullest potential; when, especially, the bowel is not moving along toxic waste as fast as it should; and when the bronchial tract and lung structures are overloaded with pollution and toxic wastes, not expelling them efficiently. The lymph system is also involved in the elimination of catarrh, and it is through the lymph system that catarrh is delivered to other parts and organs of the body. If elimination is blocked or slowed down in any of the elimination channels, the catarrh may be forced to settle in inherently weak organs and tissues and near orifices where this excess could be eliminated naturally. Chronic sinus catarrh is always associated with bronchial and lung catarrh.

SOURCES OF POLLUTION IN THE BODY

Let us remember also that the pollutants from our drinking water supply and the residues from some 2,000 food additives have been found, in some cases, to be carcinogenic. We may find these in our junk foods that are really "dollar" foods, prepared in such a way that all the life force that nature put in the original food is diminished and disarranged. Most manhandled foods are no longer natural.

The American Cancer Society claims that 35% of today's cancers could be prevented or helped through use of a proper nutritional program. Why isn't this promoted? Why isn't this health work looked into? Although the Health-damaging effects of environmental pollution were once controversial, as in the days when Rachel Carson's book *Silent Spring* first came out, scientists now agree with her. Our body is part of this environment. There are thousands of people who have found their way into health work who listen, but we find that truth seems to be for the few.

A study by medical researchers at the University of California at San Francisco has revived a turn-of-the-century idea that toxic substances produced in the bowel can have damaging health effects. The study's findings also support recent suggestions of a link between a diet high in fat and low in fiber and an increased risk of developing breast cancer. The study of 1,481 non-nursing women showed that those who were severely constipated tended to have abnormal cells in the fluid extracted from their breasts. Such cells have been found in women with breast cancer and, the researchers suggested, may indicate that the women face an increased risk of cancer. The cellular abnormalities occurred five times as often in women who moved their bowels fewer than three times a week than in women who did so more than once a day. Chronic constipation is often the result of a diet high in protein, fat and refined carbohydrates (sugars and refined flour) but low in such fibrous foods as whole grains, fruits and vegetables.

By allowing the free-flowing elimination of catarrh and toxic waste from the body, we keep in the best of health. We should take care of our elimination channels in order to be well. These include the bowel, the lungs and bronchial tubes, skin and kidneys. We should be taught how to take care of these eliminative systems.

We realize that a preventive approach to disease is in order. To persuade a person to try to prevent a problem before he is aware of it is very difficult. Western medicine is going to come out one of these days and tell you that you will develop a particular problem if you don't live a more natural life. They will also set you up in a healthy nutritional program in your home. We shouldn't wait until the horse has run away to lock the barn.

When toxic buildup exceeds the body's capacity to eliminate, we have waste absorption affecting body organs and tissues, and a person will often suffer from one or more of the many following catarrhal disorders.

CATARRH—ACUTE INFLAMMATIONS

This catarrh becomes part of our body makeup. It becomes part of our tissue makeup. It becomes part of the whole body that has to be cared for. It may settle in all organs of the body. Eventually, to get rid of it, the person will have to go through a reversal process in which that excess catarrh will be eliminated, and carried off through the various orifices of the body.

1. Catarrh of the stomach called gastritis.
2. Catarrh of the mouth called stomatitis.
3. Catarrh of the throat called diptheritis (diphtheria).
4. Catarrh of the nose called rhinitis.
5. Catarrh of the bronchi called bronchitis (hay fever, asthma, etc.).
6. Catarrh of the lungs called pulmonitis (influenza, pneumonia, consumption).
7. Catarrh of the eyes called conjunctivitis (trachoma).
8. Catarrh of the ears called otitis.
9. Catarrh of the brain called phrenitis, also meningitis.
10. Catarrh of the small intestine called enteritis.
11. Catarrh of the large intestine called colitis.
12. Catarrh of the appendix called appendicitis.
13. Catarrh of the liver called hepatitis.
14. Catarrh of the pancreas called pancreatitis.
15. Catarrh of the kidneys called nephritis (Bright's disease).
16. Catarrh of the vagina called vaginitis (leucorrhea).
17. Catarrh of the uterus called metritis.
18. Catarrh of the ovaries called ovaritis.
19. Catarrh of the bladder called cystitis.
20. Catarrh of the prostate called prostatitis.
21. Catarrh of the joints called arthritis.
22. Catarrh of the veins called phlebitis.
23. Catarrh of the arteries called arteritis.
24. Catarrh of the heart called carditis, pericarditis, endocarditis, etc.

The above list serves to show how medical institutions name inflammation symptoms according to their location and treat each symptom as a different disease while disregarding the cause. It also shows the slow and steady progress of what becomes a chronic condition that finally affects every organ, structure and function in the body.

A REMEDY WITH A RECOVERY— THE REVERSAL PROCESS AND YOU

When the health level improves as a result of changing to a right way of living, all tissues and organs cooperate in strengthening the weaker tissues in which suppressed materials have been stored. The stored toxic materials begin to be activated, moistened, liquefied again, as if the body was being reversed to the same condition of illness or disease as before. This is actually what happens in the reversal process. Sometimes we bring back our old problems because, as we have built up our body toward disease, there has to be a return towards good health.

HERING'S LAW

We follow a law *that all disease is corrected from within out, from the head down and in reverse order as we have built it up in the body.* It has been said that we suffer the sins of our past. If we have built up one shoulder on coffee and donuts and the other on creamed wheat, if we have built our left knee on pancakes and the right knee on devil's food cake, then we have to cleanse these things from the body by the reversal process before we can build better tissue with better foods.

This process is called the reversal process, and it works exactly as described.

It may seem surprising that as we get healthier, we work our way back to symptoms of old illnesses, conditions, pains and diseases, but that is nature's way of healing. Food doesn't *cure* disease. It supplies building materials to make new tissue and chemicals to restore chemical balance in the body. If a balanced supply of nutrients is provided in the proper foods, the new tissue will be healthy normal tissue, where disease cannot exist. When the body is balanced chemically, normal function is restored, and the elimination of old catarrh and wastes in the "healing crisis" is a sign that tissue renewal is taking place, as predicted by Hering's Law.

In the reversal process, we retrace our way back—from the most recent to the most distant illness—and relive old symptoms while the toxins and wastes that were suppressed years ago are finally liquefied and expelled from the body.

This is an organized system. It is no "fly-by-night" idea. This works and everyone who follows this program will find out that it works. We have used it on thousands of patients, and those who have gone through a cleansing and a purifying process have developed these healing crises. During these healing crises, patients have eliminated some of their oldest health problems and many are now living in the best of health.

One boy who came to the Ranch on crutches, had no control of his bowel or bladder. In a year's time, this boy progressed enough to get a job driving a taxi. He no longer uses crutches and, although he is not completely well, he has come to the place where, after 13 years of health problems, he was able to take care of himself and hold a job. I asked him one day, "Dick, suppose that this improvement in your health happened all in one moment's time instead of over a period of a year." He said, "That would have been a miracle!" I can't help but recall what I heard during a visit to China. *You don't have to seek a miracle—you ARE a miracle!*

This is not an isolated case in my work. I have hundreds of these successful case histories, and it has been a great thing in my life to see patients recover their health. I have many "before" and "after" pictures of these patients. They have provided their own testimonies for several of my books. My system has been *organized* in such a way that you can depend on what the program can mean to your health. It is not just a system of treatments. It is a new path, a new way of life with new goals.

In my program, you are going to learn to be satisfied with foods that may not taste as good as the foods that come from the bakery shelves. You will have to stay out of the candy store a little more. You will have to cut out some of your drinking habits. You will have to straighten up and become more natural in your living. Is this a sacrifice? No, I feel it is a noble goal to seek the best health possible.

I am proud of the work I have developed over a period of years and have proved over and over again in my sanitarium practice.

We had a lady at one time who came in with boils under her arm. Doctors had lanced them two or three times, but she said she was tired of having them lanced and wanted to know if diet could help her. She was sixty-five years of age, almost deaf. I had to yell at her to get her to hear me.

She went on our elimination program for a few days, and at 65 years, she had to go a little easy, but we gave her our potato peeling broth. This is the broth we use so much during the healing crisis. She had juices, too, but very little food for three days. Going on the reversal regimen, as brought out in this book, she improved in health until some three months later, when she broke out with boils on her breast, I asked her if she ever had boils before on her breast and she said, "Yes, three years ago." So I put her on the potato peeling broth again and told her to rest for two or three days. *(A healing crisis usually lasts three days, sometimes longer as we grow older or possibly shorter for a young person.)*

She got over her troubles very well, but about six months later she came in again with two people helping her walk. I said, "I don't understand what is happening to you. Have you ever had this trouble before?" She said, "Yes, ten years ago I had this same problem." It was a rheumatic condition. The rheumatism lasted for a year-and-a-half at that time, but this time the symptoms were more exaggerated. So I said, "Let's go on the elimination diet, the potato peeling broth again." She felt very well after the fourth or fifth day and went home.

Nothing seemed to happen for some time, until about six months later she called and said, "Do you know what's happened to me? My ears are starting to run." I couldn't understand why her ears should be running, because, after all, that wasn't the problem she came in with, but I remembered her hearing problem. She had been almost deaf. We find that as her body was going back over the reversal track, going over the path of her past, she brought back a catarrhal elimination through the ears. I asked, "Have you ever had it before?" "Yes," she said, "thirteen years before." I asked what was done for it, and she described how her doctor had used various things to suppress or stop the discharge that was coming from her ears. I told her to go on the elimination diet, rest and just let the discharge flow for a day or so and everything would be all right. I

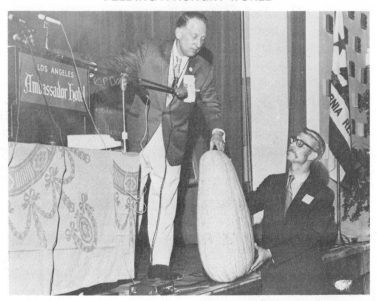

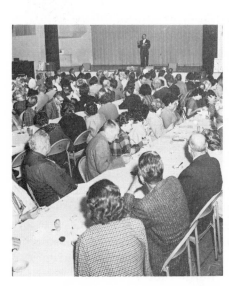

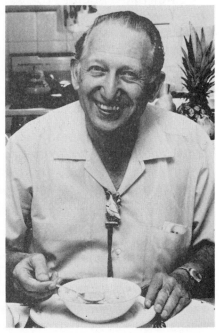

Feeding the mind is as important as feeding the body. Everyone who cares for patients should teach as well as treat.

EXERCISE AROUND THE WORLD

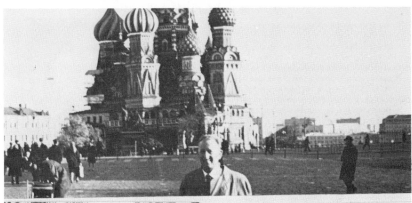

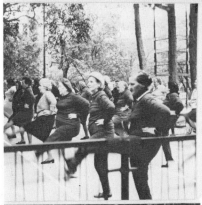

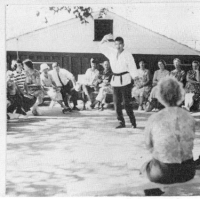

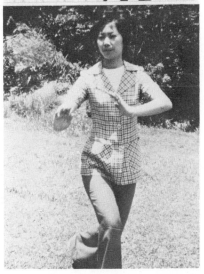

Top: Visiting the Kremlin. Mid-Left: Every morning, 150,000 senior citizens exercise around the Black Sea in Russia. Mid-Rt and Lower Left: Tai Chi is one of the most graceful forms of exercise in the world. Exercise is necessary along with proper nutrition.

LONGEVITY IN MANY LANDS

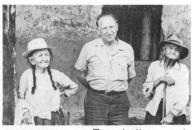

LI CHUNG YUN OF KAIHSIEN, in the Province of Szechwan, China, was born in 1677 and died in 1933, at the age of 256 years. A professor in the Minkuo University claims to have found records showing that Li was born in 1677, and that on his 150th birthday, in 1827, he was congratulated by the Chinese government. Fifty years later, in 1877, he was sent another official congratulation on his 200th birthday.

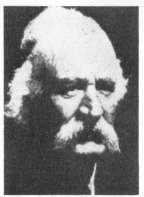

Fifty years later, at the age of 250 years, he lectured before several thousand university students for many hours at a time, on the art of living long. Men who are old today declare that their great grandfathers, as boys, knew Li as a grown man. He had 24 successive wives and 11 generants of descendants.

Early in life, Li developed an interest in herbs, and especially in genseng, and for the greater part of his long life, he wandered round collecting herbs and selling them. He was especially interested in collecting the best specimens of wild ginseng, and for two centuries, he partook of ginseng tea four times daily.

Two ladies nearly 100 years old who jogged 5 blocks every morning. Man (left of center) was 139 years old in Vilcabamba, Ecuador, where no one has heart troubles. Bottom: In winter, these ladies in Armenia, made soup of garlic and dried comfrey. The mother was 127 years old and the daughter 85 years old.

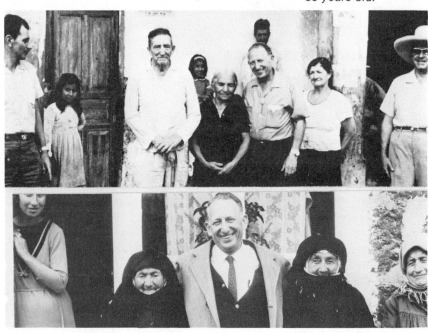

have learned that this is the program, the usual process, and I had no concern that she might be developing a disease, because she was a good patient, faithfully following the program.

The next night she called again and asked, "Do you know what I had to do? I had to take the clock out of my bedroom because I can hear the ticking for the first time in many years; it was so loud, I couldn't sleep!" Her hearing was restored after that third crisis.

Now, I did not treat the ears. I treated the whole body, and if we can realize that when we start building good health, every organ helps lift and support and build good health in every other organ in the body also.

We have had many, many cases go through the reversal process, bringing back old disease symptoms, and by the cleansing of the body, we have returned these patients to better health than they have had in years.

I think one of the worst things to take care of today is a new development called iatrogenic diseases which are diseases or health problems that have developed as a result of other treatments that have been given in the past. Doctors now often have to undo what they have done in the past. And I saw figures where some 50% of the patients going into the hospitals and clinics today have to be treated for treatments they received in the past. This is something to think about.

Why can't the treatment be right to begin with? It may take more time. We may have to change our habits of living, even change our job or get a new outlook on life. There may be many things to be done, but I think it is very worthwhile because when we develop degenerative diseases that we could have prevented in the very beginning, we have taken a foolish path. However, it isn't easy to go in and to start with a new philosophy, a new day program, one that is going to keep us clean, fresh and healthy for our future. We become set in our ways. Change is difficult, even when we know it is best for us.

WE NEED A NEW WAY OF THINKING

I would like to bring out a little thought that I heard the other day. A doctor was mentioning how many babies were dying, and there was quite an unusual program being tried out for these

397

babies that would just stop breathing. They found that there was less chance of the breath stopping when the baby was next to the mother, probably because of the mother's breathing cycle and rhythm that helped the child carry through that period where it stopped breathing. So, they developed some kind of instrument that would put out a rhythmic pulsation in time with the normal breathing cycle. The doctors said it may seem unusual to use such a different method of taking care of these babies, but as there were so many babies dying, there is always room for creative thinking. We hope that this book can help you see that with more creative thinking, we could keep ourselves in the best of health.

Almost any chemical or drug trapped in the body tissues can be eliminated through the reversal process. I feel the reversal process is a readjustment to normal in the body and a call to a better cell activity. Nutrition is the greatest aid we have in eliminating the old and taking on the new. The immune system and our resistance to disease are built up when we use the best nutrition possible, along with a good lifestyle.

I would like to mention an "imitation food" which is actually a drug and creates a side effect in the body. This drug is saccharine, a sugar substitute, over 200 times sweeter than sugar. The body can't use it because it isn't a food. It has its side effects. Western medicine calls it a carcinogenic agent—cancer forming—and there are an unknown number of other products we get in our food additives and catarrhal suppressing remedies that may also be carcinogenic. We need to stop and think about these things.

HERING'S LAW AND THE REVERSAL PROCESS

Hering's Law of Cure states:

> *All cure comes from the head down, from within out, and in reverse order as symptoms first appeared.*

This is a homeopathic law of cure. I use this as the basis for getting my patients well.

This means that as we follow the path of good health, every organ and tissue in the body begins to be strengthened and renewed. The stronger ones support the inherently weak tissues until a point is reached where the healing powers within eliminate the stored up catarrh, toxic material, old drug residues and pollutants. **Health is worked for; it is earned; it is learned.**

When we begin to eliminate this old material, we have reached what is called a "healing crisis." This is the crowning reward of our efforts, a spontaneous and natural cleansing of the tissues of the body.

Unlike a "disease crisis," in which symptoms show that a toxic acid condition is developing in the body and the body is coping with the development of a disease, a healing crisis shows that old toxins are leaving, never to return if a person continues living right. Yet, it resembles in every way a disease crisis. The healing crisis is the return of a problem you have had in the past.

Old Symptoms Return. There may be—singly or in combination—vomiting, diarrhea, fever, rash, skin eruptions, discharges from any or every orifice of the body, for about three days. Then it is gone, and our body is much cleaner. This is nature's way of cleansing and healing. During the healing crisis, you should rest as much as possible, taking only a little broth, vegetable juice or chlorophyll and water now and then. This healing crisis comes when we follow the right nutritional way and the new lifestyle path.

The main way to tell the difference between a **disease crisis** and a **healing crisis** is that a healing crisis usually comes right at a time when we have never felt better. One day we are walking on "cloud 9," the next day we are flat on our back feeling miserable. This is usually a healing crisis. It took energy to have this crisis and you have built up a body to have this elimination take place. The reason a person goes through this suffering period and elimination period is because he or she has accumulated enough energy through right living to bring on the healing crisis. At this moment, all our stored-up energy is being used for elimination, so weakness is a usual part of the process. This is an orderly program, following a natural law process. It comes after a person starts a right-living program.

A healing crisis is a blessed moment in a person's life and should be greatly valued, not considered a detrimental disturbance. I am telling you this ahead of time so you will not try to suppress your symptoms but allow nature to have its way.

We believe in the natural control of disease. But if it is impossible, if the disease has gone too far, and nature hasn't the ability to bring a return, then there is only one other way we can turn—conventional medicine, hospital, drugs, surgery, etc. But we are trying to bring out here that much can be done before we get to this extreme degeneration point. This is where preventive medicine comes in. This will come when the doctors and hospital staff will teach people how to live right, how to select, prepare and eat the proper foods before they leave the hospital. Patients will be given a course of instruction on natural hygienic care of their bodies, a series of lectures. After they leave the hospital, they should continue to attend weekly workshops or seminars where they will continue to learn how to take care of their bodies properly.

I think it is criminal that people are allowed to live a life on junk foods and never be told the consequences. I think people want to do the right things but in most cases don't know what to do. Doctors make a living on the average person's living. It is right here that we want to stop that. This is the reason for teaching, for lecturing, for writing articles and books and giving people information on eating properly, cooking properly, preserving their foods properly, raising their children properly and so forth.

There may be many healing crises or few as you continue to move onward and upward on the path of health. The wonderful advantage of nature's way of healing is that once you have retraced your way back through the symptoms of past illnesses, you need never experience them again, and you can rest assured that your body is cleansed of the toxic material associated with any of these conditions. *Disease preys on a weak and malnourished body.*

In following the way of nature, the body is cleansed of toxins, tissues are rejuvenated and the old is replaced by the new. The immune system is strengthened to resist and prevent many diseases.

A REMEDY WITH RECOVERY

The highest ideal of the sincere health professional is the well-being of his patients, but many of the remedies and therapies of our

400

time leave the patient at a lower level of health than before treatment. This is why they say, "One operation leads to another." A whole new field of treatment has been developed for iatrogenic disease, taking care of those who have developed new problems while under treatment in hospitals, clinics and by those in private practice. But every treatment eventually fails without proper nutrition.

I believe in my work very much. I have seen many hundreds of people get well and stay well for many years. You can't help but think there is something wonderful in this work when it has been applied and used properly in your life. I think the greatest criticism of the natural approach to health care is that there is no order, no organization and no place to begin. Where do we start? One person could start in this way, another could start another way. We can start with exercise and diet. We could start with any of the various treatments we have in the healing arts. But the organization seems to be left out. I would like to say that there is a very organized way of healing by using nature as an ally. The moment we turn to good food and a different lifestyle, our bodies begin to quicken, repair, rebuild and change. I call this replacement therapy because tissue replacement takes place. New tissue comes in place of the old.

In order to explain this, we find that the body is a servant to both the internal and external environment. *It is a servant to the mind and the spirit.* It is a servant to our environment, whether natural or polluted. It molds to our thinking, to our emotions. It molds to the minerals we take. It molds to coffee and donuts. It molds to a salad. The body is really a servant that doesn't ask for very much. But we have to start somewhere, and I believe this is the way the organized program should be followed. At first we should start on a nutritional program. Mechanical manipulation may be necessary. There are many treatments, including acupuncture, osteopathy and massage, that build the circulation. Good nutrition together with improved circulation means each cell will be fed better and can function better after these treatments.

We know that no one treatment has the whole answer to our disease problems. We cannot look to mechanical manipulation alone without proper nutrition. Nutrition is not enough if we are depleting our bodies taking alcohol, drugs or junk food. It is a matter of cleaning up our lives, developing new habits that are going to make changes for the better in the tissues. As we build new tissue, our body organizes and reorganizes its internal functions automatically without much help from the outside.

We find that nature does the curing, but the doctor gets the fee. Nature only needs an opportunity, and by giving it this opportunity, the body gets well. The body goes through an organized way of repair and rebuilding. We find first of all we have a renewed feeling of well-being. We have a quickened step. We feel good. We feel capable. We have more enthusiasm. Our body is making changes that help us accomplish more and feel more confident.

With better health, we can live a good life and have a better marriage, a better sex life, do better work. We find that our body is now more in tune with nature. It's more in tune with the universal laws that we should be living by in the first place. We develop a better mental acuity. Our hearing may improve. Our sight may improve. We find that our tissues are going to respond at a higher level as we seek that higher opportunity.

We must keep our body clean, because only a clean body can be well. We may go through tissue cleansing. The bowel is cleansed. All elimination channels have been attended to every day. We work with our body in our waking hours.

A sluggish, toxic body becomes a body that falls behind. It cannot keep up with the average person. It cannot do what it should be doing. When the tissues are cleansed and we are eating the proper foods, a healing crisis can be expected. You can look to a healthier body to come. You will not be raising your children as doctor bills. Your husband won't be taking something for a headache every night when he comes home from work. The wife will not have to live on suppressant drugs for catarrhal discharges in the body.

As the body becomes clean, we begin flowing in good health. No doctor should object to this state of being. Society should be interested in this. Our hospitals should be teaching this. Doctors should be having classes on how to reach this state of health. What we need more than anything else is research to see how much health we can have in life, rather than how much disease we can treat. Wouldn't it be nice to have a diagnostic method giving us our health level of every organ in the body?

I believe there is a place for surgery and drug intervention, but I feel both are used far too much when other helpful and less dangerous treatments are available. Surgery usually involves removal of a part of the body, taking away any possible opportunity for the tissue to recover. The organ removed has been cared for but 90% of the rest of the body goes on in the ill health condition. Drug therapies stimulate or depress tissue function, leaving undesirable side effects, long-term effects and time-bomb effects that may not show up in years to come. However, there are genetic effects and conditions that signal a point of no return for the natural repair and recovery of tissue. This is where surgery and drug intervention have their places.

Only through nutrition can new tissue replace the old by rebuilding and replacing underactive, toxic-laden organs and other body tissues. Toxic conditions and underactive function seem to go together. Nature's way is to get rid of the old through the healing crisis and bring in the new through balanced nutrition and right living. *We elevate our health level.*

Nutrition is the only way I know which provides a remedy with full recovery when used with any treatment. You can depend on chemical restoration through foods to bring good health, along with proper supportive treatments.

Remember, food is our best medicine!

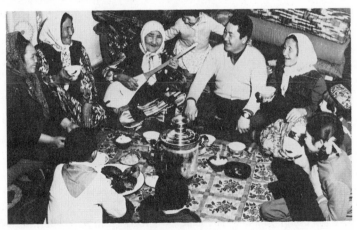

The Kirghiz SSR. Kasymbala Kanaeva (OPS) is well-known in the Tyan-Shan as a skillful performer of folk melodies playing the national instrument: komuz. In spite of her age (97 years), Kasymbala always participates in all national festivals and celebrations. OPS: Kasymbala Kanaeva (center) seen among her family.

403

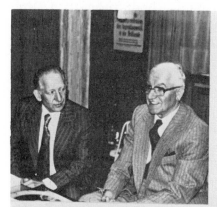

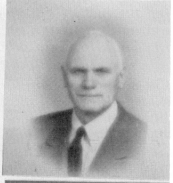

"BRING ME MEN
TO MATCH MY MOUNTAINS.
BRING ME MEN
TO MATCH MY PLAINS.
MEN WITH EMPIRES
IN THEIR PURPOSE.
AND NEW ERAS
IN THEIR BRAINS."

SAM WALTER FOSS

"THROUGHOUT THE CENTURIE
THERE WERE MEN
WHO TOOK FIRST STEPS
DOWN NEW ROADS
ARMED WITH NOTHING
BUT THEIR OWN VISION."

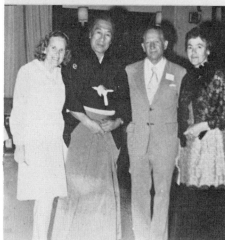

Top Left: My colleague, Dr. Josef Deck, the top iridologist of Germany. Right: Peter Maloff of the Doukobors in Canada, where I received some of my first inspiration about a good life to live. Lower Left: Dr. Kazuhiko Asai of Japan, developer of organic Germanium.

30

Alternative Healing
At Its Best—
The Story of Mrs. E.P.

After several years and some hundreds of cases of tissue cleansing using the colema method to take care of the bowel, I have seen wonderful results in shifting the body tissues in all organs to a higher level of activity, a higher level of function, through elimination of some of the toxic material formerly held in the body. We have run through many cases where we have found an underactive, enervated bowel, a bowel pocketed and ballooned, a bowel with unbalanced electrolytes and a deficiency of favorable flora such as lactobacillus acidophilus. This is associated with many kinds of symptoms throughout the body. When the bowel was taken care of, the symtoms greatly improved or left.

Changes after a tissue cleansing program are often very dramatic. Many patients have had medical tests before coming into our tissue cleansing program, and I also have blood and urine tests taken of my patients at a medical laboratory the first day of the program. Within a few weeks, new tests often confirm changes. One patient came in with a 4+ Pap smear, which changed to negative three months after her tissue cleansing. Another with an initial lab test showing blood triglycerides of 1401 mg/dl, a very dangerous level, dropped to 345 in a week's time. A patient with severe anemia, as shown by a red blood cell count of 3.84 million came up to 4.47, an increase of 630,000 red blood cells, in a little over a month after her tissue cleansing. (Normal for women is about 5 million.)

We have seen breast lumps disappear or diminish, high blood pressure drop to near normal, prostate troubles improve and psoriasis change for the better and even clear up. In one case,

405

doctors had given up on a young man who had advanced kidney disease (glomerulonephritis) but he was much improved after tissue cleansing and changing to a better diet. In another case, a man with severe infected ulcers of the ankles and feet and extremely poor circulation, whose doctors wanted to amputate his feet, obtained great relief and improvement in only 7 days. With proper diet and a good maintenance program, he was completely cured in a year. Our "before" and "after" pictures as shown in my book *Tissue Cleansing Through Bowel Management* will verify this.

You wonder, sometimes, what is really happening in the body when this particular type of cleansing is taken by a patient. The whole body is responding, I am sure. Not all patients get the same results. Some are slower in their physiological response process. But, all seem to be improved. This is the fastest working therapy I have found in the natural healing arts. Of course, there's no saying that these people couldn't get their old conditions back if they returned to the same lifestyle and food habits that brought them on in the first place.

Just by taking care of the bowel, we see many conditions that involve many organs in the body shifting and changing to a higher state of well-being. The activities of the bowel, kidneys, lungs and skin, the body's elimination channels, are greatly improved after the tissue cleansing. One organ, when it is improved, seems to help the other. Digestion is also better. I believe that drug residues and their effects on tissues are reduced because of the foul odors that often accompany this elimination, and undesirable drug side effects seem to be relieved after the colemas are used.

I took up this tissue cleansing work in the beginning as a project worth looking into. I didn't know the bowel cleansing would have such a dramatic effect in allowing the whole body to return to normal expression. It was a great revelation to me to see how the rest of the body responded so quickly from just taking care of the bowel. I haven't found any other treatments that have had such a powerful effect on people as the tissue cleansing program using the colema, which I believe is nothing more than a home treatment that a person can use just as well as an enema. It is more thorough. It takes more time to accomplish. But with patience, over a period of time, many good results will come about. I believe the results won't stay, however, unless appropriate lifestyle and food habits are adopted.

There is one case among those who have taken the tissue cleansing that comes to my mind more than any of the others over the past few years, and that is the case of Mrs. E.P. Her suffering was so great, and her relief from pain was so sudden and dramatic following the tissue cleansing, that she stands out as special.

THE BEGINNING OF SYMPTOMS

I think the best way to show what happened to Mrs. P. is to present parts of her story in her own words, as taken from an interview in my records. She was 74 years old at the time this was written and lived in Southern California. The onset of symptoms, as she describes them, began in 1981.

"One day I was swimming with my husband, I said, 'I have a tugging—it feels just like you were pulling my neck.' He said, 'Oh, it's nothing. You're always imagining.' The next day I went to swim, the tugging began again. On the third day, I had a pain. He said, 'It'll go; it'll go.' I took aspirin, Bufferin, whatever, but it didn't go.

"One night when I went to lay on my pillow, I had to scream, the pain was so bad. It was a pain that I've never felt, even in childbirth. It was dreadful! I couldn't lie down, so I sat up the whole night.

"The next day, I went to my doctor. He sent me to the finest man who does X-rays. He took the X-rays and said, 'You know, you have seven vertebrae in your neck. Five have degenerated. Only two are near normal. You have osteoarthritis. This didn't just happen—you've had it for 20 years at least. But, you overdid or were stressed and something triggered it off.'

"I said, 'What am I going to do?' He said, 'Well, you can't drive a car, and you can't be driven. Bumping is the worst thing.' He put me in a neck brace and I was in that brace for a year. I couldn't drive. We had to get a maid. I could do nothing. Absolutely nothing!"

THE SYMPTOMS GO FROM BAD TO WORSE

Mrs. P. followed her doctor's orders, but the pain grew worse. So she went to a doctor recommended as the best rheumatologist, a doctor who had treated one of our past U.S. presidents. Here is her account of what happened.

"I went to the best rheumatologist, and he said, 'You're having a terrible spasm.'

"I said, 'You've got to give me something to relieve this pain or I'm going to kill myself.' I was vomiting from the pain.

"So he prescribed Percodan, Butazolidin and Ascriptin for the pain. And, he gave me steroid shots once a week. They say arthritis is incurable, and the doctor said that drugs would bring the only relief for the terrible pains in my neck. I was told to eat anything I wanted, that coffee and diet had nothing to do with arthritis. He did all he could for me."

We find that she took these drugs for over a year without improvement in her condition. According to the **Physician's Desk Reference (PDR)**, one of the drugs she was taking, Butazolidin, is an extremely dangerous drug with many known undesirable side effects. It is not recommended for chronic use in the elderly because of its toxic effects on the blood, gastrointestinal system, kidneys and liver. In fact, her doctor was monitoring her blood and urine every week to make sure that she wasn't hemorrhaging from this drug. Altogether, the **PDR** lists at least 64 known possible side effects for this drug—including leukemia. It is really one of those "last resort" drugs used only with extreme cases.

The Ascriptin is aspirin with two alkaline salts to protect the stomach from bleeding due to the aspirin. She was taking 10 of these a day. Percodan, the third drug she was using, is a narcotic, an opium derivative with aspirin added. It is mainly a pain reliever. It acts on the brain and nervous system, depressing the respiratory system and increasing spinal fluid pressure. Possible side effects include lightheadedness, dizziness, nausea, vomiting, euphoria, constipation and pruritis.

Percodan can become addictive. The **PDR** says it should be given to the elderly only with caution. Of course, the steroid injections she was getting once a week would have a powerful effect on the functioning of her endocrine system. So, we find that in treating arthritis pain, drugs were taken that anesthetized parts of the brain and nervous system, interfered with the functioning of most of the vital organs and introduced powerful toxins into her body. This is what medicine has to offer for arthritis pain.

After a year's treatment with pain-relieving drugs for arthritis and no improvement, her husband told her, "I want you to see Dr.

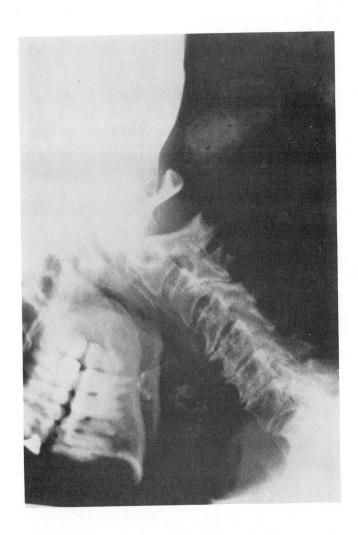

This X-ray of Mrs. E.P.'s neck (at age 74), shows the arthritis spurs that caused her such extreme pain. She got rid of the pain on a nutritional program. She experienced this pain for 3 years previously. After 5 years, the pain has not returned. There has been no need for further drugs or treatments.

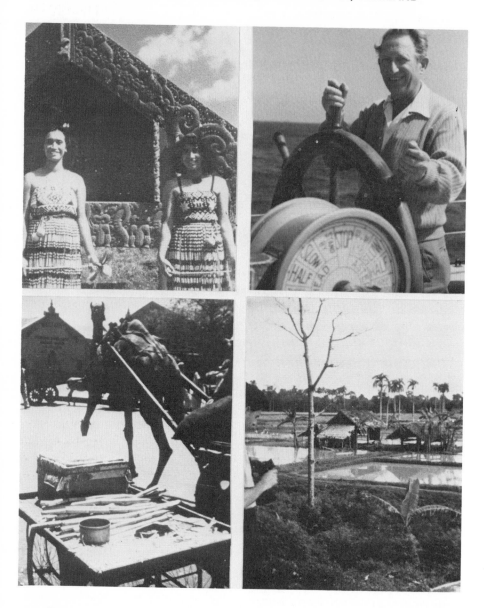

Travel and study of other peoples' customs have been one of the great experiences of my life. Upper left: Maori ladies in New Zealand. Lower left: I had to pay $5 to photograph this camel in Afghanistan. Lower right: Rice paddy in Thailand. Wherever I went, I learned many things that helped in my practice.

Jensen." At the time she came to my Ranch, she could hardly lie down or move her neck. She could walk, but not much else.

CHANGING DIRECTIONS IN HOPE OF IMPROVEMENT

During the office visit with my patient and her husband, I suggested she go on the tissue cleansing program. She didn't really want to, and I didn't really blame her. She had been through so much. But she finally decided to put herself in my hands. Her story continues.

"Well, I came to Dr. Jensen's Ranch, and he said, 'The first thing you've got to do is get off all drugs.'

"I said, 'Dr. Jensen, you can't take me off the Ascriptin, because if that pain comes back, I swear to God, I'll kill myself.' The pain had been unbearable, day and night, before the drugs. It drained me. I was so nervous, I was shaking.

"He said, 'You've got to get off of every drug or I cannot treat you. Trust me. I'm going to put you on a semi-fast.' So, he put me on the seven-day tissue cleansing program. He had a nurse come up and give me the treatment and the colemas twice a day. I took broth, teas and the supplements, but no medicines. To my amazement, the fourth day I was pain-free without drugs.

"On the seventh day, I was given some steamed carrots. Then a coddled egg and some stewed fruit. I had gained a pound on the cleansing program when he weighed me. He thought I would lose weight. After that, Dr. Jensen gave me a food regimen to follow when I went back home. He insists on a mixed green salad every day, and I also have a green vegetable daily, and for a starch, I take brown rice, millet or corn. For desserts, he'd rather I eat fruit. I have very little red meat—mostly I have chicken and fish.

"I felt well when I went back to Los Angeles, and then a month later I had a healing crisis."

THE HEALING CRISIS

I took on E.P.'s case thinking possibly it was too serious a case for me to handle through taking care of the colon alone. When she reported taking all of those drugs and as many as 10 Ascriptin tablets a day, I realized that nothing more was being done than suppression of symptoms. Her doctor was trying to take care of the

411

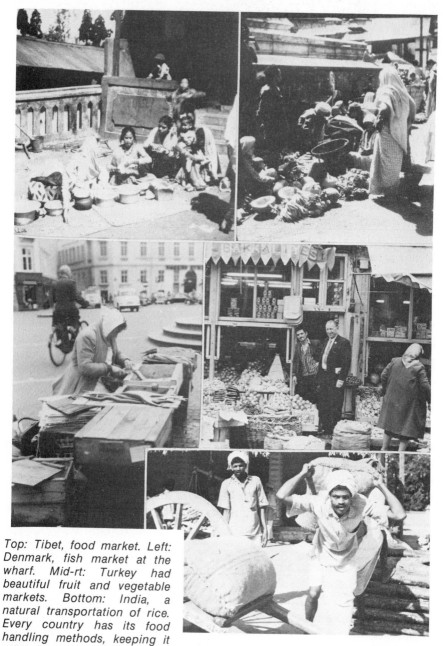

Top: Tibet, food market. Left: Denmark, fish market at the wharf. Mid-rt: Turkey had beautiful fruit and vegetable markets. Bottom: India, a natural transportation of rice. Every country has its food handling methods, keeping it natural, pure and whole is the big problem.

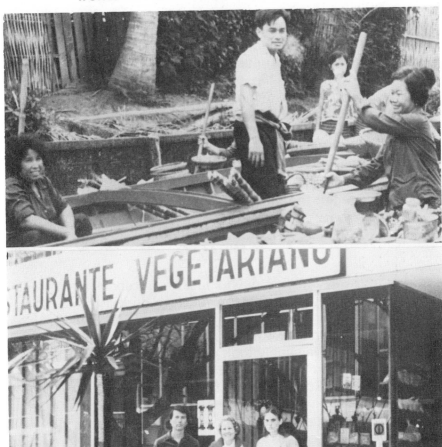

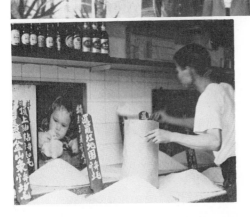

Top: River transport of foods in Thailand. Mid: A Mexican doctor started this vegetarian restaurant in Mexico City. Bottom: A Chinese merchant displays many varieties of rice. Food is a necessary requirement and to see the natural ways that food is handled around the world made me look into the processing, milling and transporting of foods in our modern-day technology.

413

symptoms, but no changes were being made in the body as a whole. She was a good patient, doing everything the doctor told her to do. Nothing seemed to help, however.

Most doctors say arthritis is incurable. I took on this case not so much to try to treat the osteoarthritis or try to cure the neck problem as to take care of the rest of the body and bring it back to the best health possible. I know that her osteoarthritis did not happen overnight and was caused by a calcium-sodium imbalance in the body, and it might have been going on for 10 to 20 years. But, I felt that the tissue cleansing program followed by proper nutrition might remove enough toxic material accumulations from her body to allow it to regain the strength and energy required to take care of the problem in its own way.

A MIRACLE

I want to say that E.P. did not receive any special treatment—no more than any other person receives during the seven-day colema treatment. When she said **on the fourth day of the program that the pain in her neck was gone it seemed like a miracle.** I didn't touch the neck. We simply took care of the bowel, and the neck pain was relieved. **THERE WERE NO MORE PAINS AFTER TAKING THE TREATMENT 2-1/2 YEARS AGO UP TO THE PRESENT TIME.**

As the body becomes stronger after tissue cleansing and a proper diet, all the organs, glands and tissues become more active. Residues of old catarrh, mucus, drugs and metabolic wastes in the tissues begin to become liquefied so they can be moved along in the body and be eliminated. The body gathers strength to throw off these toxic accumulations that weakened the body in the past and made it **vulnerable** to various disease conditions.

ELIMINATION AND THE HEALING CRISIS

By the body's own natural healing processes, a time comes when the activity level of the organs and tissues reaches the acute stage and starts to eliminate this liquefied waste. **THIS IS CALLED A HEALING CRISIS.** Hippocrates, the "father of medicine," is quoted as saying, "Give me a fever and I'll cure any disease." This is nature's way, and I believe in it very much. I say, "Balance the body

414

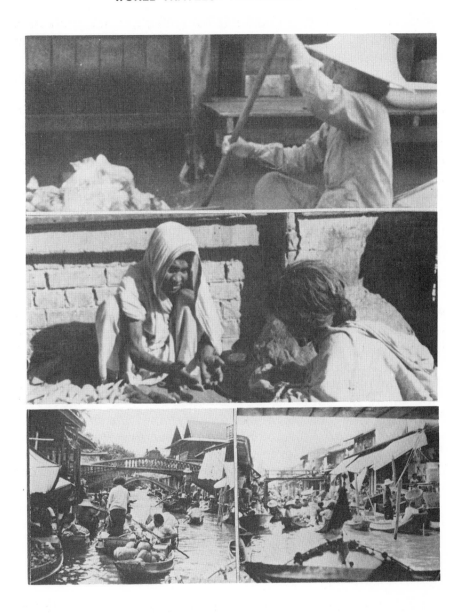

Markets in the Orient. The manhandling of food in this natural way never disturbed the balanced nutrients.

chemically, and it will eliminate its own toxic waste."

Now let us find out from Mrs. P., first-hand, what happened to her a month after she had returned to her home in Los Angeles after going through the tissue cleansing program.

"I had a terrible crisis. Phlegm coming up, but I had no cold. It started with a 105-degree fever. Dr. Jensen came to our house. And I had the 105-degree fever (intermittently) for six or seven days. I lost 10 pounds.

"Dr. Jensen said, 'I'm glad you have this fever.'

"I said, 'But I'm dying!'

"He said, 'No, you're not dying. I just want you to keep taking the colemas.'

"I thought of going to get some antibiotics from a doctor, but I had such faith in Dr. Jensen. He told me the healing crisis would pass, and *HE HAD EVEN WARNED ME EARLIER THAT I WOULD HAVE THIS HEALING CRISIS!"*

After the crisis, she was weak and listless, partly because of the weight loss. She had lost 10 pounds and was down to 85 pounds. But a month after the crisis passed, she was feeling good again.

In three months, she was doing anything she wanted to do— without pain and without drugs. Her friends told her they didn't know where she got the energy. She was able to go to the races, movies, drive her car, go shopping, everything. She came back to her normal weight of 100 pounds and she feels fine. Her neck is not giving her any trouble, even on movement. Arthritis is difficult at any age, but this patient was in her 70s, an age when it is very hard to find a treatment that will take care of arthritis.

It has been 2-1/2 years since I took care of Mrs. P., and she hasn't had any pain in her neck since she went through the tissue cleansing and she hasn't taken any more drugs.

FINAL THOUGHTS

What is so remarkable to me, and what makes this such an important case, is the realization that by taking care of the bowel, we can bring relief to another part of the body, quite remote from the bowel. This relief was a god-send to the patient, who had reached the point of suicide from the pain. What happened between the bowel cleansing and the relief of her neck symptoms is almost impossible to say, but it was most certainly a spectacular phenomenon that happened right before my eyes. Her whole body was affected.

What I have to say is this treatment produced the result that she described in her own words, and to this day, she will not go without her treatment. She takes a colema every day, once a day, She even took a trip to Europe, and we had to make her a folding colema board that would fit in a suitcase! But to her, this has meant new life—a whole new life. It is something she can depend on without the use of extreme drugs she was taking before.

FREE OF PAIN AND FEELING WELL

While we are living, no matter what age, we should be free of pain and have a sense of well-being, of good health, so that life feels worthwhile. Let me tell you one of the greatest things about this lady—she was 74 years of age when a great reversal process and healing came about in her.

As far as osteoarthritis is concerned, and the pain that goes with it at times, we have to consider the best way to take care of it. I believe drug therapy has its place, but I don't feel extreme, toxic, addictive drugs should be used until other natural and alternative treatments have been considered. This is a time when a choice has to be made. We have to consider that tissue cleansing and proper diet may be the best treatment to start out with in any chronic disease, first, to see if the condition clears up on its own with no other therapy, or, secondly, to strengthen and prepare the patient to respond more quickly and favorably to any other therapy indicated, whether surgery, drugs or other treatments.

I am not interested in claiming I have brought out something which is better than other health care therapies and approaches, but if the conditions previously presented as well as an extreme case of osteoarthritis, can be controlled by the colema treatment, I think we should not underestimate or misunderstand its potential. We should consider that maybe a greater thing is taking place here than we understand. Natural methods have a great way of bringing things to normal, if only we would choose to work with them.

417

THE REVERSAL PROCESS

It is important to understand the healing crisis that Mrs. P. went through a month or so after she took the colema treatment and stopped taking her drugs. According to the philosophy of the natural healing art, the healing crisis comes as a direct result of what we call the reversal process, which I would like to briefly describe.

From the perspective of the natural healing art, the pathway to most chronic diseases consists of wrong living habits—diets deficient in necessary nutrients, insufficient sleep, exposure to toxic chemicals in polluted air and water, high stress, worry, anxiety, bad attitudes, chronic fatigue and so forth. Disease doesn't *just happen.* We eat, drink and think it into existence. The pathway to health is just the opposite or *reverse* of the pathway to disease. This is what the natural healing art means by the reversal process—proper diet, tissue cleansing, rest, dealing constructively with stress, resolving problems that have caused worry and anxiety, improving our attitudes and turning our entire lifestyle in a healthy direction. *THE REVERSAL PROCESS IS THE PATHWAY TO HEALTH.*

To get well from a disease, you have to have energy. You have to have nutritious foods with the proper balance of vitamins and minerals. The body has to be clean enough to begin the reversal process, leading to a healing crisis. This is the way nature organizes its "get well programs." In E.P.'s case, I think the healing crisis was the saving grace that kept her from further pain and kept her life worth living.

When we take care of the bowel, we see changes in the entire body. This is why I believe we can take care of many diseases only by treating the whole body.

I have never had a patient who reported distressing or unsatisfactory results from colema treatments. If tissue cleansing with the colema method can bring relief to those who are sick and in extreme pain, relieving the problem without the use of drugs, I believe it is worth consideration for any chronic disease.

To Everyone: You cannot live right without a reversal process and healing crisis.

418

31

The
Ethel Lesher
Story

One of the greatest recoveries I have ever seen is that of Ethel Lesher, who was nearly disabled with arthritis at the age of 76. After taking up a food regimen and program I gave her, she left the arthritis behind and started playing with a dance band. She has appeared on the Johnny Carson show and played the piano on one of our shipboard cruises, at the age of 98.

Ethel's story should be a great inspiration to those who feel that chronic diseases automatically come with aging.

"I took a trip in 1961," she said, "and when I returned I was weak and my knees were swollen. I had been healthy most of my life, but I became rundown from doing too much. Besides taking care of my ranch, I was active in five different organizations. So I went to my doctor, and he told me I had arthritis. He said we all get it as we grow older. We just have to live with it.

"That kind of stirred me up. I didn't want to live with it. So I tried different things to get rid of it, but the arthritis just got worse."

Some years before I had given a lecture in Redding, California, on "The Path to Right Living," and Ethel had attended that lecture. At the time, she was having such difficulty she remembered my lecture and decided to come to my Ranch in Escondido to see if there was anything she could do for her arthritis.

The program I gave Ethel Lesher included vitamin B-12, jacuzzi baths, cold water Kneippe baths, barefoot grass walks and a food regimen that included high sodium foods such as whey, celery and okra to bring the calcium deposits in her joints back into solution in her body.

After two years of sticking to my program, the arthritis left. "I thought I would never play the piano again," Ethel told me. "But

419

gradually I was able to get back to it."

She began playing with a band which included a drummer, tenor saxophone and banjo—for senior citizen groups. One day she received a phone call from the local veterans' hall asking if she and her band would be willing to play at a Saturday night dance. Their music was so well enjoyed that they continued playing there on Saturday nights for three years. The crowd that came to dance tripled in that time.

During that time, Johnny Carson heard about Ethel's band and asked her to appear on the Tonight Show. What a wonderful thing that was for a woman in her 90s, once almost crippled from arthritis!

When she joined our shipboard cruise a few years ago, Ethel not only played the piano for us, but showed everyone she was still a good dancer. She danced with the ship's social director and had a great time on the cruise.

Ethel watches her diet carefully and follows what she learned at my Ranch, eating a variety of fresh vegetables and fruits, with eggs, poultry and fish as her main proteins. She keeps her bowels regular, is physically active and has many friends.

Recently, Ethel Lesher celebrated her 100th birthday with a gathering of friends and relatives, and this is what she had to say when she was asked to speak to the group.

"Dear relatives and friends, I love you all. I'm so happy to be here, and you have all been so nice to me. I just want you to know that my nutritional doctor, Dr. Bernard Jensen, couldn't be here. If it wasn't for him, I wouldn't have lived as long as I have.

"Thanks to Dr. Jensen, there isn't an ache or pain in my body that prevents me from enjoying everything, everywhere I go. I wish everyone could be as free of aches and pains as I am today.

"When I first went to Dr. Jensen's Ranch, my knee was swollen, my finger joints were bumpy and I could hardly use my hands.

"He told me, 'You've got to live a different life.' Dr. Jensen told me what to cut out of my diet and what should be in it. He gave me a program to follow. He said that he couldn't do a thing for me unless I made up my mind to follow a different path of living. I didn't want to be a cripple, so I made up my mind to do what he said. I had determination.

"For two years, I walked the straightest line you ever saw, until every ache and pain left me. I had no more. From that day to this one, I have felt wonderful. Today is my 100th birthday. If I had to ride a horse, I could do it.

"I want you to realize, too, what music has done for me and what I think it can do for everyone. Music is not only for the home but for the heart and for sharing with others. When you're sharing music with others, you're also enjoying it yourself. It's doing a lot for you. It's very seldom that a day goes by when I don't play the piano just a little. I don't forget playing with the dance band. I just enjoy it very much.

"I'll leave you with this thought. There's a lot of good in knowing about nutrition. But knowing won't do you any good if you don't determine to follow what you know and change your way of living. I feel so sorry when I see people crippled up with arthritis, and I believe many of them wouldn't have it if they lived right and determined to changed their ways. I believe if I can do it, most others can too."

Isn't this a wonderful story? Here is another example of a remedy with full tissue recovery, leaving a chronic disease and all its symptoms behind. The greatest thing I can say is that I agree with Ethel Lesher. If people are willing and determined to change to a right way of living, almost any health condition can be changed.

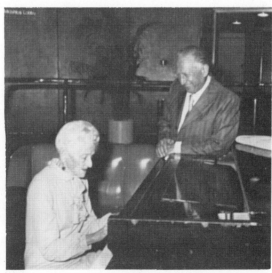

Dr. Bernard Jensen with Ethel Lesher, 98 , at the piano. To grow old and yet retain youth, we must keep active and interested in life.

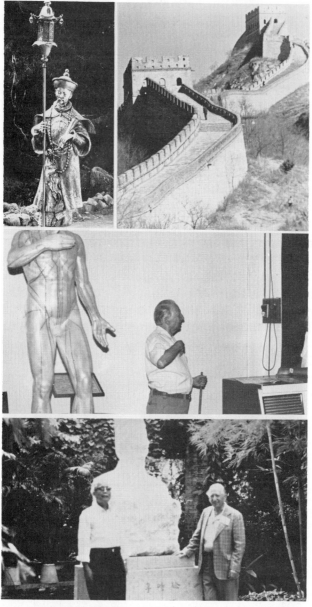

Upper: Next to the great wall of China is my own statue of a Chinese scholar with a lamp in one hand, scroll in the other. Middle: I lectured on my methods at a Canton hospital, which carried translations of my books. Below: A Chinese doctor showed me the statue of an herbalist who developed 1,500 remedies.

32

Our Sick Society
and
How to Live in It

In one of his movies, Jack Palance said to his lady costar, "This world is covered with dirt." This is very true. This old world *is* covered with dirt—with pollution, wastes, garbage, litter, drugs, denatured foods and other human excesses. We live in a sick society.

We have to learn discrimination and selectivity in this world. We have to learn to walk the path of the wise man. Maybe this is our lesson in life; maybe this is what life is trying to teach us. If we don't learn our lesson soon, the sick society will overcome us.

The "sick society," as I have called it, is sick in more ways than one. It is sick in terms of health, but also financially, marriage-wise, sexually, morally and in its attitudes toward work, human life and the well-being of our planet. We have lessons to learn in each of these areas, new discoveries to make. I have learned that beside every problem, right next to every problem, there is a solution. We can take care of these things.

A NEW DAY IS COMING

We have to recognize that in this world, this can be the day of miracles. The day has come when man's extremity is God's opportunity. This is driving more people to church than ever before.

Sometimes we find that man has to approach some kind of catastrophe before the pendulum begins to swing the other way. When a town has a terrible earthquake, everyone runs to the church. If the sun didn't come up tomorrow, everyone would seek the reason why. We are all seekers in one way or another. It is time

423

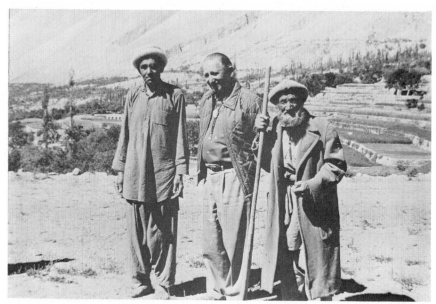

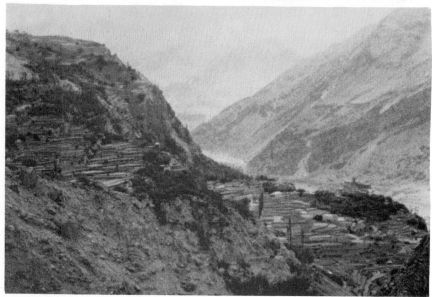

Top: Here I am with a 110-year-old Hunza man, one of many healthy Hunzas over a century in age. Their diet is mostly natural. No jails, police, hospitals, doctors or mental asylums were needed here. Their lives were free of stress.

MY VISIT TO THE HUNZA VALLEY

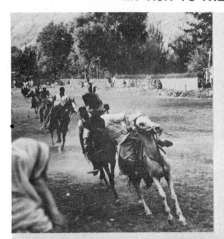

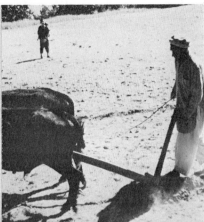

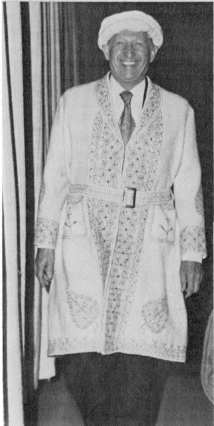

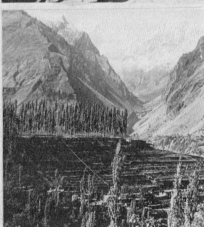

The Hunzas of Pakistan are the best polo players in the world and have used traditional methods to cultivate crops on terraced mountainsides. They planted all the way to cliff edges to save their soil. I brought back this choga coat and hat, used on royal occasions in Hunza, to lecture on right-living methods that they taught me. They get plenty of rest but also worked hard during the day. They live in beauty and serenity. They have prayers 3-4 times a day. Occasionally they fast but mainly they live a moderate life.

for a day of miracles. It is time for the pendulum to swing the other way.

The decay we see around us in our society and in civilization has come about slowly, and now we have to slowly reverse it. I believe there is a pathway to disease, but there is also a reversal pathway back to health. This reversal path is the one we must follow. It is those who take the right path who will survive.

FOLLOWING NATURE'S WAY

We find that nature's way is God's way. There is a way of pure, whole, natural living. We have to begin to say, "I walk with thee, oh Lord, with integrity." We judge not others. God does. "Vengeance is mine," sayeth the Lord.

Many people believe that our complex, expensive diagnostic machines, our laboratory tests, can tell what is wrong with man. Yet, changes are coming so fast that before a new machine or test is in use, it is obsolete and passe. New equipment is constantly taking its place, showing the cause of the problem is not quite what it seemed to be. But the problem is deeper than even the newest equipment can tell; the problem is that the **whole body** is affected, not just the part showing the symptoms. We have new machines, but they are designed to follow old concepts of disease and old concepts of treatment. They are still testing only part of the body. They are still treating only part of the body. We can put all the old tests together and they still can't tell what is going on in the **whole body.** They still can't tell what the best form of treatment would be. For this reason, we can't judge what is wrong with society by the "equipment" we have today. We are not seeing enough.

We have to ask, "Am I with God or am I working with the eyes that were given to me?" We find we are getting away from the place where we use our own eyes, our own brain. We have to have other eyes to see for us. That is why photography was born. We have to have another brain to think for us. That is why computers were born.

THE WAY OF SURVIVAL

We need to be firm believers that right will right itself. How can

426

we expect God to take care of us if we don't do the natural things? God and nature work together. Nature is the cloak of God. Our prayers go amiss if we are asking God to help us and we don't go the natural way.

We can have peace, but we are going to pieces instead. As we go to pieces, we find out somebody else has to pick us up and put us back together again. The Divine Creator is the only one who can put us back in the proper condition.

What's wrong in our time is that everyone is treating the symptoms, the end effects. Nobody is fixing up the body so it can do its own healing. Yet all the health arts acknowledge that the body cures itself; the doctor does not cure. We have to look at society, at civilization, in the same way. We have to do those things which allow society to heal naturally.

WHAT DOES AMERICA OFFER?

Too many people didn't hear what the late President John F. Kennedy said, "Ask not what your country can do for you, but ask what you can do for your country." This country offers only opportunity—without any guarantees. Your happiness is not guaranteed, but only your right to the pursuit of happiness. If you don't have a healthy body to pursue happiness with, if you don't have a clear mind to discern, think, understand and plan ahead with, then your pursuit of happiness will never succeed.

No one is doing anything for you—and why should they? You have to work out your own problems. Recall again what President Kennedy said. Consider the fact that this country is made up of people. What have you done for others? What have you done with the opportunities you have had? Too many people only think of what others can do for them. We have to have things backward.

It is the same in the health arts. We are trying to find something to take care of the virus instead of building up our health and immune system so the body can take care of the virus on its own. We are treating diseases brought on by exposure to pollution and toxic chemicals instead of cleaning up the environment. We are trying to treat the effects instead of the causes.

Good health can be torn down a little at a time, like drops of water wearing away stone. We strain our eyes working under inadequate artificial light, don't get enough fresh air, drink

427

chemicalized water, neglect to exercise, eat devitalized foods loaded with chemical additives, breathe air polluted with auto exhaust gases and toxic industrial smoke, eat foods tainted with agricultural pesticides.

We are so deluged with abnormal conditions that our bodies and minds are growing tired of fighting. It is time to go the other way. It is time to build up our bodies and minds until we have the strength and courage to throw off our health problems and our social problems. Too many are relying on money to solve their problems. Too many are relying on the government to solve their problems. Things are only going to get better as we realize that cleanliness is purity, that health is wholeness, that God works through nature and nature's laws to reveal a right way of living, a right path to follow. This is the way out of our troubles.

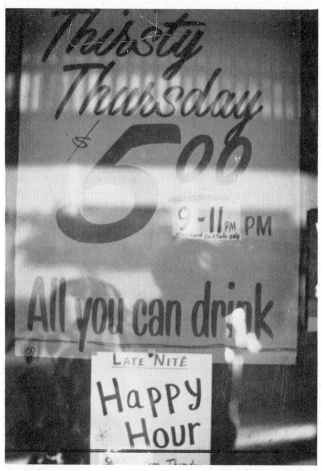

33

The Doctor Views the Latest News

The following items came to my attention in the process of keeping up with the latest news in the health arts, and I'd like to share them with you.

WHAT YOU EAT AFFECTS YOUR HEART. *43 million Americans have one or more forms of heart disease, and more than 20% have high blood pressure. Diets high in saturated fats and cholesterol contribute to heart and vascular diseases that add up to half of all deaths in the U.S. annually.*

SULFITE SCARE MAY LEAD TO BAN. *I saw in the newspaper where the FDA estimates that as many as 1 million Americans may be allergic to sulfites, a preservative used on fresh fruits and vegetables in restaurants and salad bars, in many processed foods, on potatoes, and even in beer and wine. Since 1982, 15 deaths have been linked to sulfite.*

MULTIPLE PERSONALITIES IN ANOREXIA CASES. *Psychiatrist Moshe Torem, an eating disorder specialist, found out that 10 out of 60 cases of anorexia and bulimia he studied were due to multiple personality.*

PREVENTIVE CARE IS THE WISE THING. *I read that from 65% to 75% of the 120,000 women with breast cancer are past menopause, and I feel that we need to understand that proper diet and a healthy lifestyle are very important. The best cure for cancer is to live right so we don't get it.*

IT'S NEVER TOO LATE. *Older cigarette smokers with children or grandchildren should stop smoking because of the example they set. Studies have shown that children are much more likely to become smokers when they grow up if the adults they love and look up to smoke.*

CAN FOOD BE ADDICTIVE? *Actress Judith Light of TV's "Who's the Boss?" admits that compulsive eating almost ruined her life and career. "It was the same as being an alcoholic," she says. "You name it, I ate." She was able to change her eating habits when she changed her attitude toward herself, with the help of therapy.*

429

NEW YEARS'S RESOLUTION? Although making and breaking New Year's resolutions has almost become a joke, resolution itself, the firm intention and purpose to change, is necassary before meaningful changes can take place in life. Don't make resolutions you won't keep. Don't break resolutions you make.

CHOLESTEROL AND FATS. Reducing blood cholesterol requires reducing your intake of dietary fats. Cooking and high heat destroy the lecithin in foods that normally balances cholesterol, and this raises blood cholesterol. Don't use fats in cooking.

GEORGE HAMILTON — A STAR'S HEALTH PROGRAM. Movie and TV star George Hamilton, now starring in "Dynasty," believes in fasting two days a week to cleanse his body and give his liver a rest. His regular diet includes lots of fresh vegetables and occasional meals of wild game such as deer or moose because wild game has no drugs or chemicals in it.

MANY DRUGS EVENTUALLY FATAL. I heard the story of a woman who decided to kill her husband and gave him a tiny dose of arsenic each day in his food. It took two years, but he finally died. Even minimal amounts of chemicals can become fatal over a period of time.

LYMPHATIC TROUBLE SOURCE. Whenever we find tonsil trouble, inflamed appendix, lumps in the breasts or other lymphatic system problems, diet problems are usually the cause.

PERSIMMONS FOR LONG LIFE. The Chinese believe persimmons are a longevity food, and I grow persimmons on my Ranch, freezing some to keep for year-around use.

SKIPPING MEALS IS NOT THE WAY TO REDUCE. An article in the **Journal of the American Medical Association** said skipping meals is contributing to inadequate nutrition in the U.S. Skipping meals deprives the body of needed chemical elements and causes the metabolism to slow down, increasing weight gain later.

HOW TO MAKE A STOMACH HAPPY.
1. Don't cause stomach tension by always hurrying. Plan ahead.
2. Don't talk business at mealtime.
3. Avoid controversy at meal times. Never discipline the children or scold them at the table. Don't argue while eating.
4. Don't drink any alcoholic beverages on an empty stomach.
5. Eat plenty of raw fruits and vegetables along with a balanced diet.

NUTRITION LINKED TO LEARNING IN CHILDREN. Dr. Allan Cott, a New York psychiatrist, believes as I do in regard to the importance of good nutrition in helping children learn faster in school. Balanced meals and less sugar would improve the performance of millions of so-called "problem learners."

FATS IN THE U.S. DIET. The U.S. Department of Agriculture reported that in a recent year the average American used 11.9 pounds of margarine, 4.6 pounds of butter, 18 pounds of shortening, 3.7 pounds of lard, and 22 pounds of other fats and oils.

DOCTOR ADVOCATES NATURAL DIET. Dr. Leonard Glazebrook, British osteopath, said, "Man has evolved slowly with the help of natural foods. Artificial foods could cause new cancers, new nervous disorders . . ."

CONSTIPATION SHOWS NEED FOR FIBER IN DIET. *Constipation in an otherwise healthy person is generally a sign of insufficient fiber. Fiber is a bowel "regulator," making sure wastes pass through without abnormal delay.*

MISSED MEALS CAUSE ACCIDENTS. *A British study showed that low blood sugar due to missed meals can be the direct cause of high accidents. The study added that those on low calorie weight loss diets should drive carefully.*

CHILDREN WHO EAT POORLY. *Zinc deficiency reduces the sense of taste and smell, lowering the appetite in children who do not take enough food. Seventy-five underweight children were found by government researchers to have low zinc levels.*

FAT LEVELS IN MILK. *Whole milk is at least 3.25% milk fat. Skim milk is less than 0.5% fat. Low fat milk has between 0.5% and 2% fat.*

MOODS, FOODS AND MEMORIES. *According to Dr. Alina S. Szczesniak, soft foods are liked by people who relate to them subconsciously like the baby foods that once made them feel loved and protected. Ice cream gives people good feelings because many associate it with being a reward for good behavior in childhood. Many adults hate milk because they were forced to drink it as children. Spongy foods, like cakes, are popular with ladies because they are considered feminine.*

EARTHWORMS — THE FARMER'S BEST FRIEND. *Worms, in a very true sense, are multipurposed soil enhancers. They aerate, nourish and balance the soil, resulting in greater nutritional value in foods grown. Rich soil may contain as many as 26 thousands worms per acre, and their natural wastes (castings) are 7 times higher in potash, 3 times higher in magnesium, and 5 times higher in nitrogen than the soil they live in.*

WELL-BEING LINKED TO POTASSIUM FOODS. *Did you realize that people who make potassium foods a significant part of their food regimen are seldom sick? Potassium is high in watercress, cabbage, potato skins, dandelion, dill parsley, sage, olives, bananas, blueberries, peaches, prunes, figs and coconut.*

ABORIGINES DUMP DIABETES IN OUTBACK. *Urbanized Australian aborigines who developed diabetes and returned to the bush country have often cured diabetes within seven weeks. Their low-fat, low-calorie diet was effective in controlling diabetes.*

PREGNANCY — BIGGER ISN'T BETTER. *"Remember, you're eating for two," has been a frequent remark aimed at pregnant women in past years. We now find out this has resulted in overweight mothers giving birth, with difficulty, to excessively fat babies. It is best to use a diet with high nutritional value, neither too high in calories or in fats. Nutritional counsel should be sought before pregnancy.*

THE BRAIN NEEDS EXERCISE. *Problems and challenges "exercise" brain, according to researchers, who have found out that the brain is capable of enlarging and improving its performance at any age.*

EATING OUT? EAT BETTER! *A recent survey has shown that people who eat out are ordering 57% more decaffeinated coffee in 1984 than 1982. They are also eating 48% more fresh fruit and vegetables, and 31% more salads.*

HIGH FIBER FOODS FOR HEMORRHOIDS. *High fiber foods soften stools, improve bowel tone and regularity, and relieve the pain and bleeding of hemorrhoids in most cases within two weeks, according to experts. Fiber foods can also actually shrink hemorrhoids.*

SWEET NEWS ABOUT SWEET POTATOES. *One sweet potato provides a week's supply of viatmin A. The average American eats 5 pounds of sweet potatoes per year these days, as compared to 29 pounds in 1920.*

WOMEN STAYING YOUNGER LONGER. *"A woman of 40 today is biologically equivalent to a woman of 30 or 35 twenty years ago," says Dr. Givliano Gelli, chief of obstetrics and gynecology at San Donato Hospital in Milan, Italy.*

HIGHEST CAVITY-PROMOTING SNACKS. *Snacks promoting highest cavity rates include carob bars, Welch's Grape Drink, Heath Bars, Crunchola Bars, sunflower seeds, peanut butter on cheese crackers, and the Hoffman Energy Bar, according to the Baylor University College of Dentistry in Dallas, Texas.*

HERBAL HELPS FOR BETTER CIRCULATION. *The herb Butcher's broom helps venous congestion, varicose veins, hemorrhoids, leg cramps, phlebitis and poor circulation.*

DRUGS PRESCRIBED FOR STRESS. *According to Dr. Abram Hoffer, only a patient in an advanced state of physical and mental upset should be given a prescription drug. The best approach to restoring health, Dr. Hoffer says, is balancing lifestyle, eating habits, work, play and sleep.*

GET OFF DIET. *Every popular magazine seems to have a new diet these days. If we ate more balanced meals with more fresh fruits and vegetables, more whole cereal grains, less red meat, and cut out all refined foods, we wouldn't have to diet, especially if we exercised regularly.*

HEALTHY EATING OUT RULES. *1) Choose fresh foods. 2) See if an appetizer might serve as a healthy entree. 3) Tell the waiter no butter or sauces on your food. 4) Drink water instead of nibbling on rolls before dinner. 5) Have fruit for dessert.*

UNREFINED CARBOHYDRATE POWER. *People who eat lots fiber fruits and vegetables are often high in energy and staying power, lower in weight than the average American. Fiber moves food through the digestive system faster, tones and regulates the bowel, reduces cholesterol.*

MILK AND ALLERGIES. *A study of 22 asthma patients in Israel showed that 15 improved dramatically when taken off all dairy products.*

CHILDREN AND DIET. *Children of undernourished mothers have been found to show less interest in their surroundings, less competitiveness, less persistence at hard tasks, and less initiative in group activities than children of adequately nourished mothers.*

LET'S GO BANANAS! *Bananas are high in fiber, lower in fat and high in potassium. They also contain magnesium, phosphorus, vitamins A, C, and some B vitamins.*

COOLING OFF HEARTBURN. *To cool off heartburn, avoid alcohol, fatty foods, chocolate, cigarettes, citrus juice, tomatoes and coffee. Stay away from hot spices. Also, avoid food for 3 to 4 hours before bedtime.*

PEOPLE WHO FEAR FOOD. *Many people are reportedly afraid of chemicals in food, cholesterol, refined foods and fatty foods. Increasingly, food manufacturers are packaging their products in earth-colored packages to reassure buyers of their "health value."*

DON'T CHEAT YOURSELF OUT OF BETTER HEALTH. *Many people who try to save money by cutting their food budget lose it later in doctors bills. Eat the best food you can buy.*

KEEPING THE LEAD OUT. *Pennsylvania State University researchers have discovered that adequate levels of zinc intake can prevent most lead from accumulating in the body.*

THE EFFECT OF DIVORCE ON THE CHILDREN'S HEALTH. *In a 38-state research project, scientists compared the health status of 358 children from intact families with that of 431 children of divorced parents. The post-divorce children (and their parents) had distinctly lower health ratings.*

AEROBIC EXERCISE LOWERS BLOOD PRESSURE. *Recent studies of the effects of regular aerobic exercise such as brisk walking, jogging, swimming and bicycling show a moderate lowering of blood pressure in patients with mild to moderate hypertension. Isometric exercises and weight lifting may raise blood pressue.*

THE CHEMICALS WE EAT. *"Last year each of us, on average, swallowed three pounds of flavorings, coloring, preservatives, glazes, antispattering agents, emulsifiers, bleaches, and other additives with our food."*

Joan Morgan, M.D.

HOW MUCH SUGAR DO WE FIND IN PACKAGED FOODS?
(As checked in 1985)

PRODUCT NAME	% SUGAR	PRODUCT NAME	% SUGAR
Coffee-Mate	65.4	Fruit Yogurt	13.7
Hamburger Helper	23.0	French Salad Dressing	23.0
Jell-O	82.6	Russian Salad Dressing	30.2
Kellogg's Apple Jacks	52.0	Quaker 100% Natural Cereal	17.0
Post Fruit Pebbles	48.0	Bouillon Cubes	14.8
Quaker Cap'n Crunch	39.0	Canned Corn	10.7
Kellogg's Frosted Flakes	39.0	Canned Peaches	17.9
General Mills Trix	37.0	Ritz Crackers	11.8
Nabisco 100% Bran	19.0	Ketchup	28.9

NO GREAT LOSS. *"Thirty percent of the products in grocery stores today could be thrown out and nobody would be the worse."*

Dr. Mark Hegsted
Professor of Nutrition
Harvard University

433

SALT IN FOODS. Excess salt has been linked to high blood pressure and heart disease, and while we can control the amount we sprinkle on food, often we don't know how much is in packaged and prepared foods. The body needs only 2 grams of sodium per day.

FOOD ITEM	SODIUM (mg)	FOOD ITEM	SODIUM (mg)
Tuna, canned, 3½ oz.	800	Two Hot Dogs	1100
Instant Pudding, ½ cup	404	Kellogg's Corn Flakes,	
Salad Dressing, 1 tsp.	315	1 oz.	282
English Muffin	215	Kellogg's Rice Krispies,	
McDonald's Big Mac	1510	1 oz.	267

THE POISONING OF OUR LAND AND WATER. "Each year more than 600 million pounds of pesticides of all kinds are sprayed, dusted, fogged or dumped in the United States - about three pounds for every man, woman and child in the country."

Gaylord Nelson in
"Our Polluted Planet"

GENETIC DAMAGE AND RADIATION. A study of 216 families who have children with Down's Sydrome, as published in the **Journal of the American Medical Association,** showed that the mothers had significant exposure to X-rays before the birth of their child, and a number of the fathers had been exposed to radar waves.

OUR BODIES ARE WONDERFULLY MADE. If a person bicycles ten miles an hour, he or she uses the energy equivalent to 1.4 ounces of gasoline. That amounts to our bodies getting over 900 miles per gallon, an energy efficiency no machine known to man has ever reached.

ORIGIN OF THE SANDWICH. The sandwich, now so popular in the U.S. and many countries of the world, was first invented in 18th century England. The Earl of Sandwich, a compulsive gambler who at times spent more than 24 hours at a stretch playing cards, disliked stopping to eat, so he would order meat between slices of bread. This way, he could hold his cards in one hand and his "sandwich" in the other.

I don't recommend sandwiches, because most Americans have far too much wheat in their diets, but if you must have them occasionally, include vegetables as part of the filling - lettuce, sprouts, slices of zucchini, radishes, tomato and so on. Bread, unless taken with vegetables, tends to slow the movement of food through the bowel.

STOP SMOKING! Warning: The Surgeon General Has Determined That Cigarette Smoking is Dangerous To Your Health.

Cigarette smoke introduces a powerful drug (nicotine) into your body which acts as a suppressant and causes degenerative diseases. It also lowers your immunity, your ability to ward off diseases in general. Help prevent cancer, emphysema and heart attack. STOP SMOKING!

Before he died, film and stage star Yul Brynner told friends he would like to do a TV commercial warning cigarette smokers that they must stop smoking. "I used to smoke 5 packs of cigarettes a day and that's what I believe caused my illness," Brynner said. "I was an enormously healthy and very strong man. It (smoking) is suicide, no question about it."

The American Cancer Society, The American Heart Association and the American Lung Association began an unprecedented advertising campaign against the dangers of smoking in October, 1985, to help counteract the $2.7 billion annual advertising campaign of the tobacco industry.

According to a Congressional study, the adverse effects of smoking cost the U.S. $65 billion in medical bills, premature death and lost work time. U.S. employers pay $7 to $8 billion a year in smoking-related insurance costs alone.

Any woman who smokes takes a risk of up to 3.6 times more in giving birth to an abnormal child, according to a study conducted in Japan.

I feel the evidence against smoking speaks for itself.

KIDS AND SCHOOL LUNCHES. Of kids who take school lunches, 40% are fixed by parents, 29% by the kids themselves, according to Better Homes and Gardens magazine. Foods that kids like least are lamb, beans, yogurt, sour cream, and fish. Parents fix sandwiches 86% of the time, soup 55%. Cookies or other sweets are packed in 52% of the lunches.

THINK YOUR WAY THIN. Use your head when you diet. Read recipes carefully and substitute low-calorie ingredients when possible. Trim the fat off meat before you cook it. In the past year, 60% of the U.S. adults have dieted, 76% by reducing calorie intake, 51% by exercising more.

IS OUR MEAT SAFE? The USDA inspects 127 million cattle, sheep and hogs, and over 4 billion chickens and turkeys for chemical and bacterial contamination each year. They say our meat is safe but could be safer if the inspection system was computerized and updated.

A DIET FOR THE KIDNEYS. I see that Harvard scientists have a new diet that is said to slow down or stop certain chronic kidney diseases, even making kidney dialysis unnecessary. The diet is mostly vegetarian, and in testing it on 24 patients, kidney disease was stopped in 7 cases and slowed down in 3. More than 3 years later, 7 are still on the diet instead of on dialysis machines. In some cases, all symptoms have disappeared.

ALCOHOL PROBLEMS IN THE U.S.S.R. Soviet officials say 2/3 of the traffic accidents, 80% of crimes and 60% of divorces in their country involve alcohol, and they are doing something about it. Liquor store hours will be cut and liquor prices raised, and tough fines will be given for public drunkeness.

JET-SET DIVORCEE-TO-BE OFFERS SPAGHETTI DINNERS AS EVIDENCE OF MOTHER LOVE. A jet-set mother involved in a child custody battle mentioned Sunday spaghetti dinners for her children as evidence of her caring and competence as a mother. I feel she has only proven that she knows how to raise doctor bills.

TIPS ON HEALTHY DINING OUT. When you go to a restaurant, many times you can get healthier substitutions and changes in things served. For example, ask if you can have sliced tomatoes instead of French fries. Ask for your baked potato to be served without butter, and with your sour cream in a side dish.

WHERE CHOCOLATE CAME FROM. According to an article in **Chocolatier** magazine, the Aztec emperor Montezuma II drank 50 goblets of chocolate drink (chocolat) every day. The Spanish who conquered the Aztecs brought chocolate back to Europe with them, and it soon became a popular beverage.

POTATO CHIPS MAKE BETTER LOVERS? I found a news article the other day that claimed potatoes were once considered an aphrodesiac in Europe, and then it went on to say that potato chips are high in Vitamin E, which increases male potency and boosts the love life. I can tell you that any food cooked in boiling fat is not good for anyone.

THE POPE'S DIET. Pope John Paul II is said to like natural foods, usually having a big breakfast, only a salad and fruit for lunch, with a small pieces of cheese with mineral water for supper.

AN ALMOST UNIVERSAL PROTEIN. They say that lamb is accepted as food by almost every religious sect in the world. This is because the lamb's reputation for purity is a fact, and the baby lamb is still consumed with fervor at Passover time in Israel and at Easter in Greece.

THE WISDOM OF THE OLD ONES. Some may recall a lively old man who appeared on the "Ed Sullivan Show" some years ago, a shepherd from the Andes in South America, who reached the venerable age of over 140 years by living mainly on fruits and cheese.

WHAT IS SMOG? 200,000 tons of undesirable chemical wastes are released into the air in the U.S. every year. These include carbon monoxide, sulphur oxides, nitrogen oxides, hydrocarbons, oxidized photochemicals, particulate matter, incompletely burned fuels, dust, ashes, smoke and fumes. Some cause cancer; all of it contributes to ill health in smoggy areas.

JUNK FOODS DIET FOR KIDS? WHO SAYS SO? A New York therapist is now pushing the idea of feeding children whatever they want, whenever they want it, in the hope of weaning children away from later troubles with anorexia, bulimia and obesity. The therapist, who specializes in eating disorders, says her children are choosing healthy foods under this philosophy. I would like to know just what she considers healthy foods. We find out that this philosophy doesn't take into account the heavy TV advertising of junk foods for kids, peer pressure from other children, or the tendency of children to choose "yummy" foods over healthy foods. I feel it is the responsibility of the parents to give their children a balanced diet and to teach them why a balanced diet is necessary until they understand.

CAROB CORNER. Carob is a natural chocolate substitute used in ice cream, candy, cookies, frostings—just about every way chocolate has been used. Carob lacks the caffeine, theobromine and oxalic acid which makes cocoa and chocolate undesirable to many of those who are concerned with health matters.

WHAT WILL THEY DO WITH ALL THOSE EMPTY HOSPITAL BEDS? At the national level, hospital occupancy rates in 1979 were only a little over 50% Many people are rebelling against the high cost of hospital care in the realization that many medical procedures do not prolong life or satisfactority resolve serious health problems.

436

CHANGING TIMES AND FOOD CHANGES. A recent Gallup survey for **American Health** magaine showed that 24% of Americans eat less meat than they used to. USDA figures show that the average annual beef consumption has dropped from 84 pounds in 1970 to 78.6 pounds in 1984, and many restaurants are featuring more fish and chicken entrees and fewer beef dishes.

HEALTH RISK FOR BEAUTICIANS. Studies of cancers in various occupations have put beauticians and cosmetologists at a higher risk level than the average worker. Cosmetic industry products contain about a hundred chemicals listed as suspected carcinogens by the National Institute for Occupational Health and Safety. Tests have also shown that permanent wave solutions, setting lotions and hair straighteners contain toxic chemicals that cause skin problems and allergic reactions.

TIME TO WATCH OUT FOR YOUR HEART. The most dangerous time for a heart attack occurring is between 6 a.m. and noon when physical activity, heart rate and blood pressure are all rising, according to researchers at the Harvard University School of Medicine.

WATCH THOSE ANTACIDS. Antacids containing aluminum hydroxide gel can reduce the level of blood phosphates, aggravating osteoporosis, causing any existing anemia to grow worse, and contributing to toxic reactions by the heart.

CHEMICALS AND CANCER. Over 65,000 chemicals are in commercial use in the U.S., but only 50 have been adequately tested to see if they cause cancer, according to scientists.

THE COKE AND PEPSI WAR. The Coca-Cola Company announced that its 1985 3rd quarter profits rose 11.6% to $195.7 million, up from $175.3 million the same period a year ago, while Pepsico, Inc. reported its 3rd quarter earnings increased 17% to 135.3 milllion.

A NEW LIFE FOR TONY CURTIS. Tony Curtis, star of over 140 films, has turned over a new leaf. "I don't smoke, drink or put any foreign substance in my body. I sleep at least 7 hours . . . have a little exercise routine . . . I pamper myself these days," he recently told on interview.

WHAT SMOKING DOES. Cigarette smoke irritates a smoker's lungs and bronchials, causing inflammation and catarrh. It greatly increases the time it takes for the lungs to expel toxic material. Heavy smoking often leads to coughing, chronic bronchitis, emphysema and is linked to heart disease and cancer.

WHAT WORRIES AMERICANS. The top health concern among food items in the U.S., according to a Roper survey in 1984, was salt. Cholesterol was second and sugar was third. Others named were caffeine, saccharin and aspartame (NutraSweet).

ALLERGIES HARDEST IN MIDLIFE. Of the 35 million Americans with allergies, most are bothered more in their 30's than any other time - about 35% of women from 35 to 40 and 25% of men from 30 to 35.

CHILDREN AND MILK. From 2% to 10% of U.S. children under 3 are allergic to pasteurized milk.

PRINCE CHARLES, WHOLISTIC HEALTH ADVOCATE? *Prince Charles has stated his belief in "complementary medicine . . . looking at a person not so much as a machine, but as the whole, in a classic, ancient sense." It is said that the Prince fasts and rarely eats red meat, preferring fish and fowl.*

SURVEYING AMERICAN HEALTH HABITS. *A National Center for Health Statistics survey in 1985 showed that 45% of the U.S. people view themselves as overweight and 37% are trying to lose weight; 41% exercise or engage in sports regularly; 78% get at least 7 hours of sleep each night; 39% snack between meals nearly every day; 66% rarely or never discuss nutrition with their doctors; 44% believe stress affects their health; and 34% of adults don't drink.*

THE "SOUTHERN BELLE" DIET. *Phyllis Diller says she follows the "Southern Belle" diet over the holiday season - "Well, shut mah mouth!"*

THANKSGIVING CALORIES. *Half the U.S. adults pick up 4 to 7 pounds from Thanksgiving through New Year, according to the experts. Heavy eaters can put away as much as 8,000 calories on Thanksgiving alone, 4 or 5 days worth of food in a single day.*

ASPARAGUS THERAPY. *A Pittsburgh dentist advocates using 4 Tblsp. cooked asparagus daily as a cancer preventitive, 8 Tblsp. daily to help reverse and get rid of cancer. People using this "asparagus therapy" claim to have been helped with cancers of the mouth, bladder, breast, lung, intestine and prostrate.*

WE MUST FEED OUT CELLS THROUGH THE RIGHT FOODS. *Human beings have about 200 different kinds of cells in their bodies, each requiring a sligtly different combination of nutrients. This is why we recognize the food law that we must have a **variety** of foods.*

COMBINATIONS INCREASE VEGETARIAN PROTEIN VALUE. *Many vegatable sources contain some protein, but most of them are incomplete, lacking one or more of the essential amino acids. To get the best protein values from vegetarian souces, combine legumes with whole grains, legumes with nuts and seeds, grains with nuts. The amino acids in each one supply those missing in the others.*

THE GREAT AMERICAN PUMPKIN DIET. *I have seen many diets come and go. Pumpkins are members of the squash family, high in nutritional values and always good as a low-calorie addition to a **balanced diet.** They say you can lose up to 10 pounds in 7 days on the pumpkin diet, but as with other imbalanced "crash" diets, weight lost that fast is always gained back.*

YOGURT IS FOR EVERYONE. *Yogurt is a perfect food for milk-intolerant people because its lactose is broken down by the good lactobacillus bacteria, which makes it easily digestible. Use only raw milk yogurt.*

WHO NEEDS VITAMINS? *Women, teenagers, the elderly, frequent dieters and those with a high-stress job or lifestyle are more likely to need vitamins than others.*

AMERICAN PROTEIN PREFERENCES. *In a recent year, Americans ate 214 lbs. of red meat, 53 pounds of poultry and 13 lbs. of fish. We should eat more poultry and fish, and less meat if we want to live longer.*

SHOULD WE SKIP BREAKFAST? *Tests show skipping breakfast reduces attention and level of performance in many persons. The ideal breakfast is a whole grain cereal and a piece of fruit or glass of fruit juice, according to Dr. Frederic Starl, professor of nutrition at Harvard University.*

THE JAPANESE DIET. *The Japanese include a good deal of fish in their diet, very little beef, lots of steamed vegetables and rice. They broil food on a spit or grill and cook foods lightly to preserve nutritional value. There are very few overweight Japanese, and many Americans would lose their excess weight on such a diet.*

PICKING UP THOSE ESSENTIAL NUTRIENTS. *Good sources of B-1, needed for carbohydrate and protein metabolism, are: avocados, peas, oranges, pinto beans, sunflower seeds and whole wheat flour. Folacin, needed for building the blood and tissue repair, is found in eggs, whole milk, raw cabbage and oranges. B-12, required for healthy blood cells and cell division, is found in cheddar cheese, cottage cheese, Swiss cheese, milk, eggs, tofu and fresh tempeh. Calcium is needed by every cell in the body but especially for the bones and teeth, and best sources are cheese, yogurt, tofu, spinach, sesame seeds, and other seeds and nuts. Best sources of iron needed to build red blood cells are figs, dates, parsley, raw peas, lentils, garbanzo beans, prunes, raisins, tofu, wheat bran and chlorophyll-rich leafy vegetables such as spinach. Zinc, needed for growth, tissue repair and the sexual system, is found in brown rice, wheat bran, pumpkin seeds, garbanzo beans and lentils.*

THE AVERAGE WEIGHT PROBLEM. *Fifteen percent of Americans are classified as obese. Obese males are overweight by an average of 28.5 lbs., while obese women average 30.7 lbs. overweight, according to the National Center for Health Statistics.*

OBESITY AND ETHNIC BACKGROUND. *According to a study at John Hopkins University, overweight problems can be linked to a person's ancestors in many cases. Sometimes ancestry can be traced to cold countries where fat was necessary for survival, and in other cases it is linked to cultures with traditional food patterns that produce obesity when used out of cultural context (at lower levels of work activity, for example).*

HOW SAFE IS OUR FOOD AND WATER? *In 1985, 85 persons died from eating contaminated cheese, over 200 became ill from pesticide-contaminated watermelons, several persons died from sulfide preservatives, 16,000 got sick from infected milk, and wines from several countries were returned after traces of a toxic chemical were found in them. According to the Environmental Protection Agency, 63% of rural residents may be drinking water contaminated with pesticides and agricultural chemicals. One independent study found pesticide residues in 44% of all food tested.*

Can you think of a better reason to eat only whole, pure and natural foods and stick to reverse osmosis drinking water?

STAY AWAY FROM HOSPITALS. *According to Lowell Levin, professor of public health at Yale University's School of Medicine, 20% of the 30 million Americans who enter hospitals annually come down with hospital-caused health problems, and 10% get infections while in the hospital.*

439

REJUVENATING THE CELLS. *Researchers in Israel have succeeded in reversing changes due to aging in mouse cells by reducing the amount ot sphingomyelin available to the cells and increasing the amount of lecithin. Both nutrients play an important role in cell membrane activity and integrity.*

LACK OF FIBER CAUSES DIVERTICULITIS? *Diverticulitis is an inflammation of tiny sacs that pouch outward from the bowel wall, and millions of Americans have it. In many cases, infection and bleeding result. Many human and animal research studies now link diverticulitis with a diet deficient in adequate fiber.*

MILK PRODUCTS - THE NOT-SO-IDEAL FOOD. *These days, selective breeding has produced cows that give more than twice as much milk as cows did in the early 1980s, and the result is a glut of milk products on the market along with high-pressure advertising campaigns to sell them. Milk products in general tend to cause bowel disturbances when used in the high amounts the average American consumes. (The average U.S. diet is 24% milk products.)*

WHERE DOES IT ALL COME FROM? *A large supermarket may carry as many as 25,000 items.*

DIETING TO LOWER HIGH BLOOD PRESSURE. *Recently scientists have found that diets high in calcium and potassium, low in salt (sodium), help to lower blood pressure.*

CHEMICAL FOUND IN WINES. *Traces of the chemical diethylene glycol, used in antifreeze and for industrial purposes, led to the 1985 recall of several brands of imported Riunite wines. U.S. government tests have found diethylene glycol in 45 Austrian wines, 5 German wines and 12 Italian wines. We find out that chemicals are being found in almost all man-handled foods these days.*

CONTAMINATED SALADS. *Until late 1985, most people didn't realize that many restaurants and salad bars were spraying chemicals called sulfites on their vegetables and fruits to keep them crisp. The problem is that several people have died from the chemically tainted foods, and thousands of others have had reactions to the sulfites, ranging from breaking out in a rash to severe nausea.*

BE CAREFUL WITH CAFFEINE DRINKS. *I read the other day about a National Institute of Mental Health Study which showed that caffeine can trigger sudden panic attacks, sudden feelings of doom. These feelings may also be accompanied by choking, heart palpitations and perspiring.*

AMERICANS NOW DRINK MORE SODA POP THAN WATER. *In 1960 Americans drank more water than any other beverage, but soft drinks reached the top in 1984, according to a market research firm. Soft drinks made up 25.5% of all drinks taken, while water made up 24.9%. The study also showed that Americans drank over twice as much coffee as fruit juice, and only a little less beer than coffee.*

YOUNGER CHILDREN TRYING ALCOHOL. *I see that a survey by the Parents' Resource Institute for Drug Education showed that 33.4% of 6th graders had tried beer or wine and 9.5% had tried liquor. Alcohol use also more than doubled among 6th graders from 1983 to 1984.*

HEADLINE WRITER SHOULD LOOK AROUND. *I came across a headline the other day that said, "NUCLEAR WAR SURVIVORS WOULD STARVE." I don't believe in nuclear war, but if we look around we find out that two-thirds of the*

440

people of the world go to bed starving or hungry every night, and the majority of the other third is malnourished from eating imbalanced diets, refined foods, chemicalized foods, junk foods and sugary foods.

DRINKING WATER SHRINKING. The Worldwatch Institute claims that water supplies will fall short in rich countries as well as developing nations within 20 years, citing increasing ecological damage as one of the reasons for the shortage. Waste and rising costs were other reasons given.

THE LONGEST-LIVED PEOPLE. The Japanses are now the longest-lived people on earth, according to recent statistical studies. The average Japanese woman now has a life expectancy of 80.2 years, while men are expected to live an average of 74.5 years. Could if be that the great emphasis on sea foods in Japan is responsible? (Average life expectancy for American women is 78.2 years, American men 70.9 years.)

THE DEMISE OF SUGAR. We find out from the newspapers that the refined sugar industry is suffering from overpopulation, a glut of sugar on the world market, following consumption and economic competition from chemical sweeteners. Sugar growers and refiners are looking for alternative products and services to switch to. I can hardly believe this news, but the sooner we get sugar out of our diets, the better it will be for our health. However, I don't believe artificial sweeteners are a safe substitute, and may even be worse than refined sugar.

CHOLESTEROL AND HEALTH. Amercans' average blood cholesterol levels are around 210 mg/dl, about 30 mg/dl too high. Cholesterol is the fatty substance that deposits in the arteries and blood vessels, one of the major contributors to cardiovascular disease, heart attacks and strokes. "When cholesterol begins depositing on the vessels that feed the heart," according to Dr. Basil Rifkind of the National Heart, Lung and Blood Institute, "this is the beginning of heart disease." This starts happening above 180 mg/dl, and when cholesterol readings rise above 260, people are considered high risk. For best heart health, the blood cholesterol should be between 150 mg/dl and 180.

I feel the best way to take care of the cholesterol problem is to get rid of the frying pan. At temperatures over boiling, lecithin is destroyed, leaving the cholesterol. Frying, baking and any method of cooking in heated oils (or cooking foods containing oils at high temperatures) can cause cholesterol problems. The best way to get the oils we need is to get them from oil-containing foods - nuts, seeds, grains, cheese, meat, avocadoes, and so forth.

COCAINE - PUBLIC HEALTH THREAT. I feel that imbalanced diets and imbalanced lifestyles are creating unnatural desires for drugs and alcohol, which are causing a great deal of the crimes, violence, divorces, child abuse and accidents in this country. Dr. Donald Ian MacDonald, chief of the Federal Alcohol, Drug Abuse and Mental Health Administration, has said, "Cocaine can be a killer. Emergency room admissions associated with cocaine use tripled between 1981 and 1984. The number of deaths associated with cocaine also tripled." Cocaine is now considered one of the most powerfully addictive drugs known.

NAPS NEEDED FOR HEALTH? *Over 50% of the people in the U.S take naps, according to a recent survey, and scientists say that among human beings, naps may represent a biological need. I feel there are two ways of looking at this. Most of my patients have come to be fatigued, tired, run-down, and they need rest as much as nutritional correction. A need for extra sleep may indicate health problems. Another observation is that fast lifestyles and staying up too late may create a need for naps. Finally, however, I feel a hardworking person can benefit from an afternoon nap.*

LOST WORK TIME DUE TO TOXIC CHEMICALS. *In 1981, 126,000 cases of work-related illness accounted for 850,000 lost work days, due to suspected reactions to chemicals in the work place, according to estimates by the U.S. Department of Labor.*

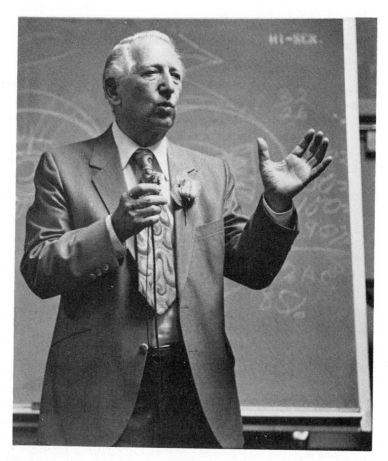

We believe the average person wants to do the right thing. Where are the teachers?

442

————34————
Endorsements —
"Flowers that Light
Up the Room"

It is so good to hear from you again with the contribution of your latest book, **"Slender Me Naturally."** I have to marvel at your creativity in bringing out so many books in natural therapeutics that have become classics in their field.

> H. John Zitko, Ph.D.
> World University
> Benson, Arizona

Your book is a masterpiece . . . I congratulate you on its publication and on receiving the Dag Hammarskjold Award. I am privileged to know you personally . . .

> Robert S. Mendelsohn, M.D.
> Evanston, Illinois

Thank you again for sharing your wisdom with all of us.

> Rhody Edwards, D.C.
> Malama Chiropractic Clinic
> Kailua-Kona, Hawaii

...the Planet is a better place because of people like you.

> Shirley Eichner
> Kennewick, Washington

I believe that natural medicine is the way to preventing the degeneration of the human being. I share totally your wholistic views of man . . .

> Luis H. Gutierrez
> Universidad Peruana Cayetano Heredia
> Lima, Peru, South America

. . . everyone needs you. You'll never know what an inspiration you've been to thousands - and how much the Natural Health Movement owes to you.

> S. Jonathan Spector, D.C.
> Wholistic Health Clinic
> Sarasota, Florida

Read *"Vibrant Health From Your Kitchen,"* and take back your right to enjoy and thrive on delicious, natural food. Your soul, your mind and your body will rejoice! Nutritional pioneer Dr. Bernard Jensen may just push the fast food emporiums past the token salad bars now emerging there, to a full menu of real food."

James J. Julian, M.D.
Author and Lecturer
Physician to Celebrities

I have known Dr. Jensen for quite a few years and I use his material as authority when I instruct my patients on diets. His observations are sound, practical and very useful. I recommend his ideas highly."

Harry A. Lusk, M.D.
Los Angeles, California

At a time when the medical doctors are suggesting that people at large are consuming too many vitamins in the search for good health, it is refreshing to see that Dr. Jensen has given us so much wisdom that we achieve, *"Vibrant Health From Your Kitchen."* Speaking personally, it is now seven years since I have had to take antibiotics or antihistamines which were so frequently prescribed for me all my life. Medical practitioners and supplements both have their place, but before using either we should be looking toward out kitchens. My own new vibrant health tells me this is true. Winner of the Dag Kammerskjold Award, Pax Mundi Society, for his work in Natural Medicine, Dr. Jensen has done it again. He has created a book that should be a kitchen bible.

Leon M. Brosnan, PhC, MPS, JP
Pharmaceutical Chemist & Nutritionist
Queensland, Austria

Your books are full of wisdom.

Grand Prior Marquis don K Vella Harbor
Sovereign Order of Saint John of Jerusalem
Gzira, Malta

Eat fiberous foods daily. The secret of beautiful, healthy teeth is having a proper diet from birth of good natural foods in proper proportion.

R.M. Gibson, D.D.S.
Honolulu, Hawaii

I remember well your visit to our college and how inspired I was to see and listen to the man whose teachings I had read so much of.

Ms. Linda Caplin
Auckland, New Zealand

We follow your healing methods and get excellent results . . . you have made a wonderful contribution to world health . . .

Mr. & Mrs. Ken Farmer
Natural Healing Centre
Rotorua, New Zealand

It was a pleasure learning from you and being with you.

Bill McKenna
Mt. Vernon, Maine

444

After thinking about the information I read in your books, I came away with a better understanding of what selective foods really can do for us. It works. And it's working for me right now.

Mr. Mike Ross
Spokane, Washington

You personally changed my life . . . the results are miraculous.

Dr. Lewis Meiring, M.D.
Pathologist, State Hospital
Pretoria, South Africa

I have become a devotee of your "Philosphy of Health."

Janusz Dernalowicz, MSc.
Instytut Biocybernetyki
Warszawa, Poland

. . . a wonderful thing for me - my bowels are better than they have ever been for forty years - and to think the doctors offered to do a colostomy a few years ago . . . I do love and appreciate all that you have shared with so many . . .

M.H.
Alberta, Canada

You are doing more good for human beings than anyone I know. I admire your work - and your energy to do it all!

C.B.
Manufacturing Executive
Melkev, Oslo, Norway

*. . . I have read practically everything you have published and consider this (**Vibrant Health From Your Kitchen**) the greatest thing on nutrition and health you have ever written.*

George Fathman
Life Research Institute
Payson, Arizona

. . . I am sure happy to have discovered you and your work.

Ricardo R. Bedoya
Neuronoetics
Lima, Peru

I have no words to express how grateful I am to you.

Karl Heinz Boldt
Cape Town, South Africa

Thank you for the week at your ranch. I am much better and learned a lot. I am applying it to my patients and we are all benefitting.

B.W.
Ontario, Canada

My stay at the Ranch did a lot of good.

M.E.M. Del Campo
Mexico City

Your whole life has always been one of touching people on some level and their lives are always enriched because of the contact.

Louis Foundation
Orcas Island, Washington

You have helped so many.

H.H. & Family
Nevada

We want you to know how important you have been to us.

Kostas & Olga Kohylas
Athens, Greece

Followed your advice - never felt better - had 2 healing crises and nodule on wrist has dissolved.

Margaret Christchurch
New Zealand

Wonderful work.

David Ai-he Zhu, M.D. (China)
Oriental Medical Institute of Hawaii, Hawaii

Your books are wonderful and you are an inspiration.

J.R.
North Carolina

I received great spiritual values.

Dr. M. Padilla
Bemidji, Montana

Appreciated very deeply the kindly constructive spirit.

Dr. B. Holstead, M.D.
California

My life has changed dramatically . . . thanks to you.

M.R.
Atlanta, Georgia

In a world increasingly clouded by sickness, crime and all manner of physical and mental uncleanliness, there exists a remnant, they being stewards of the manna who excite us to the finer and higher possibilities of life. Bernard Jensen is such a steward.

Rev. R. Donald V. Bodeen, BS,BS, MST,DC
Poughkeepsie, New York

I sense a quickening atmosphere of the whole holistic scene in America - and I know and believe that a good share of it is due to your sensitive and real work in providing the framework for so many to know which way to go.

Jack Tropp
New York, New York

My heartfelt gratitude to you, Dr. Jensen, for all you have done in the health field . . . a lifetime of wonderful service to mankind.

LaDean Griffin
Author, Iridologist and Herbalist
Provo, Utah

If I were to describe Dr. Jensen in one word, I would choose the word, PEACEMAKER. He helps his students make peace with their bodies, spirits, environment, family, and neighbors.

Clinton R. Miller
Executive Director, NHF
Monrovia, California

We are great admirers of your work.

Richard A. Katz and Patricia Kaminski, Co-Directors
The Flower Essence Society
Nevada City, California

I am getting back to normal after your fantastic visit to our country (South Africa), which has created a tremendous stir amongst the professional people who had attended your seminar.

F.V. Kraayenburg, Director
"New Dimension"
South Africa

In the beginning it was called pure hoke, and with wry amusement many in the medical-science field believed that the study of the iris would pass from view in due course. It has been Dr. Bernard Jensen who has made everything great and good come to people through his studies.

Richard K. Stacer, Attorney
San Diego, California

Your teaching is a blessing to the world. It provides a way for people to help themselves.

Dr. Hugh Wayman, D.C.
Salt Lake City, Utah

His dedication and driving force in this study reveal an unselfish endeavor to assist in a better understanding of their physical, mental and spiritual unfolding - the proper care of the whole man.

Lynne B. Johnston
An ardent student of Iridology
Mesa, Arizona

You were one of the main inspirations for the establishment of the Canadian College of Natural Healing.

J.R.M., Dean
Canadian College of Natural Healing
Canada

With admiration, from . . .

Andrew Weil, M.D.
Arizona

. . . but when we meet and listen to people like yourself, I feel that it is all well worthwhile - I wish you the best.

D.M. Robinson
Former Mayor
Auckland, New Zealand

447

I've been a research scientist, but none of my experiences have been more challenging or rewarding than the past 4 or 5 years working under your personal leadership.

Bill McMahon
Expanded Optics
Santa Ana, California

Thank you for the very detailed and helpful analysis you provided me.

L.A.
Winnipeg, Manitoba, Canada

Your course at Omega was a highlight in my life.

J.Y.L.
Maine

You revealed a non-compromising dedication to truth.

A.D. Buelton
California

I wanted to tell you how much you mean to my family.

The Hill Family
Spokane, Washington

You have been a very important influence on me and my family.

M.M.T.
Florida

Your books are useful to me and will help others.

J.B. Medellin
Columbia, South America

Your work will have profound effect on the rest of my life. Not a doubt.

B. Johnson
California

I cannot but marvel that you still adhere to your teaching schedule, not to speak of such a tiring trip as the one to China.

Dr. K. Asai
Asai Germanium Research Institute
Tokyo, Japan

I am still thrilled when I hear from a patient who has visited with you and gotten marvelous results from your dietary suggestions and counseling, despite having something which sounded quite life threatening. I commend your courage in treating these quite ill patients.

A. Simon, M.D.
San Diego, California

I am so grateful to Dr. Jensen, whom I credit with my recovery. It has been a miracle that shortly after returning home from the cruise I could walk without my crutches.

Mrs. M. Goldberg
New Orleans, Louisiana

Thank you for teaching me how to care properly for my "temple."

Katherine MacGregor, actress
Hollywood, California

448

I have a lot of respect and admiration for your work in the field of nutrition and natural healing.

B.M., M.D.
Del Mar, California

A friend of mine in the Naval Reserve let me read one of your books and I was so impressed.

Dr. C.E. De Leon, DMD, MD, CL. Psych.
Dayton, Ohio

I probably have one of the earliest copies of Dr. Jensen's book - it has been at my right hand on my desk and is a constant source of reference. I look forward to his new one.

Dr. Martin R. Filmer
Johannesburg, South Africa

Nothing after all exists unless others search, find and then educate. It is of the latter that Dr. Bernard Jensen has excelled. For over fifty years he has attempted to educate others.

Richard H. Tyler, D.C.
Editor - The Chiropractic Family Physician
New York

Dr. Jensen is a Master Teacher and very experienced lecturer on nutrition.

H.F. Michael, O.D.
Los Angeles, California

Thank you for your outstanding seminar.

Dr. R. Cooper, N.D.
Park Rapids, Montana

Thank you for the most beautiful learning experience of my life.

M.A.
New Jersey

I believe Dr. Jensen is a true healer.

Bruce Halstead, M.D.

I was once arthritic, all bent over, being promised a life of pain, crutches and wheelchair. After 40 years with your help I am straight as a die - no pain - no crutches - no wheelchair.

Eulah Null
Long Beach, California

Thank you again for all you have shared with us.

T.R. Nova Nutritional Products
California

A courageous pioneer in the health field.

K.R.
Sauderton, California

Your work and life is testimony to the beautiful truth of how we should live - in glowing health with food as our medicine.

Dr. M. Moric, M.D.
Berkeley, California

449

This one man, both friend and doctor, talented, accomplished and the complete, compassionate physician that thousands have made their guiding light, has been almost the total inspiration I have needed in long years of study, practice and raising a healthy family.

Maurice Archer, D.C., N.D., D.O.
Naturopathic Health Clinic
Editor - *"Health and Happiness"*
Auckland, New Zealand

Your books have done more than anything to focus the attention of health-minded people of the country.

Victor E. Irons
Cottonwood, California

There is warmth and honesty in his plain and clear language.

Fred Lux, Attorney
Greenich, Connecticut

Your teachings and writings are continously inspiring me.

Gerald Olarsch, N.D.
Newark, New Jersey

Neither intellectually nor character-wise do I know a man with greater assets. Study his book and let him convey to you the blessings he can thus bestow upon you.

Dr. Charles H. Gesser, Homeopath
Florida

Thank you again for sharing your wisdom with all of us.

Dr. Rhody Edwards, D.C.
Kona, Hawaii

The mental patients in this hospital have responded with great success using your nutritional methods.

Dr. Nicolaev
Director of Mental Hospital
Moscow, U.S.S.R.

We much admire all your activities. We should desire to be so active at such an age as you are now. Again, we congratulate you very much for the great success you have had in Spain, being decorated by Queen Juliana.

Dr. Zdenek Rejdak, President
International Association for Psychotronic Research
Prague, Czechoslovakia

If we could use more of your work in Russia we would have a lot less operations.

Prof. F.N. Romashov, M.D.
Chairman of Scientific Board
Yasenevo, Moscow, U.S.S.R.

Thank you for your contributions to chiropractic and your service to humanity.

Dr. Michael Flanegan
Hawaii

450

Thank you very much for your working trip both here and in the U.S.S.R., because your trip and your presence had a great impact on moving ahead the development of your work.

Dr. Zdenek Rejdak
Dr. Michael Cernousek
Prague, Czechoslovakia

At the conference held in December, 1984 in Madrid, Spain, I was very impressed by your conception of man as a whole (body-mind-spirit).

Dr. Luis H. Gutierrez
Peru

For several years I have become a devotee of your "Philosophy of Health," trying to practice it together with my nearest people.

Janusz Dernalowicz, MSc.
Institute of Biocybernetics and Biomedical Engineering
Warszawa, Poland

There are individuals who so live as to push the boundary of the known outward. Such a man is Dr. Bernard Jensen, who has made the subject of his concern the Theory and Practice of Iridology - meaning iris fiber analysis.

Paul Courtright-Whyte, O.D.
Nutritional Counselor
Oshkosh, Wisconsin

Dr. Bernard Jensen is known throughout the world as the greatest man in iridology. His work is outstanding. His books will help improve the health of many people.

H. Ray Evers, M.D.
Evers Health Center
Cottonwood, Alabama

I have a lot of respect and admiration for your work in the field of nutrition and natural healing.

Dr. Barnet G. Meltzer, M.D.
North County Holistic Health Center
Del Mar, California

The professor from Canton (China) Hospital wrote to me to say that he was impressed from your lectures and they were very pleased to acquire the knowledge from you. The doctors who attended your lectures convey their thanks to you.

S.T. Young, Homeopath
Essex, England

Dr. Jensen's many books have made it possible for me to do the seemingly impossible - to be a new mother, a housewife and a professional actor/producer -to be in good health and enjoy it. My life changed for the better when I became a patient of his.

Susan Clark, Actress
Hollywood, California

451

We need all of the knowledge, equipment and inventiveness of the medical profession. There is nothing in this book intended to be degrading toward the medical profession. This book was written to show the theory and practical measures used in helping my patients to receive the highest state of well-being. We have considered these measures as an alternative way to some of the practices that are used today. Many of these practices were neglected to be taught or the knowledge was not available at the time I went to college.

This book was not written to further my practice, as I am retired. This work is the culmination of 55 years of research, observation, theory and practice with intense study to develop the right teachings for patients.

My only hope is that this book will aid people in learning a better standard of health and prepare them for a more beautiful future.

—Dr. Bernard Jensen

35

Concluding Thoughts— An Idea Whose Time Has Come

NUTRITION AND OUR NATION

Our nation is in need of more information on nutrition.

It has come to the attention of the American public that diet and nutrition are something that we should know about in taking care of most diseases that come upon us. There is much written about the effects of diet and nutrition on high blood pressure, cancers, cardiovascular disease, obesity and weight loss. How much protein is enough? Does a vegetarian's routine diet furnish all the proper nutrients that his body should have?

Only 20% of the medical colleges in this country today are teaching separate courses on nutrition. In fact, they have shown that U.S. medical schools devote only three days to nutrition in four years. Pressure on the medical profession is being brought by the laymen and very possibly by the drugless doctors, to teach more about nutrition for the control of disease and for care of the well-being of our bodies.

Very few doctors are able to give a good diet or present the information necessary to help the average person in his daily routine at home. Unless a doctor has spent some time of his own in broadening his original training, he does not know how to take care of the average person with chronic disease such as bronchial troubles, cancers, urinary disturbances, catarrhal discharges, bone diseases, rheumatism, arthritis and bowel conditions.

In the newly published book, *Nutrition Education in U.S. Medical Schools,* we find many things we should be considering. Researchers have found a strong association between food hab-

453

its and many of the "killer diseases." Proper nutrition is the key to prevention of these diseases and to lowering the costs these diseases bring to our society. Better nutrition was the most cost-effective strategy to take care of the problem. It was brought out that disease prevention through nutrition was the best approach for us to consider.

It was brought out that specific conditions develop from hidden hungers and nutrient deficiencies in the elderly, in children, pregnant women, alcoholics and so forth. More could be added to this, I am sure. I feel that nutrition is a factor in our criminal problems, learning disorders and our mental institution population. I believe great improvements can be made in these problem areas of our society by improving the diets of prison inmates, mental patients and children with learning problems.

The authors came to the conclusion that there was a vital role that nutrition could play in the human life cycle and that there was a good deal of research that was necessary in finding out how to take care of the various complaints of health such as we find in chronic diseases, reproduction and in immune functions.

The book brought out the fact that education was necessary for both physicians and the patients, which is something for us to think about.

I have said many times that while we have a Health Department in practically every city, the Health Department is more like a "Disease Department." It doesn't teach people to prevent disease but takes care of epidemics and plagues, waiting until a serious sitution arises before doing anything.

It was brought out in a discussion of the subject of education in U.S. medical schools that there should be a sound understanding of how nutrition acts in all metabolic activities and all of our physiological processes, and how nutrition affects our reaction to the toxic conditions that exist in our environment and in our own reaction to the taking of medicine. They brought out that many children are born into this world with a lot of genetic problems and may need more nutritional care than is currently being supplied to them.

When some 52% of the population in the U.S. is considered as overweight, nutrition is one of the main subjects that should be brought out for the control of it. We saw where years ago doctors were very interested in diet and nutrition care before they got into the complexities of drugs and how to control physiological functions and to suppress the various symptoms that may come as a result of disease. Alternatives to drugs could have been developed through proper diet and nutrition.

If we look to the continuing process of man's thinking we can see where nutrition is one of the main things that people have in their minds today in considering the control of any disease. While the American public is demanding more of a program of dieting that fits with what they have to live on in society, the average person just has to know what to do. They are kept in the dark and, of course, the physician is responsible for a good deal of this darkness because he should be teaching a good deal of the nutritional work that is given out today.

I think there should be nutritional institutions where experiments could be carried on and patients could be taken care of to the extremes with nutrition, to find out what the responses are of that patient and also what the doctor can expect in using this alternative way of correcting ills of all kinds.

No one should leave a hospital without the proper nutritional information or advice given to him. Each patient should be taken through the kitchen and taught to cook properly. In their rooms they could be shown educational films so that they could go home with nutritional knowledge necessary to keeping them well.

There is very little funding to see that nutrition is part of the curriculum of the medical school, but we find on the outside people who are experimenting with every type of nutritional manipulation to see what is the best way to follow.

It has been said that there is far too little time spent on this nutritional work by those who will become doctors in the next few years. We just have to wait and be satisfied with people who have learned as we have through the "college of hard knocks" and by experimenting on our own bodies.

The worst part of this nutritional work is that most people who are teaching it, giving advice in nutritional work, are people who have been sick and found their way out through the nutritional field.

There is a lot of information in the work that is being done in nutritional endeavors that could be organized and put together by someone or some department that is not inclined to bring in only medical studies. Medical studies are good, but we have to consider that there is a natural side of this that has been omitted from the studies of nutrition. It is when the average medical school only spends 21 hours in the nutrition education for its medical doctors, then you can see what a plight we are in trying to straighten out people's nutritional problems.

WESTERN MEDICINE AND ALTERNATIVE THERAPIES

Much has been said about drugless therapy versus drug therapy. Many times we just wonder if there isn't some kind of reasoning whereby both sides should be able to come together. We find that we have two different perspectives coming together, two different paths coming together, and we find that there should be some common ground that would enable us to work together. I believe that wise men counsel, and it is only fools that argue. I believe that argument only brings out hostile attitudes in those who take part.

It has never been in my mind to condemn the medical profession; never been in my mind to condemn the man who uses drugs and surgery. There are times, however, when I feel criticism is necessary, when we should take a fair look at which is being done and see if there is such a thing as a better alternative, in many cases, to the use of drugs or surgery.

Alternatives that have been developed and used by the drugless therapy people in the healing art usually take a good deal of time to produce a good response, a new working body with new tissue. This can only come from an improved way of living. Improved nutrition and lifestyle fit the needs of the human body better than harsher treatments.

I feel we should be looking for ways to save lives. We should be looking for the good which is in everyone and in all therapies. Personally, I believe we have lengthened our lives by the therapies which we have used in both the medical profession and the drugless therapy. However, on the other hand, there are many methods we could use to help lengthen lives even more. We must consider that improvements in the quality of living are very

456

important, and when we stop and realize that possibly there are more than 30,000 patients in this country today who are in need of heart transplants, I feel we should give some thought to finding the causes and the reasons why we have need of so many transplants.

We have a medical profession today that accepts this transplant business as a standard and common thing to do, as something to take care of when an organ is defective. I feel there is not enough time put into corrections; into educating people to understand the worthwhile things in life which would make transplants unnecessary. I feel there are possible alternatives for these transplants that we haven't even thought about up to the present time. The reason we do not think about it is because we haven't been taught to look for alternative ways that would enable us to do things differently. I think we must expand our continuum of consciousness, our social consciousness and our individual consciousness, to take in more that would have to do with health. Health is not everything; but without health, everything else is nothing.

It often seems to me we are taking care of basket cases. It looks like we keep the ambulance waiting at the bottom of the cliff. It seems like we are taking care of people who have already made reservations on the other side. It is this particular type of case that I feel the medical profession, both from a drug standpoint and a surgery standpoint, is pushed to the limit to do something. I believe that 80% of the medical profession's good comes in taking care of these types of cases. Of the patients treated today who have chronic diseases, there is a large percentage, possibly 60% to 70%, that would benefit from alternative therapies such as nutrition. Many who have chronic diseases could bring about a reversal process by living an entirely different kind of life in which recovery comes by having better tissue. I feel we should be able to demonstrate the value of drugless alternatives by laboratory tests that would prove that specific changes in lifestyles were bringing improvement in cases of chronic disease.

Vile attitudes by those who are against alternative medicine and by those in alternative medicine who are against the orthodox methods are a great obstacle to communication. It is this hostile mental activity that I feel is actually keeping the two sides from coming together with any kind of agreement in order to help humanity.

To doubt that the medical doctor or surgeon has had anything but the best in training is really foolish, but we have to consider that it isn't the training that we have had, but the training omitted that causes the problem. It is what we have neglected to learn that makes the healing art incomplete, when a complete healing art is needed so much. The sin of omission in the healing art, in all branches, is important for us to look at and consider, rather than what some person is doing or not doing correctly.

The reason why we say this is we feel there is an important omission in training in the medical schools. There are many now neglected hygienic measures that can be used in the treatment of patients. This is a sin of omission. On the other hand, the drugless doctor has an important omission in his lack of training in appreciating those situations where drugs or surgery are the wisest choices. This hasn't happened because most of the drugless work is based on a natural premise. Of course, Indian medicine men who didn't go to college cannot be accepted, despite the fact that their tradition may have been taught and practiced for hundreds of years. Chinese herbology cannot be accepted by the average medical doctor in spite of the fact that books have been written about it some 2000 to 3000 years before Christ.

We find that the Indian had to find out how to treat himself with the natural remedies, and our first doctors in this country were able to use many of these natural remedies very effectively. Some of these methods were unsanitary and some of them were not quick enough to do the job. In the modern health arts, we have uncovered many mysteries, gone into things from a chemical standpoint and a mechanical standpoint to such an extent that we have developed a system whereby we are suppressing symptoms of diseases today instead of allowing for a correction and a better healing. In other words, we are now cutting off the disease without considering that 90% of the body was actually affected by that disease and needed to be cared for as well.

I feel there is no reason for anyone to believe that there isn't a place for the drugless art and that the drugless art will be with us always. And, there are some people who must practice the drugless art, otherwise, they feel that they are not as close to the Divine Principles that they were meant to follow from the very beginning. To try to get around or ignore these Divine Principles by symptom relief measures, such as drugs and many times surgery, we find that we are missing something very important. We have to consider man's mind, his philosophy, his physical training, his nutrient needs. We need to consider the proof that is in the alternative healings which can be demonstrated.

FINAL THOUGHTS

Throughout this book, I have spoken about various parts of the body, various therapies to be used, and the importance of sound nutrition in a healthy and balanced lifestyle.

Balance, to me, is essential. I like the way the English say it—that we should keep away from the "edges"—that is, that we should avoid the extremes in nutrition and treatment.

My goal in writing this book has been to offer some alternatives in nutrition, treatment, and, most of all, in lifestyle that will lead to greater health and well-being. Constantly in my mind is that man is deserving of the very best; I serve the part of mankind that is *ready* for the very best—ready to make changes in attitude, habits, diet and lifestyle to achieve greater health. It is not a matter of trying to change humanity in a day or trying to move society to a fast change, but rather of assisting in the changes that can only begin with the individual.

I realize, of course, that this work isn't complete. I did not want to offend anyone; I didn't wish to criticize anything unless it was to bring a better alternative. I have tried not to say "don't" unless I could offer you a better way to do things. However, I firmly believe that everything good will come to the person who endeavors to put into practice the principles expounded in this book.

459

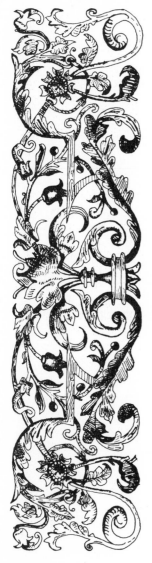

G o placidly amid the noise & haste, & remember what peace there may be in silence. As far as possible without surrender be on good terms with all persons. Speak your truth quietly & clearly; and listen to others, even the dull & ignorant; they too have their story. ❦ Avoid loud and aggressive persons, they are vexations to the spirit. If you compare yourself with others, you may become vain & bitter; for always there will be greater & lesser persons than yourself. Enjoy your achievements as well as your plans.

❦ Keep interested in your own career, however humble; it is a real possession in the changing fortunes of time. Exercise caution in your business affairs; for the world is full of trickery. But let this not blind you to what virtue there is; many persons strive for high ideals; and everywhere life is full of heroism. ❦ Be yourself. Especially, do not feign affection. Neither be cynical about love; for in the face of all aridity & disenchantment it is perennial as the grass. ❦ Take kindly the counsel of the years, gracefully surrendering the things of youth. Nurture strength of spirit to shield you in sudden misfortune. But do not distress yourself with imaginings. Many fears are born of fatigue & loneliness. Beyond a wholesome discipline, be gentle with yourself. ❦ You are a child of the universe, no less than the trees & the stars; you have a right to be here. And whether or not it is clear to you, no doubt the universe is unfolding as it should. ❦ Therefore be at peace with God, whatever you conceive Him to be, and whatever your labors & aspirations, in the noisy confusion of life keep pace with your soul. ❦ With all its sham, drudgery & broken dreams, it is still a beautiful world. Be careful. Strive to be happy.

Index

A

Acidophilus 347-350; Babies 348; Bowel 347, 348, 350; Chlorella 350; Diet 348; Digestion 349; Kumiss 348; Lactobacillus 348, 349; Matzoni 348; Underactive 347; Underactive 348

Advertising Foods; Dollar Foods 12, 65

Acne 360; Bee Pollen 308

Agricultural Chemicals 30

Agriculture 29

Allergies 31, 371, 386; Bee Pollen 309; Milk 65, 66; Wheat 65, 66

Almonds 95, 119

Almond Nut Milk 77

Alternative Healing 405-418; Free of Pain 417; Healing Crisis 411, 414, 416

Alternative Therapy 456-459

Amino Acids 90

Analytical Food Guide 225-244

Animal Experiments: Pigeon 38, 39; Rats 40

Arthritis 293; Ethel Lesher 420

Edwards 5, 6, 7, 10

B

Babies 138, 139, 394, 398; Acidophilus 138; Bowel 348; Mother's Milk 138; Weaning 136, 137; Weaning Menu 138

Barley 73

Bee Pollen: Analysis 310, 311; Health Research 307-310; Natural Food 307; Nutritional Value 311, Prostrate 324; Treats/Treatment 307

Beri-Beri 13, 24

Blackberries 103, 108

Body Feeding 223

Body Hints 294

Body Systems Chart 219-222

Bones, Teeth and Joints 22; Teeth 44

Bowel 104-106, 143, 150, 224, 292, 350, 354, 388, 406; Bee Pollen 308; Elimination 367-378; Tissue 416; Tissue Cleansing 371, 375; Underactive 348

Brain and Nerves 327-342; Analysis/Soy Lechithin 338, Bee Pollen 340; Black Pepper 329; Brain 332; Brain Center 332; Cerebellum 333; Cholesterol 339; Choline 338, 339; Congestion 333; Diet 331, 337; Disease 339, Disease and Conditions 329; Eggs 337, 338; Feeding 337; Fever 333, Foods 333, 334; Gallstones 339; Heating Foods 337; Lecithin 335-337, 339; Medulla 334, 336; Nerve Pain 327; Nerve Salts 329; Nervousness 330; Neural-Optic Analysis 341; Neuralgia 330, Neurasthenia 331; Neuritis 332; Phosphorus 332; Seed and Nut Butter 340; Sex Center 334; Sulphur 334; Supportive Foods 328; Tea 334; Workers 333

For Your Good Health—
The Writings of Dr. Jensen

Build a Library of Right Living—Look for Dr. Jensen's many books sharing the natural principles of happy, healthy living. If they are not available in your local bookstore or health food store, you may order direct from the address below.

Food Healing for Man—A wonderful primer of nutrition and food facts for everyone, especially for those starting out in the nutrition field, exploring the role of deficiencies in disease and the restorative power of a balanced food regimen.

The Healing Mind of Man—Wholistic healing principles for the body, mind and spirit, including the roles of inspiration, wisdom, peace and beauty in healing. The many stories here from Dr. Jensen's experience will not only uplift but delight readers.

World Keys to Health and Long Life—Secrets of health and longevity from around the world, collected in Dr. Jensen's journeys to over 55 countries of the world, visiting the oldest people on earth, including the Hunzas, the Caucasus mountain people of Russia, the strong old men of Turkey, the long-lived Rumanians and the Vilcabambains of Ecuador.

Creating A Magic Kitchen—How to turn your kitchen into a magic place where health and vitality flow into the entire family.

Vital Health from Your Kitchen—Many recipes and convenient menu plans to put you and your family on the path of healthful living.

A New Lifestyle for Health and Happiness—How to begin living a more natural lifestyle to prevent disease and enhance well-being in an age of fast living, stress and anxiety.

OTHER BOOKS BY DR. JENSEN: *Breathe Again Naturally, How to Deal with Catarrh, Bronchitis, Asthma; Survive This Day; Blending Magic; Doctor-Patient Handbook; Tissue Cleansing Through Bowel Management.* **WRITE FOR FULL LIST AND PRICES.**

THE SPOKEN WORD OF DR. JENSEN—His Best Lectures
(60-90 minute cassette tapes)

Dr. Jensen's entire Nutrition Course is available on tape: *Nutrition I*, *Nutrition II* and *Clinical Nutrition*, each set 10 hours.

The Chemical Story, Building a Better Way to Eat, Replacement Therapy, Regularity Management, Key to Inner Calm, Nature Has a Remedy, and many more. **Three Latest Tapes:** *Food Healing for Man, Nutrition for Longevity* and *Nutrition for Youth*. WRITE FOR FULL LIST AND PRICES.

VIDEO TAPES OF DR. JENSEN'S TALKS

At last, available in VHS, Dr. Jensen's greatest lectures before live audiences:

Rejuvenation Program: American Series: 5 tapes, including **The Healing Mind of Man, The Chemistry of Man** and **Nature Has a Remedy**, recorded "live" in California.

Joy of Living: Australian Series— 9 tapes, including **Nutrition for Youth, Vital Foods for Total Health** and **Food Healing for Man (I & II)**, recorded "live" in Brisbane, Australia.

World Search for Health and Long Life— Dennis Weaver narrates this beautiful "around the world" health adventure with Dr. Jensen.

Tissue Cleansing—Three hours of Dr. Jensen's teachings on colon health, so important in today's world, including one tape on *Tissue Cleansing* and one tape on *Nutrition.*

For further information on books, cassette tapes, video tapes and prices, contact your local health food store, or write to:

DR. BERNARD JENSEN
Route 1, Box 52
Escondido, CA 92025